# CRC SERIES IN AGING

Editors-in-Chief

**Richard C. Adelman, Ph.D.   George S. Roth, Ph.D.**

VOLUMES AND VOLUME EDITORS

**HANDBOOK OF BIOCHEMISTRY IN AGING**
**James Florini, Ph.D.**
Department of Biology
Syracuse University
Syracuse, New York

**HANDBOOK OF IMMUNOLOGY IN AGING**
**Marguerite M. B. Kay, M.D. and**
**Takashi Makinodan, Ph.D.**
Geriatric Research Education and Clinical Center
V.A. Wadsworth Medical Center
Los Angeles, California

**SENESCENCE IN PLANTS**
**Kenneth V. Thimann, Ph.D.**
The Thimann Laboratories
University of California
Santa Cruz, California

**ALCOHOLISM AND AGING: ADVANCES IN RESEARCH**
**W. Gibson Wood, Ph.D.**
Clinical Research Psychologist
Geriatric Research, Education, and Clinical Center
VA Medical Center
St. Louis, Missouri
**Merrill F. Elias, Ph.D.**
Professor of Psychology
University of Maine at Orono
Orono, Maine

**TESTING THE THEORIES OF AGING**
**Richard C. Adelman, Ph.D.**
Director
Institute of Gerontology
Professor of Biological Chemistry
University of Michigan
Ann Arbor, Michigan
**George S. Roth, Ph.D.**
Research Biochemist
Gerontology Research Center
National Institute on Aging
Baltimore City Hospitals
Baltimore, Maryland

**HANDBOOK OF PHYSIOLOGY IN AGING**
**Edward J. Masoro, Ph.D.**
Department of Physiology
University of Texas Health Science Center
San Antonio, Texas

**IMMUNOLOGICAL TECHNIQUES APPLIED TO AGING RESEARCH**
**William H. Adler, M.D. and**
**Albert A. Nordin, Ph.D.**
Gerontology Research Center
National Institute on Aging
Baltimore City Hospitals
Baltimore, Maryland

**CURRENT TRENDS IN MORPHOLOGICAL TECHNIQUES**
**John E. Johnson, Jr., Ph.D.**
Gerontology Research Center
National Institute on Aging
Baltimore City Hospitals
Baltimore, Maryland

**NUTRITIONAL APPROACHES TO AGING RESEARCH**
**Gairdner B. Moment, Ph.D.**
Professor Emeritus of Biology
Groucher College
Guest Scientist
Gerontology Research Center
National Institute on Aging
Baltimore, Maryland

**ENDOCRINE AND NEUROENDOCRINE MECHANISMS OF AGING**
**Richard C. Adelman, Ph.D.**
Director
Institute of Gerontology
Professor of Biological Chemistry
University of Michigan
Ann Arbor, Michigan
**George S. Roth, Ph.D.**
Research Biochemist
Gerontology Research Center
National Institute on Aging
Baltimore City Hospitals
Baltimore, Maryland

Additional topics to be covered in this series include Cell Biology of Aging, Microbiology of Aging, Pharmacology of Aging, Evolution and Genetics, Animal Models for Aging Research, Detection of Altered Proteins, Insect Models, and Lower Invertebrate Models.

# Testing the Theories of Aging

Editors

Richard C. Adelman, Ph.D.
Director
Institute of Gerontology
Professor of Biological Chemistry
University of Michigan
Ann Arbor, Michigan

George S. Roth, Ph.D.
Research Chemist
Gerontology Research Center
National Institute on Aging
Baltimore City Hospitals
Baltimore, Maryland

**CRC Series in Aging**

Editors-in-Chief

**Richard C. Adelman, Ph.D.** **George S. Roth, Ph.D.**

**CRC Press, Inc.**
**Boca Raton, Florida**

**Library of Congress Cataloging in Publication Data**
Main entry under title:

Testing the theories of aging.

(CRC series in aging) (CRC uniscience series)
Bibliography: p.
Includes index.
1. Aging. I. Adelman, Richard C., 1940-
II. Roth, George S., 1946- III. Series.
IV. Series: CRC uniscience series. [DNLM:
1. Aging. WT 104 T344]
QP86.T35 612'.67 82-1276
ISBN 0-8493-5829-9 AACR2

This book represents information obtained from authentic and highly regarded sources. Reprinted material is quoted with permission, and sources are indicated. A wide variety of references are listed. Every reasonable effort has been made to give reliable data and information, but the author and the publisher cannot assume responsibility for the validity of all materials or for the consequences of their use.



Direct all inquiries to CRC Press, Inc., 2000 Corporate Blvd., N.W., Boca Raton, Florida, 33431.



International Standard Book Number 0-8493-5829-9

Library of Congress Card Number 82-1276
Printed in the United States

## FOREWORD

The mechanisms involved in the aging process have intrigued mankind from antiquity. Only in the past few decades, however, has the scientific method been employed in attempts to unlock the secrets of this universal phenomenon. Still, the ratio of theories to experiments remains unacceptably high in bio-gerontology when compared to other scientific disciplines.

Mindful of this deficiency, and in an attempt to work toward overcoming it, we have compiled the present volume. Although it is not practical to deal with all the proposed theories of aging, some of the more popular have been addressed. It is our fervent hope that scientists interested in the aging process will be able to utilize the information contained here as a basis for both critical analysis and the designing and execution of further experiments in this exciting field.

George S. Roth
Richard C. Adelman

## EDITORS-IN-CHIEF

**Dr. Richard C. Adelman** is currently Director of the Institute of Gerontology and Professor of Biological Chemistry at the University of Michigan, Ann Arbor, Michigan. An active gerontologist for more than 10 years, he has achieved international prominence as a researcher, educator, and administrator. These accomplishmments span a broad spectrum of activities ranging from the traditional disciplinary interests of the research biologist to the advocacy, implementation, and administration of multidisciplinary issues of public policy of concern to elderly people.

Dr. Adelman pursued his pre- and postdoctoral research training under the guidance of two prominent biochemists, each of whom is a member of the National Academy of Sciences: Dr. Sidney Weinhouse as Director of the Fels Research Institute, Temple University, and Dr. Bernard L. Horecker as Chairman of the Department of Molecular Biology, Albert Einstein College of Medicine, Bronx, N.Y. His accomplishments as a researcher can be expressed in at least the following ways. He is the author and/or editor of more than 70 publications, including original research papers in referred journals, review chapters, and books. His research efforts have been supported by grants from the National Institutes of Health for the past 10 consecutive years, at a current annual level of approximately $300,000. He continues to serve as an invited speaker at seminar programs, symposiums, and workshops all over the world. He is the recipient of the IntraScience Research Foundation Medalist Award, an annual research prize awarded by peer evaluation for major advances in newly emerging areas of the life sciences. He is the recipient of an Established Investigatorship of the American Heart Association.

As an educator, Dr. Adelman is also involved in a broad variety of activities. His role in research training consists of responsibility for pre- and postdoctoral students who are assigned specific projects in his laboratory. He teaches an advanced graduate course on the biology of aging, lectures on biomedical aspects of aging to medical students, and is responsible for the biological component of the basic course in aging sponsored by the School of Social Administration. Training activities outside the University include membership in the Faculty of the National Institute on Aging summer course on the biology of aging; programs on the biology of aging for AAA's throughout Pennsylvania and Ohio; and the implementation and teaching of Biology of Aging for the Nonbiologist locally, for the Gerontology Society and other national organizations, as well as for the International Association of Gerontology.

Dr. Adelman has achieved leadership positions across equally broad areas. Responsibilities of this position include the intergration of multidisciplinary programs in research, consultation and education, and health service, as well as advocacy for the University on all matters dealing with aging. He coordinates a city-wide consortium of researchers from Temple University, the Wistar Institute, the Medical College of Pennsylvania, Drexel University, and the Philadelphia Geriatric Center, conducting collaborative research projects, training programs, and symposiums. He was a past President of the Philadelphia Biochemists Club. He serves on the editorial boards of the *Journal of Gerontology, Mechanisms of Ageing and Development, Experimental Aging Research,* and *Gerontological Abstracts*. He was a member of the Biomedical Research Panel of the National Advisory Council of the National Institute on Aging. He chairs a subcommittee of the National Academy of Sciences Committee on Animal Models for Aging Research. As an active Fellow of the Geronological Society, he is a past Chairman of the Biological Sciences section; a past Chairman of the Society Public Policy Committee for which he prepared Congressional testimony and represented the Society on the Leadership Council of the Coalition of National Aging Organizations; and is Secretary-Treasurer of the North American Executive Committee of the International Association of Gerontology. Finally, as the highest testimony of his leadership capabilities, he continues to serve on National Advisory Committees which impact on diverse key issues dealing with the elderly. These include a 4-year appointment as member of the NIH Study Section on Pathobiological Chemistry; the Executive Committee of the Health Resources Administration Project on publication of the recent edition of *Working with Older People—A Guide to Practice;* a recent appointment as reviewer of AOA applications for Career Preparation Programs in Gerontology; and a 4-year appointment on the Veterans Administration Long-Term Care Advisory Council responsible for evaluating their program on Geriatric Research, Education, and Clinical Centers (GRECC).

**George S. Roth, Ph.D.,** is a research chemist with the Gerontology Research Center of the National Institute on Aging in Baltimore, Md., where he has been affiliated since 1972. Dr. Roth received his B.S. in Biology from Villanova University in 1968 and his Ph.D. in Microbiology from Temple University School of Medicine in 1971. He received postdoctoral training in Biochemistry at the Fels Research Institute in Philadelphia, Pa. Dr. Roth has also been associated with the graduate schools of Georgetown University and George Washington University where he has sponsored two Ph.D. students.

He has published more than 70 papers in the area of aging and hormone/neurotransmitter action, and has lectured, organized meetings, and chaired sessions throughout the world on this subject.

Dr. Roth's other activities include fellowship in the Gerontological Society of America, where he has served in numerous capacities, including chairmanship of the 1979 midyear conference on ''Functional Status and Aging.'' He is presently Chairman of the Biological Sciences Section and a Vice President of the Society. He has twice been selected as an exchange scientist by the National Academy of Sciences and in this capacity has established liasons with gerontologists, endocrinologists, and biochemists in several Eastern European countries. Dr. Roth serves as an editor of *Neurobiology of Aging* and is a frequent reviewer for many other journals including *Mechanisms in Aging and Development, Life Sciences, The Journal of Gerontology, Science,* and *Endocrinology*. He also serves as a grant reviewer for several funding agencies including the National Science Foundation. In 1981 Dr. Roth was awarded the Annual Research Award of the American Aging Association.

## CONTRIBUTORS

**Arthur K. Balin, M.D., Ph.D.**
Assistant Professor and Associate Physician
Laboratory for Investigative Dermatology
The Rockefeller University
New York, New York

**Richard G. Cutler, Ph.D.**
Research Chemist
National Institute on Aging
Gerontology Research Center
Baltimore City Hospitals
Baltimore, Maryland

**Vincent J. Cristofalo, Ph.D.**
Professor
The Wistar Institute
Professor of Biochemistry
University of Pennsylvania
Philadelphia, Pennsylvania

**Susan R. S. Gottesman, Ph.D.**
USPHS Postdoctoral Fellow
University of California
Los Angeles, California

**Evan C. Hadley, M.D.**
Geriatrics Branch
National Institute on Aging, NIH
Bethesda, Maryland

**Gerald P. Hirsch, Ph.D.**
Geriatric Research Educatorial and Clinical Center
Veterans Administration Wadsworth Medical Center
Los Angeles, California

**Robert R. Kohn, Ph.D., M.D.**
Professor of Pathology
School of Medicine
Case Western Reserve University
Cleveland, Ohio

**Gairdner B. Moment, Ph.D.**
Guest Scientist
National Institute on Aging
Gerontology Research Center
Baltimore City Hospitals
Baltimore, Maryland

**Denise G. Ragona, Ph.D.**
Shipley School
Bryn Mawr, Pennsylvania

**Roy L. Walford, M.D.**
Professor of Pathology
School of Medicine
University of California
Los Angeles, California

## TABLE OF CONTENTS

Chapter 1

# THEORIES OF AGING: AN OVERVIEW

**Gairdner B. Moment**

## TABLE OF CONTENTS

# I. INTRODUCTION

Theoretical gerontology has entered a period with a vast and rapidly accumulating body of data and a plethora of ideas and theories. In other words, it is in the familiar "jig-saw puzzle" stage which often precedes major advances such as the discovery of the circulation of the blood. At the present time it is impossible to tell whether all the pieces of the aging puzzle are at hand or even if all those lying around belong to the aging puzzle. Until a general theory appears that will unify the facts and make trustworthy predictions possible, no one can offer more than an informed guess as to where the key facts lie. In such circumstances it is well to remember that the history of science records many surprises of which the discovery of X-rays and other radiations is only the latest.

In the recent past, thinking about the biological basis of aging could be divided rather roughly into three general types. First there is a rather naive approach, based on little hard evidence and almost purely empirical, which does not necessarily mean that the ideas are false; all science is at base empirical. Into this group falls the interest in the longevous populations found in the supposedly healthful conditions in far away mountain villages. A second major view is based on the common sense realization that everything ultimately wears out. This "wear and tear" theory, in the form of damage to the DNA code by radiations, heat, and other agents, has been dominant ever since proposed by Szilard and Orgel nearly 20 years ago. There is also a third group of investigators who hold that the course of aging is "programmed" from the beginning of life until the end in senescence. It is now beginning to appear that these two last views are not as different as it at first seemed.

# II. GENERAL PROBLEMS

## A. Terminology

For those unfamiliar with the field of aging research a word on terminology is in order. *Gerontology* is the scientific study of aging. *Geriatrics* is the branch of medicine concerned with the treatment of the elderly. *Senescence* designates the condition resulting from the more or less degenerative changes that characterize the terminal stages of the life span or the processes that produce those changes. *Aging* designates the developmental sequence of changes that begin before birth and continue throughout the life span. The evidence for this view of aging, originally proposed by C. S. Minot[5] in 1908, is compelling and will be discussed later.

## B. The Problem of Which is Cause and Which is Effect

One of the most pervasive and stubborn problems facing any investigator of the mechanisms of aging is the familiar cart vs. horse puzzle. There is a long catalogue of carefully studied anatomical, physiological, and biochemical changes that occur with normal aging, notably as a result of the investigations in the Gerontology Research Center of the National Institute on Aging carried out by Nathan Shock and his associates. Characteristic changes have been found not only in humans but in mice, rats, and other mammals in collagen, endocrines, the immune system, brain, mitochondria, nucleic acids, and in response to a wide variety of stresses such as cold, exercise, glucose ingestion, and immunological challenges. Important changes have been documented that occur during aging in the number or effectiveness of receptor sites in the liver, brain, and other organs for hormones and other physiologically active molecules. The key question then arises. Are any of these events separately or together the underlying cause of aging or are they one and all the results of some pacemaker process which governs the events and rate of aging?

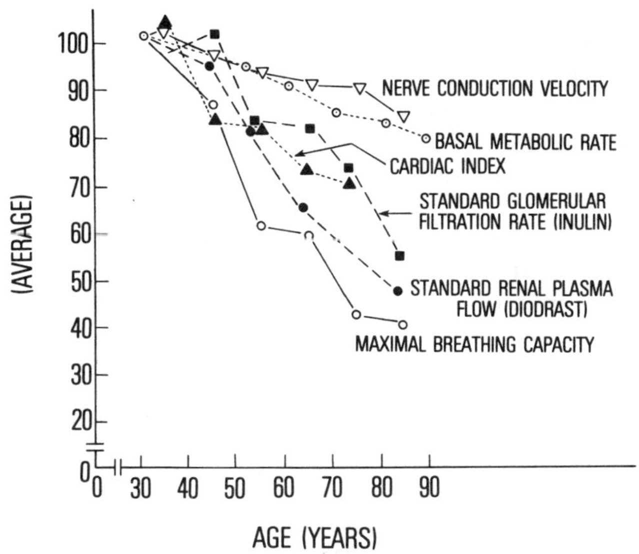


FIGURE 1. Decrement with age in selected physiological parameters of men. Note that the means at age 30 are taken as 100%. For data on another well-studied vertebrate, i.e., the hen, where the data are shown from the onset of maturity at age 1 year and decline steadily see Figure 2.

The great differences in average rate of decrement, i.e., aging, of the physiological parameters measured by Shock,[7] some of which are shown in Figure 1, plus the dramatic differences he found in the decremental rate of the same parameter in different individuals has been used as an argument against the hypothesis that the rate of aging is governed by any central or single basic process.

However, there is no compelling reason to believe that all organ systems would respond at the same rate to the same influence. These organ systems develop in the embryo and later mature at very different rates. Furthermore, different stresses, e.g., starvation, clearly do not affect all organ systems equally. The adult nervous system, for example, is far more resistent to starvation than other systems. Moreover, the different aging rates of particular systems in different people is exactly what would be expected in the light of the enormous genetic heterozygosity of the human race.

### C. Extending Mean Life Span Vs. Extending Maximum Potential Life Span

An equally pervasive and intractable problem lies in the criterion which is commonly used to determine whether or not any specific intervention into the life of an animal, whether dietary, surgical, biochemical, or other, is really touching the aging process itself or is permitting the animal to come closer to living out its full maximum potential life span. For example, a given dietary manipulation or a stimulation of the immune system which increases the mean life span of a group of laboratory mice or rats may do so by enabling them to postpone the onset of the tumors and the renal and pulmonary afflictions which so commonly end the lives of these rodents. If this is the case, the situation is no different from increasing the mean life span of a group of people by eliminating some childhood disease. In any basic sense, such treatment may have nothing to do with aging. It would be no different from increasing the mean life span of a population of sea turtles by providing them with protection during the first hour after hatching. During this period, when they scramble down the beach into the surf, the mortality may be 50% or higher from hungry sea gulls and fish. Consequently, in looking at a survival curve for a group of test animals, it is important to compare the maximum attained age with that of the controls.

## D. Human Relevance and Irrelevance

It should be emphasized that whether or not any particular course of action touches the basic aging pacemaker processes is irrelevant from the practical human and public health point of view. After all, the symptoms of malaria were controlled and in many cases the victims made permanently symptom-free by quinine in the form of cinchona bark for 350 years by Europeans and prior to that by Peruvian Indians long before the cause of malaria or the molecular structure of quinine was known. The relevant and important consideration is how effective any specific regimen or procedure is in extending human life that is healthy physically, mentally, and emotionally. No sane individual wants to continue a mindless vegetable existence. It is not the objective of the National Institute on Aging to turn us all into Methuselahs but to enable men and women everywhere to enjoy the active and useful life exemplified by such individuals as Verdi who composed what many regard as his greatest opera, *Otello,* when he was 75. That the NIA is not pursuing some will-o'-the wisp ideal is clear from the number of individuals who not only lived long and healthy lives but were outstanding achievers. Churchill was 66 when he became Prime Minister at the start of World War II and the history-making Pope, John XXIII, was elected Pope at 77. An outstanding example among biologists is Darwin's only slightly younger friend, the botanist Sir Joseph Hooker, who continued to publish for almost 30 years after Darwin was under the floor of Westminster Abbey.

## E. Selection of Appropriate Animals as Models

### *1. Limits to the Unity of Life*

The deepset unity of life is undeniable. Consequently there is no animal and, in theory at least, no plant from which information might not be gained which would be applicable to human aging. All the cytochromes are much the same throughout the plant and animal kingdoms with the same general structure, properties, and function in the terminal steps of aerobic respiration. The DNA spiral is the same everywhere and its behavior is the same whether in spore formation between the gills of a mushroom or in gamete formation within the gonads of a mouse.

Nevertheless, there is no *a priori* reason to believe that the underlying mechanisms of aging must be the same in all animals much less in both animals and plants. Both on the anatomical and the biochemical level, the same functional requirements are met in very different ways. The wings of insects are structurally and genetically very different from those of birds or bats. Oxygen is transported in the blood of vertebrates and certain invertebrates by hemoglobin, an iron-containing porphyrin complexed to protein. In many mollusks and arthropods oxygen is carried by hemocyanin, a blue copper-containing protein without any porphyrin, while in three families of marine annelids oxygen is transported by a green pigment, chlorocruorin which contains iron and porphyrin but the porphyrin is quite different from that found in hemoglobin. In fact some animals do not appear to senesce but live indefinitely, e.g., certain hydroids and flatworms.

### *2. Uncertainties of Animal Classification*

The 18th century binomial system of placing a group of similar species in a genus and then arranging several genera into a family and so on up through orders, classes, and phyla forms the indispensible frame of reference of biological research. These relationships represent the more or less subjective views of taxonomists working largely with anatomical traits but since the structure of any animal is the read-out of its genome, it seems likely that the present views are valid in the main. The trouble is that it is impossible to determine how closely any two animals are related. A family in one phylum may or may not correspond to a family or a class or even an order in some other phylum. Vertebrates cannot really be compared with arthropods nor arthropods to mollusks or protozoa. Recent methods of comparing amino acid sequences (another read-out of the genome), in cytochromes[18] for instance, and methods for comparing DNA sequences across species, should yield firm answers.

*3. Diversity of Aging: Vertebrates and Invertebrates*

To a zoologist it seems a virtual certainty that the aging mechanism within taxonomic groups such as the mammals will turn out to be the same throughout the entire group. Within larger groups such as the vertebrates it appears probable that the basic processes would be closely similar. However, the diversity of "aging" among fish raises questions. The atrophy and death of salmon after breeding with hyperplasia of adrenals and pancreatic islets[38] clearly implicates the endocrine system in the aging of vertebrates in general, as indeed, some recent investigators suppose to be true of mammals.[18a,19,21,23] Some fish are very short-lived with a longevity dependent on temperature. Other species of fish are not known to grow old. What aging involves on the cytological or biochemical or any other level in frogs and other amphibians apparently remains completely unknown.

Invertebrates constitute such an enormously diverse array of forms that it is hard to believe that there is one and only one aging mechanism to be found among them. Unless of course it is some form of Orgelian wear and tear on the DNA of the genetic code. Consider such contrasting animals as the octopus which breeds but once and then dies within hours and some of the larger sea anemones which live for decades in aquaria and only seem to die when something unfortunate happens to the pumping system for the sea water.

Clones of ciliated protozoans such as *Paramecium* and human cells cultured in vitro both have limited and characteristic clonal life spans. However, whether the limiting mechanisms are the same, similar, or entirely different remains uncertain.

*4. Nematodes and Rotifers*

Some investigators, such as B. M. Zuckerman,[57,58] believe that nematodes are destined to become "the *Escherichia coli* of the metazoan world" as tools for basic research. Other nematode enthusiasts like Edgar[20] and Wood point out that "attempts to find mutations that directly alter life span so far have failed and progress in this general area has been minimal."

Nevertheless nematodes possess certain highly important advantages such as ease of culture under controlled conditions with accurately synchronized age groups. Their life span is helpfully short so that results can be obtained relatively quickly and readily replicated. At 20° some species live approximately 2 weeks with a generation time of 3 to 4 days. Nematodes are moderately complex anatomically with gut, body cavity (though it is structurally different from the coelom of vertebrates), a prolific reproductive system, a muscular body wall enclosed within a largely impervious cuticle, and a surprisingly complex nervous system compared with earthworms, in some species accounting for about 50% of the somatic cells. In addition, nematodes have a fixed number of cells as adults, all permanently postmitotic, except of course for the germ cells. For current work see Swanson and Riddle.[48]

There are many variations in life histories, especially among parasitic species. The common vinegar eel, *Turbatrix* (formerly *Anguillula) aceti,* which has been used in many biochemical studies, exists as separate males about 1.4 mm and females about 2.0 mm in length. *Caenorhabditis elegans* (perhaps a variety of *C. briggsae*), widely used in aging research, is a self-fertilizing hermaphrodite. Nematodes typically molt thrice. If starved, a second stage larva of some species becomes a "dauer larva" in a state of arrest until favorable conditions return. The effect suggests an inhibition of something comparable to the molting hormone, ecdysone, of insects which is necessary for insect molting.

Several species are readily available from biological supply houses, such a *Rhabditis* and *Cephalobus* species which can be grown easily on potato plugs. A permanent culture of a semitransparent species, probably of *Rhabditis,* about 5 mm long, can easily be obtained by plating out 10 mm pieces from the posterior end of several earthworms on a Petri plate of 2% agar. Remove the gut to avoid soil nematodes. Juvenile *Rhabditis* are commonly within the nephridia and brown bodies. If transferred regularly to fresh agar, fed bits of ground beef and kept at 20 to 23°, such a culture will flourish indefinitely.

Large parasitic species are also available. *Ascaris,* some species of which attain over 30 cm, i.e., a foot, in length can usually be obtained from a friendly slaughter house. It was gametogenesis and fertilization in *Ascaris* that were used by Boveri in his classic work to unravel chromosome behavior. Cell lineage of *Ascaris* during embryonic development is well known from both classical and modern work. Because aging and reproduction are linked in at least some nematodes, it might be worthwhile to kill the primordial germ cell which is a single cell in the 16 cell stage and which gives rise to all the reproductive cells and none others. Modern medical laser equipment seems designed for such an experiment. The kidney worm, *Dioctophryma renale,* of dogs and other carnivores reaches well over 30 cm in length and a centimeter in width.

No group of metazoans is farther removed taxonomically from rest of the animal kingdom than the Aschelminthes to which both nematodes and rotifers belong. Rotifers offer the same sorts of advantages for aging research that nematodes do — a short life cycle, relative ease of culture, a very small and fixed number of postmitotic cells. In addition, rotifers are parthenogenic so clones of identical genotypes are available, indeed in some species males are unknown. Their life span can be altered by a number of dietary and other manipulations and some very interesting and potentially important results have been attained by Lansing, and by Meadows, Fanstil, and Barrows.[33]

*5. Insects*

Insects have been extensively used in aging research, notably several species of *Drosophila* ever since the pioneer investigations of Pearl in the 1920s. Several kinds of larger flies have been extensively used by Rockstein et al.[6] The detailed anatomy, life history, and culture methods are well known for *Musca domestica,* the house fly and for various blue bottle and other blow flies. *Drosophila* offers the special advantage of an immense amount of data of the most detailed kind on its genetic and cytological makeup and its embryological development. Benzer et al. have published methods permitting the precise localization in developing eggs of the cells destined to form specific structures in the adult including parts of the brain responsible for the control of behavioral traits such as "drop dead". There is also extensive work on clonal domains in *Drosophila* development by Garcia-Bellido in Spain and Lawrence and Morata in England and Bryant in the U.S.[15]

The very short life of adult mayflies, which belong to one of the most primitive groups of insects, the Ephemeridae, is well known but almost all scientific work has been limited to Dipterans such as those mentioned above. There are, of course, many other orders of insects which are very different in life histories and much larger. Much is known about their endocrine systems and the biochemistry of the hormones which govern insect development. No group of animals shows greater diversity in nutritional requirements, size, and longevity. A queen honey bee commonly lives about 6 years. A worker, which like the queen is a diploid female, lives for about 2 months during the nectar-gathering summer season and up to 6 or 7 months of semihibernations over the winter. The life span of the 17-year cicada contrasts not only with that of the mayfly which lives a year as a larval nymph and part of one night as a sexually mature adult, certainly not more than 24 hr, but also with other species of cicadas having a much shorter life cycle. There are insects which cannot complete their development, i.e., aging, until after they have experienced a period of intense cold. There are ants over a centimeter and a half long and other species barely visible at a scant millimeter in length. There are additional diversities of life span including haploid adults among the social insects both in the Hymenoptera, which are the most "advanced", and the Isoptera (termites), which are placed among the most "primitive". It is of some interest that the termite workers, which are sexually and otherwise undeveloped males as well as females, are maintained in this youthful state by one or more hormones exuded by the queen which are licked by her attendants from her abdomen and transmitted to the rest of the colony. If any individual fails to receive this potion, it is then free to develop into a sexually mature adult of the chromosonally appropriate sex.

*6. Protozoans: Ciliates*

Ciliates, notably the various species of *Paramecium,* are the classic animals in aging research. They are readily available, easy and very inexpensive to grow, and found in a very wide variety of forms. More than 6000 species have been described. It is a common fallacy to regard ciliates as simple or primitive animals. They have been evolving fully as long as the vertebrates and there is at least as much diversity among ciliates as among birds or mammals. The difference is that the metazoans have achieved complexity and specialization by grouping many cells together with each separate nucleus governing a discrete mass of specialized cytoplasm with muscle fibers, cilia, or pigment in separate cells. The ciliates in contrast have evolved a system with one or more macronuclei producing contractile fibrils, pigment, cilia, trichocysts, and other organelles within a single cellular envelope.

The striking fact is that most species of ciliates have a definite clonal life span (a kind of Hayflick equivalent) of a characteristic number of cell generations before cell division slows down, many of the cells show degenerative changes, and finally the clone dies out. The number of possible cell generations is different in different species and may be as few as about 50 to as many as 300. Species with long clonal life spans do not or cannot mate with close relatives. *Tetrahymena* is exceptional because it is able to propagate asexually for many years without clonal death. This genus lacks, however, a micronucleus which is the reproductive nucleus, and is regarded as "genetically dead".

It is almost exactly a century since Maupas and Hertwig discovered that if senescing clones were enabled to mate, then they were rejuvenated for another clonal life span as long as the previous one. The explanation has been under investigation continuously but a good answer has only very recently come to light and will be discussed later (see Section V.A).

*7. Fish*

Fish, specifically the bony teleosts, presents economical and very diverse research material which has yielded some highly interesting results. We have already mentioned the salmon[38] which die very quickly after spawning with at least many of the stigmata of senescence. The immediate cause appears to be a run-away adrenal gland. There are large kinds of fish like carp which do not appear to age and small species which are known to be annuals. Comfort found that the rate of tail regeneration in fish declines with age but that fish which had been retarded in growth by food restriction regenerated the tail like young fish. The octopus also senesces rapidly after spawning.

*8. Amphibians*

What little is known about aging in amphibians is mostly the result of maintaining frogs or salamanders for some other purpose. This might change. The techniques for keeping amphibians healthy under laboratory conditions are widely known. Methods for breeding special strains have been developed in the University of Michigan Amphibian Facility at Ann Arbor and elsewhere.

There are two features of amphibian development that give them unusual interest as models for aging research. If, as some gerontologists believe, aging in vertebrates is under some kind of general control by the hypothalmic pituitary axis, then amphibian metamorphosis may hold an important clue to the overall mechanism of aging. Due largely to the work of Etkin, it now appears that in the early premetamorphic period in the life of a frog tadpole the thyroxine level is very low. In the initial stages of metamorphosis the hypothalamus acquires a sensitivity to positive thyroxine feedback. Perhaps new receptor sites appear. In any case, more thyroid stimulating hormone (TSH) is released which results in higher levels of thyroxine. In this way an accelerating positive feedback is established with thyroxine levels rising higher and higher. Simultaneously prolactin levels in the blood fall as the TSH goes up with the result that growth rate decreases. The emergent question is what causes the hypothalamus to become different?

Second, neotenous salamanders such as the Mexican axolotl do not appear to age. Neoteny, sexual maturation while still in a morphologically juvenile condition, frequently with growth retardation, is associated with primate evolution and a longer life span. In different perennibranchiate salamanders neoteny has been attained by different methods, a circumstance which might be useful experimentally.

*9. Birds*

Birds appear to offer several important advantages for gerontologists. Not only are they warm blooded, easily available, and relatively cheap to maintain, they also exhibit a vast range of life spans. At least one species, the domestic chicken, has been the subject of repeated longitudinal studies. Because of the economic importance of egg production this aspect of these birds has been intensively investigated.[27] The result has been a dramatic demonstration of the theory advocated by C. S. Minot[5] in 1908 that aging is a continuous part of development beginning in the blastula stage of the embryo and ending with senescence. As early as 1923 Brody, Henderson, and Kempster showed that the number of eggs laid by a hen in any one year is a fixed percent of the number laid the previous year. This fact has been repeatedly confirmed in several different laboratories. The percentage found in most laboratories ranges from 70 to 80%. The differences are presumably due to breed and conditions (Figure 2).

The regular fall in egg production can be regarded as the hands of an aging "clock". If the hands of the "clock" were removed, i.e., if the bird were overiectomized, aging would presumably take place at approximately the same rate if the experience with mammalian castrates is any guide to what could be expected. The life span of chickens, which is somewhat over a decade, is long enough to study aging over a considerably longer period than the 2½ to 3 years of rats and mice and is consequently in that respect more comparable to the human condition as well as affording a longer time to observe changes in a wide variety of parameters. At the same time, unequivocal results could be observed within much less than a decade. At the end of the third year egg production has fallen to only about half of its first year value and by the end of the fifth is only about a third of that value. Among the questions that arise are those about other changes in chickens which show a regular change, increasing or decreasing with time and, of course, what it is that sets the pace.

The effect of dietary manipulations on longevity in chickens was explored some 20 years ago by workers at the Monsanto Chemical Company. Apparently nothing about this was ever published in any scientific journal but newspaper accounts did appear with photographs of the chickens and claims of large increases of life span. The

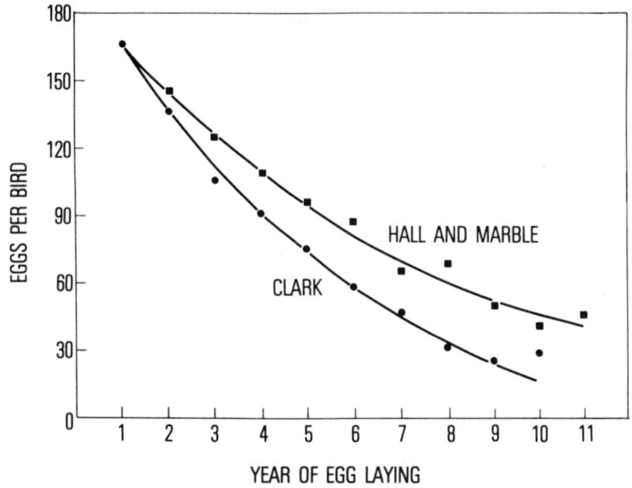


FIGURE 2. Annual egg production for hens as reported from two different laboratories. Note that aging begins at the start of the life span and continues in a regular way throughout life.

method that had been used was to feed the birds on a diet lacking tryptophan. This procedure may have been inspired by the work of Osborne and Mendel who found that a tryptophan-free diet inhibited the growth of rats if not indefinitely at least for many months after which they would resume growth to normal size on an adequate diet.

Chick cells have been standard material for research with cell cultures since the very beginning of tissue (i.e., cell) culture. Very few other studies of aging in chickens have been made although it has been found that blood pressure in chickens increases with age much as in humans.

*10. Dogs*

The use of dogs, mostly beagles, in aging research, has been relatively minor. They are cheaper to maintain than primates but very expensive compared with rodents. The life span of beagles averages about 15 years which offers advantages in studying long-term effects of diet and other factors compared to the very short-lived rat. The physiology of dogs is well known, another significant advantage.

In some breeds of dogs the maximum life span is said to be as much as 40 years. C. M. McCay[31] claims "large breeds age much more rapidly than small ones." This difference might prove a promising area for investigation. However, the brain-body weight ratio favors the smaller dogs and it might be that the very large breeds have endocrinological or other differences from smaller ones which amount to disadvantageous abnormalities. With the great interest in dogs and in aging it ought to be possible to secure support for such an investigation.

*11. Rodents*

Rats and mice are, of course, the animals of choice for most basic research in the field of aging and for good and well-known reasons. In recent years it has become increasingly clear that strain differences in both rats and mice in response to diets and other experimental parameters are sufficiently great to make it imperative that the strain be specified in any published account of investigation. Minimal use has been made of the abundant variety of species of rodents although the contrast has been studied which exists between the life span of *Mus musculus,* the diminutive house mouse and presumptive ancestor of laboratory strains of mice and the longer lived *Peromyscus,* the deer or white-footed mouse, of which there are at least 14 species in North America.

Exceptional opportunities are opening up for analyses of aging in a new way by the development of successful methods of making aggregation chimeras, or multiparental, mice and rats. These techniques combined with the newer ideas about the clonal basis of development have already yielded striking results in the analysis of inherited differences in behavior patterns (rope climbing, alcohol preference, cricket killing) in mice with mosaic brains (Nesbitt, Butler, and Spence[35]).

*12. Nonhuman Primates*

Primates, except man, share with the birds the distinction of being the most unused group of warm-blooded animals in the study of aging. There is no disagreement about the potential value of studies on primates which would be second in importance only to investigations of the human organism itself. The acquisition, breeding, and care of even the smaller primates is expensive, especially when compared to the costs of a rat or mouse colony. Furthermore, workers with monkeys have experienced dietary and behavioral, i.e., psychological, problems which there is every reason to believe affect aging adversely, or at least life span, under laboratory conditions. However, anyone who has visited the colony of several hundred macaques in the Madison Wisconsin Zoological Park and which live under the auspices of the University Department of Psychology will be convinced that the problems of working with large numbers of rhesus monkeys are far from insurmountable. Fortunately there is a recent (1979) and comprehensive book on aging in nonhuman primates edited by D. M. Bowden.[13]

## III. DIE HARD IDEAS: A FEW CLUES AMID THE ILLUSIONS

### A. Beneficial Effects of Remote Uplands

The most widely known and certainly most popular theory about human aging revolves around the Shangri-La fantasy. It is the belief that in certain high mountain valleys in remote parts of the world people live in good health to extraordinary ages, 140 or even older. The theory is that if we could only discover the secret of this longevity the rest of us could live equally long and, fully as important, equally vigorous lives. The factual basis for these fantasies is the existence in at least three remote mountainous regions of small communities where the air is pure, life is hard, and there are lots of obviously old but vigorous people some of whom claim to have attained astounding ages, 140 or more.

One such place is the village of Vilcabamba in the Chilean Andes, another area lies in the Caucasus mountains in southern Russia between the Black and Caspian Seas, and a third has been found in a high valley in the Karakorum mountains at the Western end of the Himalayas in north westernmost Pakistan. All three have been visited by knowledgeable people, anthropologists and biomedical scientists, and the people of Vilcabamba and the Caucasus have been intensively studied. Alexander Leaf of the Harvard Medical School faculty has published a handsomely illustrated book about all three.

The evidence now at hand makes it impossible to believe the claims of unusual longevity for the inhabitants of the Andes or the Caucasus and the burden of proof certainly lies with those who make similar claims for the mysterious Hunza people in the Karakorum mountains. Leaf originally relied on the appearance and the word of the people and, in the Andes, on ancient church records. But a more recent careful reexamination of the records revealed that they are highly unreliable. This is not at all surprising because there are many repeating names in South American towns which are common as John Smith in the U.S. Furthermore, any records kept over a century ago in a remote village of illiterate peasants seem bound to have inaccuracies. The whole problem is further compounded by the fact that in many parts of the world, including the U.S., country people take a special delight in fooling the city slicker. In the spring of 1978 an international conference was convened in Bethesda, Maryland attended by Leaf, the Minister of Health of Ecuador, and others who had investigated the Vilcabamba people. Based on the re-examination of the records and a study of the skeletal condition of the people the conclusion reached was that the oldest living inhabitant was probably over 90 but clearly not over 100. A large part of the reason for the unusually high percentage of the aged appears to be that there are extremely limited economic opportunities in a place like Vilcabamba and younger people move away.

The evidence regarding longevity in the Caucasus is equally negative. Zhores Medvedev, a leading Russian authority on the Caucasus inhabitants, reports that falsification of birth records has been going on there for many years to avoid military service, both under the Tzars and the Soviets. "The best way" he concludes, "to get a reputation for being very old is to lie a little." Sula Benet, Emeritus Professor of Anthropology at Hunter College, lived among the Caucasians and left convinced that many of them must be at least 125 years old. When challenged about her evidence she replied that she had found these people to be friendly and entirely reliable, which is no doubt true, and that in many cases there were five generations living together. However, if it is assumed that the parents in such families had averaged 19 year of age when their first child was born, surely not an unreasonable assumption, and that the fifth generation was made up of children under 10, then the oldest member of the group would be 86, a ripe old age but a long way from 125 not to mention 140.

The recently developed method of determining age by measuring the degree of spontaneous racemization of the amino acids in any protein, such as that in teeth, which is not replaced during life, should end this entire controversy permanently.

### B. Gonads as Biochronometers

Another well-publicized theory postulates that aging is paced by the gonads. As long ago as 1889 Brown-Sêquard of the University of Paris believed that he had discovered a rejuvenation factor in testis extract. Then in the 1920s Serge Voronoff of the Collêge de France and others in other countries reported success in grafting sex glands from young nonhuman primates into aging humans with positive results.

These claims cannot stand against rational scrutiny. The lack of any control for psychological factors invalidates this work at the very start. Furthermore, as Robert Butler, M.D., the Director of the National Institute on Aging of the NIH has pointed out, the idea that elderly men and women are without sexuality is a myth, provided they enjoy good health, are are not using drugs including tranquilizers, and are free of psychological impediments.

Modern experience with the enormous difficulties of getting a heart or kidney graft to be accepted by the host for more than a very few weeks makes it virtually impossible to believe the claims of the Voronoff School. This is all the more true because their work antedated knowledge of the importance of matching blood groups and repression of the immune system. If the gonads governed the rate of aging, then eunuchs and other mammalian castrates of both sexes would be expected to show a very different life span from intact individuals which is not the case. A statistical study of institutionalized human eunuchs showed that they live on the average a bit longer than intact men on the outside. However, the medical supervision within institutions was probably better than in the general population and the risk of accidents of all sorts including contageous diseases was probably less. In addition, there is now good evidence that functioning of at least the ovaries is controlled in some way from a precise center in the brain.

### C. Intestinal Flora

At the turn of the century a young associate of Pasteur, Elie Metchnikoff, the discoverer of phagocytosis, advocated the theory that aging is due to the cumulative effects of toxic products produced by bacteria in the intestine and absorbed into the blood stream. As a consequence, constipation was thought to be highly deleterious, an idea by no means dead. An interesting aspect of the Metchnikoff theory is that prominent among the toxic substances named are skatole and indole, molecules largely responsible for the characteristic odor of feces, and both slightly modified derivatives of tryptophan, an amino acid which is implicated in the control of growth and aging.

An additional reason for mentioning this old theory is that there is now good evidence from both human and animal studies that intestinal bacteria of various kinds exude vitamins and possibly other substances of importance to the host. Metchnikoff himself advocated the ingestion of *Lactobacillus bulgaricus,* an organism present in yogurt, as a corrective for the toxic products of other bacteria. In fact, it was discovered in 1908 that germ-free chicks and ducks benefited from innoculation with intestinal bacteria. This work was almost forgotten until modern investigators began using gnotobiotic animals. This relatively recent work showed that such germ-free animals, both birds and mammals, suffered from vitamin deficiencies, especially vitamin C and the vitamins of the B group.

### D. Rejuvenative Elixers

Anyone who comes forth with a cure for old age is sure to be called a charlatan by the medical profession. Unfortunately there is usually excellent reasons for such a judgment. At the same time it should be recognized that historically the medical profession has been notorious for ignoring or even bitterly opposing innovative ideas of which the doubly tragic case of Semmelweiss is only one of the best known.

The only case relevant suggesting reluctance to try the new with an open mind (scientific skepticism should work in *both* directions) in recent times is that of Anna Aslan and her clinic in Romania. For the past two decades she has been claiming very significant rejuvenating results in human patients from injections of "Gerovital H3" which is procaine (novocaine) modified by the action of benzoic acid and potassium metabisulfate. The discovery of the surprisingly beneficial effects was a serendipitous one made in the course of treatment for peripheral vascular disease, a common ailment in the aged.

There are two noteworthy aspects to this affair. The procaine used has been found in this country to be a weak inhibitor of monoamine oxidase. Mono- and other amines, it will be recalled, serve an important function in the central nervous system including within the hypothalamus which some suspect is the site of an aging "clock". The other aspect to note is that although there is no evidence that this procaine treatment increases the natural human life span, indeed Aslan[9a] herself says that it does not, there is evidence that in a large number of cases it aids greatly in the alleviation of ills of old age. Despite a lot of emotionalism both pro and con, there have been a number of tests both on rats and humans with Gerovital H3 or closely similar substances in this country without any conclusive results one way or the other.

## IV. GENETIC PARAMETERS

### A. Heredity and Environment in Aging

For anyone at all familiar with modern genetical science, there can be no doubt that the maximum potential life span of any species, within a given environment, is set by the genome. It is the nucleic acid code that turns one egg into a mouse and another look-alike egg into a starfish. The overriding fact is that environmental factors can only vary the phenotype within its genetic limitations.

The questions that do arise are, first, how flexible the genetic limits are, that is how far environmental influences can modify the phenotype, and second, how the genome determines those limits, set by the rate of aging. Is it by regulating the effectiveness or quantity of DNA repair and protective enzymes? Is it by setting some limit on the number of cell generations possible in any multicellular organism? Is there some master pace-setter for the whole course of aging, possibly within the brain? Because environmental factors such as disease, pollutants, diet, drugs, and life styles play such an important role in determining how much of its genetically possible maximum life span any individual actually achieves, the relative importance of heredity and environment in aging presents an extremely challenging problem.

The degree to which genetic factors control the differences in the rate of aging or the presumed maximum potential life span between two individuals of the same species has proven to be difficult indeed to measure. In the case of the wild, i.e., nonlaboratory animals (and this includes *Homo sapiens*) the environment cannot be controlled, so it is extremely difficult even to estimate much less to measure extent of its influence. Among laboratory animals variation is commonly so large that sometimes an "L. D. 50" of caged life on a specific diet is about as precise as it is possible to be.

### B. Geneological Analysis

The degree to which differences in length of life between human individuals are due to biological inheritance has been investigated in several ways. As early as 1922 Pearl published a breakdown of the data on a population of 1594 individuals. The result shows a "dose-related" response in the offspring to the age attained by both parents. The completed massive study, published in 1934, supports the old adage that "the best way to a long life is to select long-lived parents".

Recently Abbott, Murphy, and their associates[43] have reinvestigated this entire problem including special attention to the descendants of Pearl's original nonagenerians. They found a "clear and almost uniform familial component in the length of life" of the population studied. However, in the words of Murphy, "Expressed as a regression, this does not seem to amount to more than a 1 year increase in survivorship in the progeny for every 10 years in the parent." Since the original Pearl studies nearly half a century ago, the great advances in medicine from antibiotics to cholesterol-low diets have rendered any comparisons between the descendants of Pearl's nonagenerians and the descendants of those who died in their 60s or 70s almost meaningless. Modern medicine has certainly helped individuals with a weak genetic constitution to overcome that handicap.

The caution of Murphy's conclusion is amply justified on two grounds, first, the genetic heterogeneity of any group of sexually reproducing organisms is immense unless strict inbreeding has been practiced which was obviously not the case with these populations. Not only are sibs very different genetically but when more than one generation is involved genetic heterogeneity is greatly multiplied, first by meiosis and then multiplied again by fertilization. The human race is notoriously heterozygous and on top of that are other factors such as heterosis which is known to produce hybrid vigor even when one or both parents (as in Drosophila) carry deleterious genes.

Equally important, it is impossible to control the environment and without such control, even the most sophisticated statistical methods leave room for legitimate doubt as to the relative importance of genetic and environmental factors in aging.

### C. Twin Comparisons

In marked contrast to the Pearl-Abbott geneological type of study is the comparison between monozygotic (MZ) twins. Because such twins have developed from the same fertilized egg both carry the same genotype give or take a possible somatic mutation or two. Indeed a pair of MZ twins belong to the same clone, a clone of two. Consequently an enormous thicket of statistical computations is reduced to a much more manageable size.

The diagnosis of monozygotic twins once presented a certain residuum of uncertainty. When there was any doubt, diagnosis depended on medical records of the relationship of the twins to their fetal membranes. Sometimes such records were not available, sometimes the membrane-fetal relationships are difficult to interpret. The problem of diagnosis has all but vanished now that over a dozen genetically determined blood groups are known and there are immunological and other pertinent techniques.

The classic study of the genetic component in aging as revealed in twins is the work of F. J. Kallman and G. Sander published in 1949. They reported that in a group of 58 twin pairs the mean intrapair differences in lifespan for MZ twins was 36.9 months while it was 78.3 months for same sex dizygotic (DZ) twins and 126.6 months for opposite sex DZ twins. Thus the difference in age at death of a pair of MZ twins was less than half as much as between same-sex DZ twins. Subsequent work by L. F. Jarvik et al.[43] have confirmed this result and shown that the intrapair differences between MZ twins in performance and other parameters increase somewhat with age, a change that could easily be due to environmental factors.

The outstanding advantages of MZ twins in the study of aging, especially in longitudinal programs, has been largely overlooked. Such twins offer the only hope of dissecting genetic from environmental factors even roughly. Such a dissection is essential, if the effects of environmental factors such as diet, climate or life style are to be assayed with confidence.

## V. AGING RATE: THREE LEVELS OF CONTROL

### A. Primary Level: Unicellular

August Weismann, founder of the germ cell theory of inheritance, launched scientific thinking about the biology of aging almost precisely a century ago at the 1881 meeting of the Association of German Naturalists held in Mozart's little city of Salzburg. Weismann presented two propositions. First, the characteristic life span of any species has been determined by natural selection like other traits such as length of ears or the claws of a tiger. Up to a point this has to be true because natural selection acts as a sieve and only those traits that produce a viable organism can pass through. It also agrees with those contemporary ecologists who hold that selection, whether K or r selection, is one of the determinants of life span (see Section V.B).

Weismann[53] also suggested "that the restriction [of life span] may conceivably follow from the limitation in number of cell generations for the somatic [body] cells of each organ and tissue." He specifically disclaimed any "ability to indicate the molecular properties of cells" upon which such a restriction in the possible number of cell generations might depend. Both of these proposals have been under investigation ever since.

Shortly after Weismann, several investigators — notably Maupas in Algeria and Richard Hertwig in Germany — not only confirmed the fact of a limited clonal life span for certain protozoans, ciliates specifically, but combined it with a theory about the function of sex, i.e., rejuvenation. In the years since a mountain of data has accumulated in many laboratories most fruitfully by Sonneborn and his associates.[1,46] It is now clear that each of a number of species of ciliates possess a finite number of possible cell generations before cell division slows down and finally stops completely. It is important to note that this clonal life span is different for each species and ranges from about 50 cell divisions in some species to 300 or more in others. It is also clear that if, shortly before a clone stops dividing, it is permitted to undergo sexual exchange, it is revived and can begin another series of mitotic cell divisions until the clonal life span is again reached.

Unfortunately these remarkable results were thrown into deep shade by the work of Carrel on chick cell cultures which he claimed would continue to divide indefinitely subject only to proper medium and lack of infection. It was decades later that Hayflick discovered that Weismann had been correct all along and that normal human diploid cells did have a finite clonal life span, one of about 50 cell divisions. The result was a rebirth of interest in this old but central biological problem. Significantly Hayflick has demonstrated that if you reciprocally transplant nuclei from young generation cells into cytoplasm of old generation cells and vice versa, the cell generation age follows the nucleus.

The question then arises as to what aging means in terms of a clonal life span. How do the cells count the cell generations? Obviously the counting mechanism, the aging clock if you will, must be ticking during the early cell generations or the vigorous 30th cell generation would be the same as the vigorous 20th and aging of the clone would not occur. In other words, Minot's theory that aging begins at or really before birth clearly holds on the cellular level.

One widely accepted answer to the *how* of cellular aging was provided in the 1960s by the Szilard-Orgel theory that aging in animals is due to damage to the DNA from radiations, from thermal disturbances, and oxidative damage. Such an idea is completely plausible because animals subjected to radiation appear senescent and die earlier than controls. Furthermore, radiation is well known to damage the DNA code. This theory is an extension of the older wear and tear theory of aging based on the common sense view that everything ultimately wears out. Certainly when one organ, heart, kidney, liver, or whatever is damaged it throws added strains on others which in turn function less well and so a cumulative cascade of damage is built up. But repair is a widespread characteristic of injury or wear in a young animal. Wear on a stone is not repaired, wear and tear on the skin is.

It may be that clonal life span for cells is determined by the accumulation of DNA damage. Those species of ciliates able to avoid or repair such damage better than others have a longer life span. However, the DNA damage theory has been hard to prove. One of the most recent failures to find support for such damage was reported by Goldstein of McMaster University. He and his associates plated a small piece of tissue in the center of a large Petri plate, allowed a very large halo of outgrowth nearly to fill the plate, and then added labeled substrate to identify the dividing cells. Only those around the periphery took up the label. The remainder of the cells, descendants of cells which had undergone fewer and fewer divisions as the center of the culture was approached, were quiescent and comparable to the cells Hayflick kept in a refrigerator. When Goldstein cultured cells taken from different regions of the circle of outgrowth, the number of divisions they underwent depended on the distance they had been from the original tissue in the center, the closer the more cell divisions they showed. Put differently, the counting mechanism, the aging clock, had stopped when these cells stop dividing so they "remembered" how many additional mitoses they were capable of. The surprise came when the cells at different distances from the center of outgrowth were tested for amount of DNA damage. There was no statistically significant difference, if anything a bit less in the cells at the periphery.

If DNA damage does not clock the cells to a standstill, what does? In recent years a number of quite different counting or aging mechanisms for cells have been proposed and developed by Holliday, Medvedev, Nanney, Sonneborn, Martin, Olodnikof, amid others (see Martin[32] for a review.). One favored by Goldstein holds that there are reiterated DNA sequences on the end of one or more chromosomes. With every mitosis one is lost and when the last of the 50, or however many there are, is lost, cell division stops. It is in meiosis, when homologous chromosomes are tightly paired, rather than fertilization that the rejuvenation of a clone occurs. Presumably at synapsis there is a full compliment of genes and repair takes place. Goldstein has found such reiterated DNA segments in his material.

### B. Secondary Level: Generalized Endothermal Metazoans

Whether clonal life span of a line of cells is set by the accumulation of DNA damage or by some chromosomal counting mechanism is still uncertain. Whichever turns out to be the case, it is clear that a limited clonal life span exists for the cells of metazoans. Does this clonal life span set the life spans of multicellular animals, specifically the endothermal birds and mammals? If so, does an accumulation of damage to nucleic acids set the upper limit of life span?

The weight of the evidence is against a Weismann-Hayflick clonal life span of the cells setting the actual maximum potential life span of animals. It would probably set an ultimate upper limit but one far above the actual one. The cells of a number of important organ systems in birds and mammals are permanently postmitotic, notably in the nervous system, and hence not directly involved in clonal life spans. The cells of the blood, mucosal cells of the gut, basal cells of the skin, etc., are proliferating populations which are continuously replaced. However, there have been shown to be a number of ways in which stem cells for these populations can be sequested so that a stem cell does not begin to divide until others in the same population have already almost reached their clonal limit, in humans of about 50 generations.

The fact that clonal life span seems not to be the timing phenomenon for aging in higher animals militates against the theory that the rate of aging is the result of the rate of accumulation of radiation and other injury to nucleic acids. It is not proof, however. Evidence can be cited on both sides of the question. Patients with progeria, a disease due to a single gene mutation which produces apparent senescence of a severe type in children, have been studied for evidence of DNA damage in their cells. The first studies reported higher levels of damage than in normal individuals. Later work has failed to confirm this. Tice has reported that DNA repair enzymes did not decrease with aging but that long-lived animals have better repair ability, something found also by Cutler.[1,17,49] Collagen in tendons of old rats is different from that in the young. However, collagen formed in the old is not appreciably different from collagen formed in the young.

Although the cells of metazoans retain the limited clonal life span found in unicellular organisms, it is clear that other controls over the rate of aging, and hence life span, have been superimposed on the clonal life span just as the ability to form a multicellular organism has been superimposed on them. In a somewhat similar way, in the course of evolution the neopallium has been superimposed over the ancient paleopallium to make the mammalian brain.

The evolution of aging in birds and mammals was evidently a complex process, although compared with the grand total of genes in the vertebrate genome, it may well have been accomplished by only a few genes with profound and widespread effects. That this is possible is shown by the existence of progeria and other genetic syndromes that closely simulate senescence in the very young and are known to be due to one or at most a very few genes. The various forms of neoteny in which organisms become sexually mature in a juvenile morphological condition appears due to one or a very few genes. It produces a delayed development which Cutler[1,17] and Gould[26] have pointed out is related to an extension of life span.

Amid the complexities of aging in birds and mammals a number of relevant facts stand out. Enough studies have now been made to show that many if not all species of birds and mammals in the wild fail to live out their full maximum potential life span which is seen only when these animals are kept in cages or other protected environments. The chaffinch, for example, in captivity has a life span of 12 or more years.

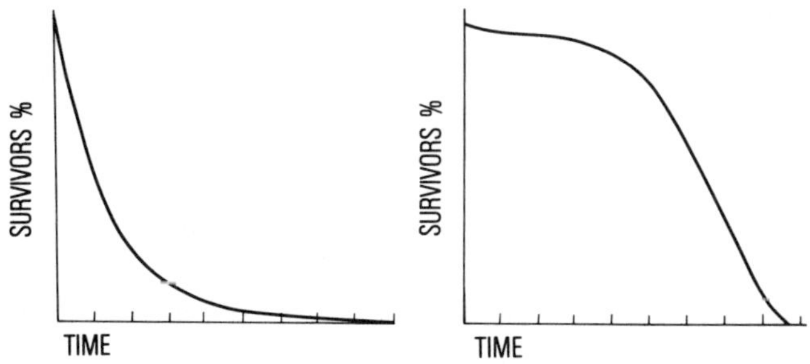


FIGURE 3. Left: survivorship curve for a population of animals most of which die long before attaining their maximum potential life span. Right: survivorship curve for a population of animals or objects such as glass dishes which senescence, i.e., become more brittle or otherwise more vulnerable with time, but also approach a putative maximum age in large numbers.

In the wild few live more than 10 months. The survivorship curve for wild birds and mammals, with few exceptions, is shown in Figure 3 left. Animals which age long enough to senesce like humans and elephants describe a survivorship curve having a long flat top followed by a rapid plunge as shown in Figure 3 right.

Both curves can be misleading by obscuring the presence of genetic aging or, perhaps better, genetic developmental program extending throughout the entire possible life span. Because an animal fails to live for more than a small fraction of its maximum potential life span does not prove that it lacks a developmental program but only that it was killed somehow before its full development was expressed. Likewise because the survivorship curve is almost level for many years does not indicate that such a population has not been aging steadily from the very start. Figure 2 shows the decline in number of eggs laid per year throughout the life of a hen. Figure 1 shows the regular decline in a number of physiological parameters in men. During these declines in both birds and men, the survivorship curve would have been virtually flat.

The view now widely accepted among ecologists and evolutionists is that selection is of two types, K and r. K selection occurs when the population has just about reached the carrying capacity of its environment. K selection favors large body size, long life span, and fewer young at a birth. r selection favors the opposite and occurs when the population is well below the carrying capacity of its environment or when its environment is subject to great fluctuations.[47] Note that the K-r theory does not state that any one of those traits is the result of direction selection, as for the chronological age at death, but only that they are associated.

In the early years of the present century Max Rubner[40] showed that the specific metabolic rate of a warm-blooded animal is proportional to its size. This follows from the simple geometrical fact that the larger an animal the smaller the surface area per gram of body and since all but a negligible amount of body heat is lost through the surface, a large animal can maintain the standard avian or mammalian body temperature with relatively less metabolic effort. Rubner went on to suggest that the reason elephants and large animals generally live longer than small ones is because they have a lower metabolism and therefore their rate of living is slower. So there may be some gerontological significance to the often stated fact that during their life spans the heart of an elephant and of a mouse will have beaten approximately the same number of times. If a large number of mammals ranging in size from mice to elephants are plotted to show the relation between specific metabolic rate and size, it will be found that they fall nicely along a curve from smallest with the highest and largest with lowest rate, except for a number of partial exceptions. The same is true if maximum potential life span is plotted against specific metabolic rate. Of course Rubner knew nothing about different degrees of oxidative damage to DNA as an explanation.

Much more recently Sacher has found that a better fit to the curve is seen if brain size in relation to body size is taken into account. A proportionally larger brain is thought to provide more redundancy in homeostatic mechanisms which promote a longer life.

In addition, it has been established, largely by the work of Fridovich,[24] that superoxidases appeared very early in the evolution of life and have ever since played an essential role in converting highly destructive the superoxide radicals of oxidative respiration into harmless products. Cutler[1,17] has now shown that the ratio of specific superoxide dismutase activity to specific metabolic activity is precisely correlated with life span maximum.

**C. Tertiary Level: Specialized Hypothalamic-Pituitary Control**

There is an active group of investigators who believe that the factors so far discussed, and additional ones such as the immune system and macromolecular cross linkages, are not sufficient to account for all the facts. The timing of the attainment of sexual maturity and of menopause, the even course of the aging changes revealed by "longitudinal" studies of hens and men, all seem too smoothly regular to be fully explained in terms of Rubner's original theory even with its sophisticated contemporary modifications in regard to DNA damage, protection, and repair.

Prominent among those sharing this skepticism is Gould[26] who has presented evidence showing that neoteny — development of sexual maturity in an otherwise juvenile body — has played an important, perhaps even dominant role in primate and especially human evolution. With this life span has been increased, perhaps due to the relatively larger brain produced by neoteny, perhaps from some effect of slowing the rate of development, perhaps in some other way such as changes in the activity of the hypothalamus and its organ the pituitary.

The belief that the central nervous system may exert an overriding control of the course of aging is supported by the fact that many, and possibly most animals possess circadian or 24-hr rhythms and some lunar or monthly rhythms as well. These rhythms or oscillations of respiration and activity of many kinds are able to run freely for long periods of time in environments from which all known clues for time have been excluded. Transplantation experiments in insects have demonstrated that the rhythm is located in a specific portion of the brain. In mammals it has been shown that the circadian oscillations follow a transplanted pineal body if the host pineal is removed. None of this is meant to imply that the course of aging is paced by the same biochemical mechanism as circadian rhythms or even a similar one but rather to note that long sustained and effective biochronometers are in fact possible.

In addition, there is ample evidence that at least some aspects of the postembryonic developmental program in vertebrates is under the overall control of the central nervous system. It will be recalled that the timing of metamorphosis in a frog tadpole is determined by events in the hypothalamus. Mammalian reproductive rhythms have also been shown to be regulated by the brain. Meites et al. found that estrous cycles can be reactivated in the postreproductive rat by electrical stimulation of the preoptic region of the brain and by dopa, epinephrine, and other sympatheticomimetic monoamines. Denckla[18a] has shown that hypophysectomy in rats accompanied by thyroxine replacement will "rejuvenate" many anatomical and physiological parameters, at least temporarily. There are even some indications that the prolongation of life by dietary restriction may be due to a deleterious effect on the pituitary, "nutritional hypophysectomy."

C. E. Finch,[1,23] a leading advocate of the role of the nervous system in the control of aging, maintains that age-related changes in catecholamines, especially in the hypothalamus and preoptic areas of the brain, are in a prime position to initiate widespread events in hormonally regulated cell functions throughout the body. Both V. M. Dilman[19] in the USSR and A. V. Everitt[21] in Australia have marshaled impressive evidence along similar lines. Specifically Dilman holds that "the genetic program of development and aging is a gradual elevation of the threshold of sensitivity of the hypothalamus to feedback suppression." Finch has put the present situation very well in saying that more basic information must be gathered about aging changes in the central nervous system in order that testable hypotheses can be formulated.

## VI. NUTRITION AND AGING

Dietary restriction is the only known method for dramatically increasing the life span of mammals. First noticed in rats by Osborne and Mendel[36] in 1915, it was not until 25 years later that McCay[31] confirmed and greatly extended that work. The following years saw only a trickle of research in the field of aging and nutrition until the 1960s when Ross,[39] then Berg and Simms[12] and then Barrows[10] again took up this problem.

This long lag period is more puzzling than the 35-year delay in the rediscovery of Gregor Mendel's laws of inheritance because of the clear human importance of every aspect of nutrition. From the point of view of public health it makes little difference whether a dietary regimen, that can increase the mean age at death by 50% or more, acts by placing less wear and tear on the DNA, slowing some neuro-endocrine pacemaker for aging, postponing the onset of diseases characteristic of old age, or by some other method. At the same time, a knowledge of the mechanism can be expected to throw light on the underlying phenomena of aging from birth through adolescence to adulthood and senescence. In addition, knowledge of the effects of both quantitative and qualitative food restriction has important implications in a world where millions of people live in pitiable semistarvation. It may very well turn out that the so-called well-fed populations are in fact overfed for their own best health. More is not necessarily better.

Among the more recent results is the discovery that dietary restriction can begin as late as early adulthood and still be effective, although not as dramatic. Among the flock of unsolved problems is whether caloric restriction is the important factor or protein restriction is a key aspect of this phenomenon. Goodrick[25] has shown the importance, in work of this kind, of using genetically homogeneous strains.

Ross[39] has presented a vast amount of data showing that if rats are given a choice of different diets, the results on longevity are different from those seen after presenting the rats a single diet. At about the same time both he and Berg and Simms found that the diseases of older rats can be postponed by diet. The possible human importance of this fact is independent of whether such dietary maneuvers increase mean life span by influencing some basic aging chronometer or are comparable to increasing mean life span by discovering a cure for some childhood disease.

A number of theories have been proposed to explain life prolongation by food restrictions.

Food restricted rats have "younger" immune systems, with thymic growth slowed and the timing of its involution postponed. However, as Weindruch,[52] Walford,[51] and their collaborators have pointed out, the immune system is not autonomous but is influenced by hormones which in turn are influenced by diet.

A theory adopted by Barrows as a reasonable working hypothesis postulates that a restricted diet means less wear and hence damage to the DNA by retarding genetic information transfer. This obviously is a form of the Orgel hypothesis as are the working assumptions of Cutler's ideas on the role of superoxide dismutase. As we have already indicated (Section IV.B.I) there is no doubt that DNA damage accumulates but it is far less certain that such damage in itself paces aging from birth to senescence. In animals on restricted diets Barrows and his coworkers have found decreased levels of activity for a number of enzymes, succinoxidase, phosphatases, malic dehydrogenase, increased $O_2$ consumption, and lower body temperature but the old question of whether causes or effects of some basic pace setter remains. Recently J. E. Johnson, Jr. has found that the effects of nutritional restriction on the rat kidney closely resemble those of surgical hypophysectomy. The idea that life extension by dietary restriction is mediated by the pituitary was adopted by Comfort in 1964 from the work of Mulinos and Pomerantz[34] who had shown that "undernutrition" resulted in "pseudo-hypophysectomy". Subsequently, Everitt[21] showed that hypophysectomy delayed the aging of collagen and suggested that the "retarded aging in the food restricted animal may be due to the diminished secretion of pituitary hormones."

The implications of this observation of Johnson extend in two directions. Hypophysectomy is the primary means used by Denckla[18a] to produce rejuvenation in rats (Section IV.B.2). Furthermore, it has been known for some years through the work of Wurtman[56] and his collaborators Fernstrom,[22] Lytle, and others that diet has a pronounced effect on the level of tryptophan in the blood and through it on brain tryptophan and serotonin of which tryptophan is the precursor. A diet, in fact a meal, rich in carbohydrates raises the ratio of tryptophan to competing amino acids for transport through the blood-brain barrier and results in an increase in brain serotonin. A protein meal acts in the opposite direction and lowers the level of serotonin. Changing levels of serotonin, are known to change behavior in mammals, including food consumption. More important, the secretion of some pituitary hormones is correlated with brain serotonin. It is in serotonin and other monoamines in the hypothalamus that Finch sees the possibility of age-related changes "that produce a regulatory cascade of changing neural, endocrine and target-tissue interactions" expressed as aging.

Here then is a mechanism through which the profound effect of diet on aging might be explained. It not only fits the observations of Denckla on hypophysectomy but also the work of Ross[39] which showed a difference in results between rats given a choice of diets and those with no choice, and the difference in caloric intake after forced and after free will exercise in rats reported by Mayer and others. "Nutritional hypophysectomy" would explain the sterility commonly seen in rats whose lives have been extended by prolonged nutritional restriction. It is worth noting that Osborne and Mendel prolonged their rats' life span by feeding zein; the protein in corn as the only source of protein since it is very deficient in tryptophan. The work on extending the lives of chickens by the staff of the Monsanto Company over 20 years ago seems to have been inspired by the observations of Osborne and Mendel.[36] The published reports of the Monsanto experiments do not say but in the photos of their longevous chickens the birds appear very gawky and even unwell.

Lastly it should be said that Winick and Brasel[55] have shown in rats and human infants that some if not all of the damage to the brain, or at least to behavior, from early "malnutrition" can be overcome by enriching the environment. In rats, handling the animals for 2 min a day for the first 21 days after neonatal deprivation suffices.

## VII. CONCLUSIONS

The bottom line of all these considerations is the importance of the open mind. The history of science, not only in physics but in biology as well, has seen many shattering surprises. It is often said that fortunate accidental discoveries are made by prepared minds. There is, however, an important proviso, the minds must not be over prepared.

The end result of theoretical investigations into the biological basis of aging will yield a double harvest. It will assuredly make it possible for more people everywhere to live a full human life span with a sound mind in a sound body. It will also add to the sum of human understanding.

## REFERENCES


### General

1. **Behnke, J. A., Finch, C. E., and Moment, G. B.,** *The Biology of Aging,* Plenum Press, New York, 1978.
2. **Comfort, A.,** *Ageing: The Biology of Senescence,* Holt, Rinehart and Winston, New York, 1964.
3. **Dietz, A. A., Ed.,** *Aging - It's Chemistry,* American Association for Clinical Chemistry, Washington, D.C., 1979.
4. **Finch, E. E. and Hayflick, L., Eds.,** *Handbook of the Biology of Aging,* Van Nostrand Reinhold Co., New York, 1977.
5. **Minot, C. S.,** *The Problem of Age, Growth and Death,* G. P. Putnam's Sons, New York, 1908.
6. **Rockstein, M. and Sussman, M.,** *Biology of Aging,* Wadsworth Publishing Co., Belmont, Calif., 1979.
7. **Shock, N. W., Ed.,** *Biological Aspects of Aging, 5th International Association of Gerontologists,* Columbia University Press, New York, 1960.
8. **Strehler, B. L.,** *The Biology of Aging,* American Institute of Biological Sciences, Washington, D.C., 1960.

### Special

9. **Adelman, R. C.,** Loss of adaptive mechanisms during aging, *Fed. Proc. Fed. Am. Exp. Biol.,* 38, 6, 1968.

9a. **Aslan, A., Vrabiescu, A., Domiliscu, C., Campeanu, L., Costiniu, M., and Stanescu, S.,** Long-term treatment with procaine (Gerovital $H_3$) in albino rats, *J. Gerontol.,* 20, 1, 1965.

10. **Barrows, C. H., Jr. and Kokkonen, G. C.,** Diet and life extension in animal model systems, *Age,* 1, 131, 1978.
11. **Barrows, C. H., Jr. and Kokkonen, G.,** Protein synthesis, development, growth and lifespan, *Growth,* 39, 525, 1978.
12. **Berg, B. N. and Simms, H. S.,** Nutrition and longevity in the rat. II. Longevity and onset of disease with different levels of food intake, *J. Nutr.,* 71, 255, 1960.
13. **Bowden, D. M., Ed.,** *Aging in Non-Human Primates,* Van Nostrand Reinhold Co., New York, 1979.
14. **Brody, S., Henderson, E., and Kempster, H.,** The rate of senescence of domestic fowl as measured by the decline in egg production with age, *J. Gen. Physiol.,* 6, 41, 1923.
15. **Bryant, P. J.,** Pattern formation, growth control and cell interactions in Drosophila imaginal discs, in *Determinants of Organization,* Subtelny, S. and Konigsberg, I. R., Eds., Academic Press, New York, 1979.
16. **Cutler, R. G.,** Evolutionary biology of senescence, in *The Biology of Aging,* Behnke, J. A., Finch, C. E., and Moment, G. B., Eds., Plenum Press, New York, 1978.
17. **Cutler, R. G.,** Evolution of longevity in ungulates and carnivores, *Gerontology,* 25, 69, 1979.
18. **Dayhoff, M. O. and Eck, R. V.,** Atlas of Protein Sequence and Structure 1967-68, National Biomedical Research Foundation, Silver Spring, Md., 1968.

18a. **Denckla, S. M. and Bolla, R.,** Age-related changes in immune function of rats and the effect of long-term hypophysectomy, *Mech. Aging Dev.,* 11, 127, 1979.

19. **Dilman, V. M.,** Age-associated elevation of hypothalamic threshold to feedback control, and its role in development, aging, and disease, *Lancet,* 1, 1211, 1971.
20. **Edgar, B. C.,** Elegans Workshop (The Worm Breeder's Confabulation) I. Woods Hole, Mass., April 1977. II. (Worm Breeder's Gazette Vol. 2 and 3) University of California, Santa Cruz, June 1977.
21. **Everitt, A. V. and Burgess, J. A.,** *Hypothalamus, Pituitary and Aging,* Charles C Thomas, Springfield, Ill., 1976.

22. **Fernstrom, J. P. and Wurtman, R. J.**, Control of brain 5-HT by dietary carbohydrates, in *Serotonin and Behavior,* Barchas, J. and Usdin, E., Eds., Academic Press, New York, 1973.
23. **Finch, C. E.**, The regulation of physiological changes during mammalian aging, *Q. Rev. Biol.,* 51(1), 49, 1976.
24. **Fridovich, I., McCord, J. M., Michelson, A. M.**, *Superoxide and Superoxide Dismutases,* Michelson, A. M., McCord, J. M., and Fridovich, I., Eds., Academic Press, New York, 1977.
25. **Goodrick, C. L.**, Body weight increments and length of life, *J. Gerontol.,* 33(2), 184, 1978.
26. **Gould, S. J.**, *Ontogeny and Phylogeny* Belknap Press, Harvard University, Cambridge, 1977.
27. **Hall, G. O. and Marble, D. R.**, The relationship between the first year egg production and the egg production of later years, *Poultry Sci.,* 10, 194, 1931.
28. **Hastings, J. W. and Schweiger, H. G., Eds.**, *The Molecular Basis of Circadian Rhythyms,* Life Sciences Research Reports #1, Bernhard, S., Ed., Abakon Verlags, Berlin, 1976.
29. **Hayflick, L.**, The cell biology of human aging, *Sci. Am.,* 242(1), 58, 1980.
30. **Lytle, L. D. and Altar, A.**, Diet, central nervous system, and aging, *Fed. Proc. Fed. Am. Soc. Exp. Biol.,* 38(6), 2017, 1979.
31. **McCay, C. M.**, Frustrations of a senescent, in *The Biology of Aging,* Strehler, B. L., Ed., American Institute of Biological Sciences, Arlington, Va., 1960.
32. **Martin, R. A.**, A possible genetic mechanism of aging, rejuvenation, and recombination in germinal cells, *Human Cytogenetics: ICN-UCLA Symposium,* Vol. 8, Academic Press, New York, 1977, 356.
33. **Meadow, N. D. and Barrows, C. H., Jr.**, Studies on aging in a bdelloid rotifer. Effects of various culture systems on longevity and fecundity, *J. Exp. Zool.,* 176, 303, 1971.
34. **Mulinos, M. G. and Pomerantz, L.**, Psuedo-hypophysectomy, a condition resembling hypophysectomy produced by malnutrition, *J. Nutr.,* 19, 493, 1940.
35. **Nesbitt, M. N., Butler, K., and Spence, M. A.**, Clonal analysis of behavior in mice, in *The Clonal Basis of Development,* Subtelny, S. and Sussex, I. M., Eds., Academic Press, New York, 1978.
36. **Osborne, T. B. and Mendel, L. B.**, The resumption of growth after long continued failure to grow, *J. Biol. Chem.,* 23, 439, 1915.
37. **Palmer, J. D.**, *An Introduction to Biological Rhythyms,* Academic Press, New York, 1976.
38. **Robertson, O. H., Krupp, M. A., Thomas, S. F., Favour, C. B., Hane, S., and Wexler, B. C.**, Hyperadrenocorticism in spawning migratory and nonmigratory Rainbow trout (*Salmo gairdnerii*); comparison with Pacific salmon, *Aging in Cold Blooded Animals,* MSS Information Corp., New York, 1974.
39. **Ross, M. H.**, Nutritional regulation of longevity, in *The Biology of Aging,* Behnke, J. A., Finch, C. E., and Moment, G. B., Eds., Plenum Press, New York, 1978.
40. **Rubner, M.**, *Das Problem der Lebensdaur und seine Beziehungen zu Wachstum und Ernahrung,* Munchen, 1908.
41. **Rusak, B. and Zucker, I.**, Neural regulation of circadian rhythyms, *Physiol. Rev.,* 59(3), 449, 1979.
42. **Samis, H. V., Jr. and Capobianco, S.**, *Aging and Biological Rhythyms,* Plenum Press, New York, 1977.
43. **Schneider, E. L., Ed.**, *The Genetics of Aging,* Plenum Press, New York, 1978.
44. **Shock, N. W.**, Age changes in physiological functions in the total animal: the role of tissue loss, in *The Biology of Aging,* Strehler, B. L., Ed., American Institute Biological Sciences, Arlington, Va., 1960, 23.
45. **Shoemaker, W. J. and Wurtman, R. J.**, Effect of perinatal undernutrition on the metabolism of catecholamines in the rat brain, *J. Nutr.,* 103(11), 1537, 1973.
46. **Sonneborn, T. M.**, The origin, evolution, nature, and causes of aging, in *The Biology of Aging,* Plenum Press, New York, 1978.
47. **Stearns, S. C.**, Life-history tactics: a review of the ideas, *Q. Rev. Biol.,* 51(1), 3, 1976.
48. **Swanson, P. and Riddle, D.**, *C. Elegana Newslett.,* 5(2), 1, 1980.
49. **Tolmasoff, J. M., Ono, T., and Cutler, R. G.**, Superoxide dismutase: correlation with life span and specific metabolic rate in primate species, Gordon Research Conference "Genetic and Evolutionary Aspects of Aging", Santa Barbara, Calif., 1979.
50. **Tolmasoff, J. M., Ono, T., and Cutler, R. G**, Superoxide dismutase: correlation with life span and specific metabolic rate in primate species, *Proc. Natl. Acad. Sci. U.S.A.,* 77, 2777, 1979.
51. **Walford, R. L.**, *The Immunologic Theory of Aging,* Williams & Wilkins, Baltimore, 1969.
52. **Weindruch, R. H., Kristie, J. A., Cheney, K. E., and Walford, R. L.**, Influence of controlled dietary restriction on immunologic function and aging, *Fed. Proc. Am. Soc. Exp. Biol.,* 38(6), 2007, 1979.
53. **Weismann, A.**, The duration of life, in *Collected Essays Upon Heredity and Kindred Biological Problems,* Poulton, E. B., Ed., Clarenden Press, Oxford, 1889.
54. **Williams, G. C.**, Pleiotropy, natural selection, and the evolution of senescence, *Evolution,* 11, 398, 1957.
55. **Winick, M. and Brasel, J. A.**, Early malnutrition and subsequent brain development, *Ann. N.Y. Acad. Sci.,* 300, 380, 1977.

56. **Wurtman, R. J.,** Nutrients that modify brain function, *Sci. Am.,* 246(4), 50, 1982.
57. **Zuckerman, B. M.,** *Free-Living Nematodes as Models to Study Biological Aging,* University of Massachusetts, East Wareham, Mass., 1975.
58. **Zuckerman, B. M., Ed.,** *Nematodes as Biological Models,* Academic Press, New York, 1980.

Chapter 2

# LONGEVITY IS DETERMINED BY SPECIFIC GENES: TESTING THE HYPOTHESIS

**Richard G. Cutler**

## TABLE OF CONTENTS

## I. INTRODUCTION

The aim of this chapter is to describe the general and special hypothesis of aging and longevity and to present experimental support and means by which they can be evaluated further. In describing the hypothesis, only the major elements will be stated. For more detailed information on the development, rationale, and supporting data, the reader will be referred to previously published papers. Consequently, the scope of the presentation is not comprehensive or exhaustive.

The first publication describing the general and special hypothesis of aging and longevity appeared in 1972.[1] Later publications[2-14] presented details and a few alterations, and more changes are expected as dictated by future experimental and theoretical results from this and other laboratories. Much of the hypothesis is based on the work of others, and thus a characteristic of the hypothesis is that it represents an integration of a number of separate hypotheses of aging and related concepts suggested by other authors. However, many aspects are unique, particularly the prediction that specific genes exist whose sole function is the preservation of general health of an organism.[1-4] It is, of course, well known for example that the function of the immune system is the preservation of general health of an organism, and that specific genes are involved in coding for its function. But what is meant by this prediction is more global in nature, in that the duration of optimum vigor and the maintenance of good health of the entire organism is governed by a limited and specific set of genes, which includes the maintenance of function of the immune system. This prediction implies that aging is a process sufficiently separate from other life functions so that its rate of occurrence is subject to control by a specific set of genes without serious alteration of these life functions. Aging rate is not, as is still the common belief, determined by the entire set (or most) of the genes required to produce an organism.

To make this point clear, the life span of an organism is commonly thought to be the result of processes determining the entire biological nature of an organism, much like the functional life span of an automobile, where most parts are designed to last about the same length of time. To increase the functional life span of the automobile, one means would be to improve the quality of all the parts and not just a few specific ones. Using this analogy, the prospect of understanding the biological nature of aging would in turn require a knowledge of all processes involved in differentiation and development of an organism. Consequently, the prospect of ever enhancing the normal life span of an organism would be quite futile, and such is the belief of many biologists.

In contrast, what the hypothesis presented here predicts is that all mammals are made up of the same quality of parts, regardless of their differences in maximum life span potentials (MLPs), and that the differences in their MLPs are determined by how well these parts are maintained, protected, and repaired. These protection and repair processes are the functions of the postulated longevity determinant genes (LDGs). Their degree of expression are predicted to be regulated by a relatively few genes. Thus, a longer lasting automobile could also be obtained by better maintenance.

It should be obvious what the consequences this prediction would have on the health-related sciences if it were found to be generally true. A different perspective on the cause of age-dependent diseases and dysfunctions would be gained and used to develop new methods for their prevention and treatment. Also, means might be found that are extraordinarily simple to postpone in time and in a uniform manner many human age-related diseases and dysfunctions and thus provide a longer more functional life span for individuals. In addition, many persons may be deficient in some of the health maintenance properties controlled by the LDPs. An identification of such deficiencies might lead to corrections and thus help ensure a more normal life span.

Although the specific gene prediction is the most far-reaching aspect of the hypothesis, this prediction is only part of a general hypothesis of aging and longevity which is devoted to all forms of life and a special hypothesis, which is the application of the general hypothesis to the mammalian species.

The general hypothesis was developed from an investigation to determine what insight might be gained on the biological nature of aging and longevity processes in humans from evolutionary theory on the origin of life and species. Typical questions raised where answers were derived are as follows: (1) are aging processes involved in the origin and evolution of life, (2) is aging an inherent characteristic of life, (3) why and how did aging evolve, (4) is aging necessary for life to exist, (5) what value might aging play in the evolutionary success of species, (6) what is the genetic and biochemical complexity of the aging process, (7) are the processes determining aging and longevity different or common in nature, (8) why and how did longevity evolve, (9) did longevity play an important role in the evolutionary success of species, (10) what is the biological nature and complexity of longevity, and (11) what value does longevity have for the evolutionary success of humans?

The special hypothesis was developed to extend such questions specifically to the mammalian species, particularly to the primates.

It would be surprising if any of the answers provided by the hypothesis as it stands now were correct, but it is hoped that at least some are on the right track. However, the main function of the hypothesis is to go beyond descriptive gerontology and to present a reasonable rationale for the design of experiments to answer the above and related questions.

## II. GENERAL AND SPECIAL HYPOTHESIS OF AGING AND LONGEVITY

### A. Background

The hypothesis was developed from an evolutionary viewpoint. Many of the ideas were derived from the writings of Haldane,[15] Medawar,[16,17] Williams,[18] Hamilton,[19] Maynard Smith,[20-22] de Beer,[23] Schultz,[24-29] Wilson,[30-35] Gould,[36-40] Sacher,[41-48] Monod,[49] and Wilson.[50] It should be emphasized, however, that it was the disagreement with some of these authors' conclusions that stimulated the development of an alternative hypothesis. For example, Williams[18] and Hamilton[19] concluded that, because of the vast complexity of pleiotropic-acting genes involved in determining aging, further enhancement of life span is clearly impossible. This author agreed with their concept that developmentally-linked genes of a pleiotropic nature played a role in aging but suggested that, in spite of their complexity, increased life span could have evolved by changes in a few genes reducing the rate of development and thus resulting in a further postponement of their expression.[4,6]

Sacher interpreted the biological basis of the correlation relating MLP to the relative brain-to-body weights of mammals as indicating that qualitative aspects in homeostatic control (where the brain was postulated to be the organ of longevity) governed aging rate and not quantitative biochemical factors. It has been argued that the body weight term reflects the level of harmful or toxic pleiotropic metabolic products being produced and not the level of wear-and-tear.[1] In addition, it has been argued that the brain is not likely to be an organ of longevity and that relative brain-to-body weight instead reflected evolutionary pressures to evolve longevity beyond that dictated by body weight or specific metabolic weight.[1] From such arguments, was proposed a hypothesis directly opposed to that of Sacher suggesting that quantitative biochemical processes were primarily involved in governing aging rate, not qualitative homeostatic processes.[1,4,6]

It should be pointed out also that an important feature of this hypothesis is concerned with what governs aging rate of mammalian species. Sacher was the first to seriously ask this question[41,44,45] and spent much effort in investigating different areas of the brain which might be the most responsible for governing aging rate and thus in maintaining homeostatic levels in animals.[48] The experimental method he developed for this was the comparative approach, using species having different MLPs. Most other hypotheses of aging do not account for longevity differences between species.[51-54] For example, proponents of the error hypothesis,[55-58] free radical hypothesis,[59-62] somatic mutation hypothesis,[63,64] or the immunological hypothesis[65] of aging did not describe mechanisms of how their hypothesis could account for species differences in aging rates. They are accordingly hypotheses only of aging, not longevity. As far as this author is aware, Sacher's homeostasis hypothesis[47] and the hypothesis described in this chapter are unique in this respect by offering an explanation that does account for species differences in aging rates.

**B. General Hypothesis**

The survival of life is based on the living system being capable of preserving information which ensures the system to be able to continue to preserve this same information.[1,6,8,12] This information is encoded within a physical structure which has a finite life span. The essential characteristics of living systems is the means they use to preserve this information. One means has been the duplication of the information before it is lost and the use of protection and repair processes to make this possible. Related supporting elements provide and maintain these functions. Any time-dependent alteration in the information-containing physical structure and/or its supporting elements leading towards an increased probability of a loss of its essential properties of self-preservation is considered in a broad sense to be an aging process. On the other hand, all processes which have evolved to preserve this information and the information-containing structure are considered in a broad sense to be anti-aging processes. From the above proposal, a definition of life can be derived, of what life is and why it exists.[1,6,8,12]

DNA is an example of a physical structure where such information is stored, and the replication of DNA is an example of one of the most primitive and still most essential information preservational processes which have evolved. It should be noted that life is a process involving entities having a physical makeup. The function of life (why it exists and what keeps it going) is the maintenance and propagation of information. This information is contained in but is not part of a physical entity. Thus, a fundamental characteristic of life is the ability to propagate an unlimited life span of sets of information within physical entities having themselves a limited life span. Only by these means are living processes potentially immortal.

It should be clear that the arguments given for the evolution of life and what its innate characteristics are serve as a definition of life. This definition was first described in 1972[1] and in other later publications.[6,8,12] For example, it defines an endogenous virus genome, even though it may never be induced as a separate free entity as a living system in its own right. Furthermore, any system whose existance depends on the preservation of information which acts to preserve itself is a living system. This definition would also include as potential living systems the so-called jumping genes or transposon elements that may make up a considerable portion of nonessential DNA in mammalian species,[66,67] episomal particles, and all other intracellular information-containing entities, regardless if their evolutionary development is governed by molecular events within the cell or by macroevents involving the whole organism. Thus, it is to be expected that one may find independent living systems within living systems, where their individual evolution may or may not be interrelated — but where their survival is.

From the origin of life and throughout the following evolution of all living systems, the interaction of aging and antiaging forces has prevailed. That life still exists on Earth indicates that antiaging processes so far have succeeded, but this may be more from accident than by design. Thus, the entire biological makeup and behavior of all forms of life existing today are taken to reflect the complex history of the interactions and trade-offs molded by the actions and counteractions of these two forces. Consequently, it would be impossible to obtain a complete understanding of an organism's behavior, morphology, or its genetic and biological makeup such as it is today without also an understanding of the interactions of these aging and antiaging forces.

The longevity of an individual of a given life form is only one of many different types of strategies that have evolved to ensure a continued preservation of its characteristic set of information.[68] A great number of other strategies exist, such as an increase in the number of individuals (sets of information). Clearly, however, the success of a species is not measured by its number but by the length of time its particular set of information has been able to survive and evolve.

Since the origin of life, longevity determinant processes have evolved. These processes insured the continuity of life and were therefore selected for, not senescent or aging processes.

In most organisms today, the cause of aging is considered to be mostly of an endogenous nature and is the result of by-products of the structural, developmental, and metabolic processes which have evolved to maintain the continuity of the living process in time. A primary cause of aging does exist. It is pleiotropic in nature and usually arises from the harmful side effects of otherwise essential processes needed to maintain the organism. Examples of the pleiotropic aging process are energy metabolism (producing the hydroxyl radical) and differentiation and developmental processes requiring the use of steroids and growth factors which may have nonspecific detrimental effects.

### C. Special Hypothesis

#### *1. Interaction Between External and Internal Environmental Hazards*

On studying the evolution of aging and longevity in mammalian species, it was calculated that, on the average, longevity of species has steadily increased.[3,4,9] It was also determined that few if any individuals of a given species living in their natural ecological niche were able to live much beyond a chronological age where their physiological aging processes seriously decreased their health status or physiological functions.[8,12] All individuals regardless of their chronological ages were essentially vigorous and healthy and were killed only by natural external factors, and rarely by internal dysfunctions.[69] This evidence is consistent with the conclusion that longevity rather than aging evolved. For example, the biological potential of a species to maintain good health and high vigor rarely appears to have been in vast excess or deficiency in relation to its environmental hazards. A high aging rate may act to enhance survival of an evolutionary line by increasing the turnover in the population for natural selection processes to operate, but apparently natural hazards were sufficient to provide such turnover. Moreover, it appears that for most species living in the wild, death occurred well before signs of senescence began to show. It was not just the old, feeble, or sick that were killed by predators. Individuals at all ages had a similar probability of death. Thus, it is considered unlikely that aging genes or a genetic program of aging existed to age individuals for the good of the species.[70] Instead, longevity of the individual has evolved, and this was not the result of less genetically-programmed death for, as noted before, life span potential was never in vast excess.

Of course, for biological longevity potential to have evolved, it must be possible for an organism to benefit by actually being able to live longer in a given environmental hazard. For this to occur, the effective biological hazards have to decrease. This can be achieved by the evolution of appropriate morphological and behavioral characteristics resulting in a higher probability of survival, and thus a lower effective environmental hazard. Another way of looking at this is that the innate ability to survive longer against external environmental hazards is considered to have co-evolved with the innate ability to survive longer against an internal environmental hazards. Support for this argument is obtained from animal populations today, where a good correlation is seen between biological longevity potential of a species (as measured in captivity) and its longevity in the wild.[4,6,8,69,71]

*2. Evolution of Learned-Adaptive Behavior*

The driving force behind the evolution of increased longevity for the mammalian species is considered to be the extraordinary success of a new intellectual trait, learned-adaptive behavior.[4,72] Because of an apparent biological limit of how fast a brain can mature and the necessity for an extended time period for learned behavior to function (obtainment of information and its processing), increased longevity was essential for the realization of the potentials of this new trait. The evolutionary success of mammalian species is viewed as representing largely the success of learned-adaptive behavior over instinctive behavior. Learned-adaptive behavior evolved in its most advanced state during the evolution of primates. Humans represent the species taking the most advantage of this new trait, having the highest degree of learned-adaptive behavior, minimum degree of instinctive behavior, and the longest potential life span of all mammalian species. In terms of energy consumption per unit gram of tissue over life span, human probably has the highest of any species ever existing on earth. *Thus, a fundamental characteristic in the evolutionary success of human involved not only the brain, hand, the ability to walk upright, and biosocial aspects, which are frequently emphasized by anthropologists, but also his remarkable long innate longevity potential.* The unusual life span of human is not considered to have just happened as a by-product of other biological processes that were more essential.[73] Instead, the evolutionary success of the human required an unusually long period of good health and vigor to take advantage of the newly evolved potential of the brain in terms of intelligence or learned-adaptive behavior. Both adaptive behavior and longevity did not likely increase over the past two million years along the hominid-ancestral descendant pathway to any significant extent without a corresponding increase in intellectual capacity.

A number of different biological mechanisms are likely to underlie the evolution of longevity. One key development has been the increase in body size, which is of particular interest because it is likely to have evolved with only a few gene changes. These changes resulted in a coordinate decrease in the effective external environmental hazards for the organism and an increase in innate longevity due to a decrease in internal environmental hazards by the decrease in metabolic rate per unit amount of tissue. Many other examples of change in a single factor, resulting in both a decrease in effective external environmental hazards and an increase in biological longevity potential, are likely to exist.

The characteristic aging rate of a given mammalian species is determined by the environmental hazards of its ecological niche. For example, the effective external hazards for the field mouse are determined by its innate physical morphology, learned-adaptive behavior-to-instinctive behavior ratio, and the physical environment hazards. This results in a probability of death for this species to approach 100% in about 1 year. If the animal is raised in captivity, the mouse is observed to undergo significant decline in vigor and general health status at an age of about 1 year or perhaps a little sooner. Because longevity is considered to have a biological cost in terms of energy (food requirements), a longer innate biological potential to maintain vigor and health than 1 year would be of no advantage and thus did not evolve. By this process, a species' mean life span in the wild defines the point where further longevity would have little benefit for the preservation of the information which defines that species.[4,6,8,12] Of course, for a given environmental hazard, other means in addition to increase of longevity evolved to insure a species' survival, such as an increase in reproduction rate or population number. However, for primates and a number of other mammalian species, there is data showing a good correlation between the actual survival of the species in the wild, its innate longevity potential, and its dependence for survival on learned-adaptive behavior as opposed to instinctive behavior. In fact, there is a remarkable consistency for those mammalian species which have become extinct (their evolutionary line no longer continues) and a period prior to their extinction where no increase in encephalization quotient or longevity potential evolved.[4,9]

*3. Biological Complexity of Aging and Longevity Processes*

In an effort to determine the biological and genetic complexity governing aging rate, the evolutionary rate of longevity during the evolution of the mammalian species was estimated.[1-4,9] This estimate of the evolutionary direction and rate of evolution of longevity of extinct species was made using two methods. One was the use of the equation developed by Sacher,[41] which has shown a remarkable ability to predict the MLP of both progressive and living fossil species on knowing only the adult body and brain weights of that species. Using published results of body and brain weights for extinct species, MLPs were calculated and an evolutionary tree of longevity for mammals was constructed. The results clearly indicated that (1) longevity increased throughout the evolutionary period of all mammalian species and (2) longevity increased at an ever-increasing rate along the hominid ancestral-descendant sequence leading to human.

The second method to estimate the direction and rate of evolution of longevity compared the MLPs of living primate species. Through a knowledge of the evolutionary tree relating their extinct ancestors at different geological time-points, a rough estimate of how longevity changed during evolution could be calculated. Similar results were found using both methods; that is, longevity increased and at a very high rate during the recent evolutionary history of human. On comparing the rate of increased longevity in the hominids 100,000 years ago (which was about 14 years of increased innate biological life span potential per 100,000 years of evolution) to how fast new genes had been estimated to appear or can appear as determined by a critical mutational load size, an estimate was calculated on how many new genes might have appeared during the evolutionary changes taking place in the hominid species at this time. These calculations gave the surprising result that at most only about 0.6% of the hominid genome could be involved in the recent evolutionary changes taking place in the hominids. Of course, many morphological and intellectual changes were also occurring 100,000 years ago, but one of these was likely to be an increase in innate biological longevity potential. Thus, the genes involved in longevity alone, if they are mostly different from the other genes involved in the evolution of the hominids (some genes are probably overlapping in their effects, such as increase in body size and decrease in developmental rate), are likely to represent even less than 0.6% of the total genome. Consequently, if there are say 100,000 genes functioning in a typical human cell, then 600 genes at most are estimated to be involved in determining life span or, most importantly, the period good health, vigor, and disease-free life span is maintained.

There are a number of reasons suggesting that a decrease in the rate of development played a causative role in the evolution of longevity. Through arguments reviewed recently by Gould,[36-40] the evolution of larger brain size and many other aspects of human morphology are governed by scaling factors. Such scaling factors appear to place a limit or constriction on what patterns of development can evolve in terms of being the most probable. Thus, certain changes in morphology and developmental rate appear to be governed by a few hormonally related processes and the qualitative nature of the changes taking place determined by scaling factors.[24-27] In this regard, the process of neoteny,[23,37,38] involving an increase in relative brain size, and the increase of longevity all appeared to be linked together by common scaling factors and as such are governed by common genes and are accordingly more likely to evolve coordinately at high rates. The prediction of MLP of all mammalian species by brain and body weight, using only three constants, also suggests very rigid constrictions on how longevity relative to morphology can evolve.[1,2]

*4. Longevity Determinant Genes*

The remarkable similarities of the primate species in terms of morphology, physiology, general biology, biochemistry, and genetics, suggested to Wilson and co-workers[30-35] that the evolution of morphology of species was accomplished mainly through changes in the timing and degree of expression of changes in regulatory genes and not through changes in the information content of structural genes. Such regulatory genes may then govern a common set of structural genes found in all mammals and, through regulating a difference in timing during development and degree of expression, determine the developmental patterns and morphology of all mammals.

Our results indicating the unusually high rate in the evolution of increased longevity, coupled with the work of Wilson's group on the genetic mechanisms involved in the evolution of morphology, de Beer, Gould, and Schultz's work on the role of neoteny and developmental rates in the evolution of morphology and development, led this author to predict the existence of a special class of genes, the Longevity Determinant Genes (LDGs) which would be similar in nature and controlled by a few regulatory genes. The unique role postulated for these LDGs was to provide the necessary duration of good health and vigor to ensure the evolutionary success of the species. It is important to emphasize that such LDGs do not assure longevity; that is, they are not longevity assurance genes, but rather genes which determine the biological potential for longevity.

Like the evolution of morphology and development, it was suggested that these hypothetical structural genes governing life span were to be found in all mammalian species, regardless of their biological life span potential. It was only the timing and degree of their expression that made the difference of whether a species would live 10 or 100 years. The genes governing the timing and degree of expression of the structural component of the LDGs would be their corresponding regulatory genes. It is these genes that were calculated to be few in number and less than 0.6% of the genome in hominids. This prediction clearly emphasizes that, in mammalian aging processes, the aging rate of the entire organism as well as intelligence and learned-adaptive behavior are controlled in a coordinated manner by a relatively few genes that are of a regulatory nature.

*5. Continuously-Acting and Developmentally Linked Biosenescent and Longevity Processes*

The evolutionary data does not suggest, however, what causes aging or how aging rate might be controlled. Therefore, to be able to initiate a search for these hypothetical LDPs and their corresponding regulatory genes, predictions were formulated, mainly from genetic and biochemical considerations of the roles of specific metabolic rate, detoxification, and DNA repair processes. From these considerations, the primary causes of aging were predicted to be of a pleiotropic nature; that is, they are by-products of normally beneficial metabolic and developmental processes.[1,4,5,6,8] Two basic types of pleiotropic aging processes were postulated: (1) continuously acting biosenescent processes (CABPs) and (2) developmentally linked biosenescent processes (DLBPs). The evolution of longevity in the mammalian species is predicted to have occurred by reduction of these two major classes of biosenescent processes. This prediction is considered to be fundamental in any efforts to lengthen life span, for it may be that without a coordinated reduction of both, a significant increase in life span may prove to be impossible.

Examples of the DLBPs are the various hormones and growth factors associated with growth, cessation of growth, and sexual maturation (the aging of the Pacific coast salmon, eels, and octopus being good examples). Examples of the CABPs are by-products of oxygen metabolism, such as the superoxide free radical $O_2^-$, the hydroxyl radical $\cdot OH$ and hydrogen peroxide $H_2O_2$.

To counteract these two classes of biosenescent processes, corresponding longevity determinant processes (LDPs) evolved, their genetic components being the LDGs. Many of these LDPs were probably in existance in early prokaryotic and eukaryotic cells. For the primate species, it is predicted that, at this point in evolutionary development, the biochemical processes involved in their differentiation and development were so strongly entrenched in the makeup of the organism that few simple alternatives were available for reducing their long-term pleiotropic aging effects. Therefore, the primary means for the effective reduction of the DLBPs was largely a postponement in time of their appearance during development. The decrease in developmental rate with increased longevity observed in the primates and other mammalian species is support for this concept and is likely to involve only a few regulatory genes.[3,4,6,8] In turn, as a result of the constrictions of what changes are most likely to occur, decreases in developmental rate are coupled with the morphological changes observed in neoteny processes; that is, the general morphology of present-day human, such as the relatively large brain and unusually slow rate of development, could be a result of changes of the same regulatory genes. All of these changes could therefore be genetically and functionally linked together serving, in a synergistic manner, the same objective and all occurring by changes in the timing and regulation of a common set of genes.

The reduction of the CABPs during the evolution of mammalian longevity is predicted to have occurred by the increased expression of genes (more enzymes or products being produced) which evolved over millions of years to counteract the pleiotropic side effects of the living processes other than those associated with development. For example, the superoxide free radical $O_2^-$, a pleiotropic by-product of oxygen metabolism, would be predicted to be counteracted more effectively in longer-lived species by higher levels of the enzyme superoxide dismutase (SOD) being synthesized.[1,6,11] Another example is higher DNA repair levels in longer-lived mammalian species to remove more completely and in less time the damage that did occur. In general, longer-lived mammalian species would be expected to have higher levels of antioxidants and higher levels of DNA repair than shorter-lived species, but all living forms of life would require a certain level of antioxidants and DNA repair to survive.[1,2]

### 6. *Aging is Dysdifferentiation*

The two major classes of pleiotropic biosenescent processes (CABPs and DLBPs) are predicted to cause aging through the mechanism of dysdifferentiation. Basic to this prediction is that aging is considered to be the random disorganization of the same orderly processes that gave rise to the creation of the organism. Starting with a single cell, an organism is created by differentiation and developmental processes, one event followed by another in a highly organized manner. The mechanisms determining when and how a cell differentiates during development are not known but are thought to involve position effects, ionic strength gradients, electrical effects, cell-to-cell contact, hormones, growth factors, and concurrent intracellular changes in the processing of information contained within the genome of each cell. Whether different differentiated cells have qualitatively and/or quantitatively different sets of DNA in terms of amount, composition and/or organization is not known. Although all cells in an organism are currently thought to have the same DNA content, chromosome structure, and chromosome number, as far as it is now possible to determine, the possibility is now seriously being considered that DNA may change during development at least in linear organization patterns.

But what happens after the adult reaches maturity? Is the differentiated state of the cells locked in and irreversible or is a positive energy-requiring effort required to maintain a given differentiated state, some states being more energy-requiring than others? Does the differentiation and developmental program really come to an end, followed by a steady-state period (a genetic program with a beginning and an end) or are developmental processes still operative in an open-ended type genetic program (a genetic program with a beginning but no end)? Such an open-ended program would be more consistent in view that individuals seldom live much beyond the age of sexual maturity, so little selective pressure would exist to evolve an end to the program. This would be true particularly if compensational processes could operate effectively for sufficient time period.[74-79]

With these considerations in mind, it was postulated that the primary effect of DLBPs and CABPs was dysdifferentiation,[7] that the maintenance of proper differentiated states does require a positive energy effort, and that the genetic program of development is open-ended in nature.[8,12] *This reduces the problem of understanding the biological mechanisms of aging to that of understanding the dysdifferentiative processes and its effects at the cell, organ, and organism levels and the biological mechanisms of longevity to that of understanding the processes governing the time-dependent stability of differentiated cells.*

New questions then arise as to what mechanism(s) maintain the stability of the differentiated state, if they are related to the processes determining the state of differentiation, and how might these processes be best studied. Since much of biology is now concerned with differentiation and development and the genetics and biochemistry of gene-controlling processes, an understanding of dysdifferentiation processes and the processes governing the stabilization of differentiation may not be too distant in the future. Unfortunately, the question of the stability of the differentiated state of cells once the state of differentiation has been achieved has not received much attention except in the field of cancer research.

Examples given as potential LDPs have been increase in body size, postponement of development, increase in DNA repair, and the increase in superoxide dismutase and a number of other antioxidants and protective processes in the cell. These processes could be interpreted as differentiation state-stabilizing factors. It is likely, however, as our understanding of the molecular biology of differentiation and development increases, we will become aware of mechanisms now unknown that may be most important in determining the stability of the differentiated cell.

Recent experimental evidence has suggested that at least some LDPs may be genetically linked and/or under control of a common regulatory gene element.[80,81] Genes associated with the major and minor histocompatibility complex region in mice and human may be sites where LDPs and/or their regulatory genes exist. This has been suggested by the presence of different alleles within or near the histocompatibility gene affecting tissue levels of DNA repair, SOD, catalase, and cAMP, as well as the immunological competence and life span of H-2 congenic mice strains. A genetic or regulatory linkage also appears to be present for the genes involved in DNA repair and protective fucntion in prokaryotic (*E. coli*) and eukaryotic (*Neurospora*) cells. It is also of interest in this regard that changes in the alleles within the human major histocompatibility complex (MHC) are known to affect the onset frequency of a number of different human diseases not easily explained as being of an immunologically related type of dysfunction. These data have suggested that the major and minor histocompatibility gene clusters in mammalian species may represent the genetic location of structural and/or regulatory genes for the LDPs. The LDGs associated with the histocompatibility regions may then have a common evolutionary and functional basis. This would be the maintenance of proper self (proper differentiated self) through self- and nonself recognition processes.

A major prediction of the general hypothesis involves the concept that aging and antiaging processes were in play during the evolution of life. As a consequence, many biological aspects of all forms of life cannot be explained without a knowledge of the biological determinants of aging and longevity. In this sense, the biology of aging and longevity should be considered as one of the basic life sciences. Also, most diseases and dysfunctions of humans today are a result of endogenous and not exogenous processes. Thus, studies in the field of aging and longevity are necessary to provide the scientific basis for the future development of the medical sciences in the effort to postpone age-dependent disease and dysfunctions.

The special hypothesis also offers a basis for a new experimental method in aging and longevity research. This is the investigation of the genetic and biochemical processes governing the general maintenance of health by comparing genetically closely-related species having substantial differences in their aging rates. This method differs from that proposed by Sacher by suggesting that a search be made of quantitative biochemical differences.[47]

Finally, the special hypothesis has led to the prediction of a specific set of genes called longevity determinant genes (LDGs) which act to govern life span. These genes appear to be governed by a relatively few regulatory genes and function primarily to stabilize the differentiated state of the cells of an organism.

## III. TESTING THE SPECIAL HYPOTHESIS

### A. Overview

The special hypothesis was developed from the concepts formulated in the general hypothesis to apply specifically to the aging and longevity processes of mammals, in particular the primates. The major predictions of the general hypothesis which are applied to the mammalian species are (1) all aging processes are pleiotropic in nature. There are no aging genes or a genetic program of aging. Death genes and a genetic program of death do occur, however, in a number of nonmammalian organisms, (2) antiaging processes evolved only to the extent necessary to ensure a species' survival, and (3) an understanding of why much of the morphology, biology, and behavior of animals is as we find it requires an understanding of the evolutionary history of the origin of aging and LDPs.

The major predictions of the special hypothesis are[1,2,5,6,8,12] (1) longevity increased in general during the evolution of mammalian species, (2) the increase of longevity was accompanied by a decrease in environmental hazards and an increase in learned-adaptive behavior, (3) most mammalian species living in their natural ecological niche exhibit an exponentially decreasing survival curve, implying that the aging process plays little role in determining mortality rate and consequently that aging genes or genetically-programmed aging are not likely to exist, (4) the rapid rate of increased longevity along the hominid ancestral-descendant sequence implies that relatively few genetic alterations were required to achieve this change, (5) the remarkable similarities in morphology, scaling factors, physiology, biochemistry, molecular biology, and genetics, as well as in the qualitative nature of the aging processes, suggest that common principles of a simple and quantitative nature are involved, (6) the evolution of longevity in mammals occurred by the same type of genetic changes responsible for the evolution of morphology; that is, the principle changes are occurring in regulatory and not structural genes, (7) all mammalian species have a common set of LDGs and the evolution of longevity occurred principally by a change in their timing and degree of expression, (8) the timing and expression of the LDGs may in part be linked or coupled to the regulation of physiological, developmental, and metabolically related genes such as those determining relative body dimensions, developmental rate, specific metabolic rate, rate of blood flow, and protein turnover rate, (9) the genes involved in governing the changes involved in the developmental model of neoteny and the control of rates of development are related, governed by a common set of regulatory genes; these genes played an important causative role in the evolution of longevity in mammalian species, and (10) developmental processes are likely to act significantly as causative factors in the aging process.

Within this framework of the special hypothesis, it was then necessary to ask (1) what the biological process(es) of aging could be and what might be their number or genetic and biochemical complexity, and (2) what the biological processes governing aging rate could be and what might be their number or genetic and biochemical complexity?

To answer these two questions, it has been proposed that: (1) the aging process in mammals has a primary cause and this is the by-products of essential developmental and metabolic processes (CABPs and DLBPs), (2) this primary cause has a primary effect, and this is to accelerate the drifting-away of the cells making up an organism from their most optimum and proper state of differentiation. This process is called dysdifferentiation, and (3) there are primary processes governing aging rate and these are the processes acting to stabilize and decrease the rate of dysdifferentiation. These primary processes are the LDPs provided through the expression of the LDGs. These LDGs are in turn governed by a limited set of longevity determinant regulatory genes.

Very little is known about processes which act to stabilize or to destabilize the differentiated state of cells. However, there is substantial experimental evidence of what factors might stabilize differentiation and what factors might act to destabilize it.

## B. The Dysdifferentiative Hypothesis of Aging

### *1. Overview*

Aging is proposed to be the result of a slow time-dependent loss of proper differentiated state of cells in an organism.[14] The word dysdifferentiation, also called disdifferentiation,[82] is used to distinguish this process from retrodifferentiation,[83] undifferentiation,[84] or dedifferentiation.[82] These latter terms are used to describe cells that have reversed their development to return to an earlier life stage, such as to an embryonic developmental state. Dysdifferentiation is more general. The same developmental and differentiation processes involved leading to a proper differentiated state of a cell in the mature adult animal are proposed to then slowly become relaxed in a random manner such that the cells drift away genetically and phenotypically from their proper differentiated state. This process could result in a cell having some embryonic-like characteristics, but the cell could also acquire characteristics of a new cell type completely foreign to the organism.

A cell's proper differentiated state is not considered to be locked in, in an irreversible manner, but instead to require some positive energy-consuming effort by the cell for its maintenance.[85] For example, a number of arguments have been put forth that DNA repair may play an essential role in effecting or stabilizing patterns of gene expression required for differentiation.[86] Also consistent with this postulate is the argument that much of evolution involves energy-saving strategies to reduce error and then to preserve the proper differentiated state of cells.[87] All cells, even with the expression of hypothetical stabilizing factors, processes, or structures, nevertheless still have a finite probability of changing to a slightly different differentiated state. The stabilizing effort only act to reduce this probability of transition, and this in turn governs the rate of aging of the organism.

One of the characteristics of the dysdifferentiation hypothesis of aging is that the cause of aging is not necessarily the result of an accumulation of damage in cells, resulting in impairment of vital functions that would eventually lead to cell death. Most aging hypotheses, such as the mutation hypothesis,[63] the error catastrophe hypothesis,[56] the altered protein hypothesis,[88] or the free radical hypothesis,[59-62] are based on the concept that aging is the result of an accumulation of damage within a cell, resulting in a cell which no longer can function properly because of this damage.[89] The dysdifferentiation hypothesis of aging proposes that a time-dependent accumulation of damage is not necessary. Cell impairment, in terms of not being able to synthesize sufficient energy (ATP),[90] the presence of altered proteins, or the inability to transcribe or translate key genes does not need occur. In fact, vital processes such as energy generation, DNA replication, transcription, as well as protein synthesis ability in cells from old animals, could be completely intact and as functional as in cells from young animals. An accumulation of damage could occur of course, but most likely this would be an effect of dysdifferentiation.

The loss of proper differentiation could be caused by a mutational and/or an epigenetic mechanism. Although normal changes in differentiation during development were thought to be of an epigenetic nature,[91,92] this view is now being seriously challenged by new insights implicating the high dynamic nature of DNA and chromatin.[93] Gene amplification or migratory DNA elements such as the transposon elements may play an important role in differentiation and developmental processes, and thus also in dysdifferentiation.[94-97] Clearly, we no longer have to propose rare mutations or errors to accumulate during DNA, RNA, or protein synthesis to create a nonfunctional cell to explain aging. Indeed, the problem now appears how to explain the great stability of the differentiated cells in light of the significant dynamic and fluid nature of a cell's genetic apparatus.

Also, in view that a substantial amount of DNA in mammalian cells (the intermediate repetitive class) may be of the selfish type,[66,67,98] its migration could conceivably interfere with proper gene regulation. Thus, longer-lived species might have selected against this type of DNA parasite in terms of reducing its rate of migration or amount of this DNA per genome. This is a prediction that can be tested with present techniques. It is also possible that both epigenetic and mutational events play an important role in aging, similar to the mechanisms proposed for cancer induction.[99] For example, the CABPs are more mutational in nature (like the initiating agents) and the DLBP resemble the epigenetic or promoter agents.

The wear-and-tear or rate-of-living hypothesis of aging was primarily based on the interpretation that everything must wear out in time with use.[100,101] Such hypotheses were supported by experimental data indicating most mammals do appear to consume a given amount of energy per unit body weight throughout their life span.[41] But how does energy metabolism cause aging? Is it actually a physical wear-and-tear process, which was suggested by the proponents of this hypothesis? Instead of wear-and-tear, this correlation most likely reflects oxygen-consuming reactions producing toxic by-products[102-110] which then act to destroy the essential processes of a cell.[1,2,6] The most sensitive components in a cell to these toxic by-products of energy metabolism are then predicted to be the genetic components involved in maintaining the proper differentiated state of the cells.

It is conceivable that an equilibrium exists within a cell between the rate of damage produced by such pleiotropic aging processes and the rate this damage is removed by degradation and repair processes (see schematic below).

**Dysdifferentiational Model of Cellular Aging**

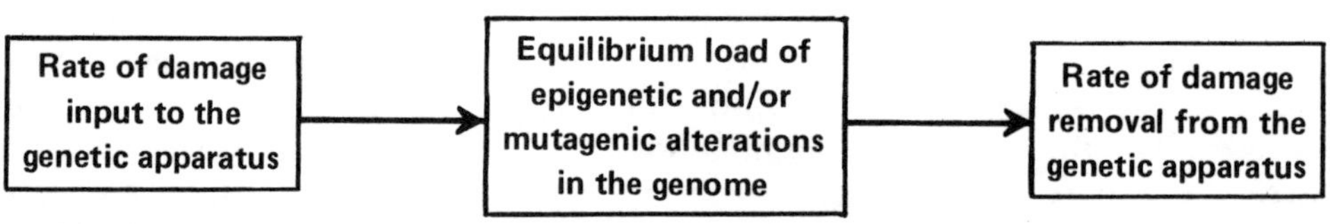

The equilibrium mutational load carried by a cell would then be determined by the difference between the rate of damage input and the rate of damage output. On this basis, it would be predicted that the cells from longer-lived species would not necessarily accumulate less damage with time. Instead, cells from longer-lived species would have a lower equilibrium mutational load than shorter-lived species due to a relatively lower ratio of damage input to damage output. The level of a cells mutational load could determine the aging rate of an organism if the probability of a cell drifting away from its proper state of differentiation is proportional to its steady-state mutational load.

In summary, it is proposed that dysdifferentiation of cells can be affected by the pleiotropic by-products of development and metabolism. These pleiotropic by-products act by mutational and/or epigenetic mechanisms primarily on a cell's differentiated state-stabilizing processes, thus creating cells with improper states of differentiation.

*2. Experimental Support*

Some of the experimental support for the dysdifferentiation hypothesis of aging is as follows:

1. Age-dependent decrease in rate of cell proliferation. Control of cell division is known to be regulated to a large degree by extracellular factors.[111] The age-dependent decrease in cell proliferation rate known to occur in most dividing cells of mammals[112,113] is not likely to be intrinsic in nature but due to altered extracellular signals to maintain this state of differentiation. An accumulation of DNA errors, abnormal proteins or damaged mitochondria, for example, seems less likely as an explanation.
2. Age-dependent changes in hair growth. A decrease in growth rate of hair, the appearance of different types of hair, the loss of hair in some areas, and the gain of hair in other areas occur with increasing age.[114,115] Most of these changes are known to be governed by extracellular hormones and not by intracellular factors. For example, testosterone is known to be associated with balding, and this balding could be an example of a developmentally linked pleiotropic aging process, the undesirable side effect of an otherwise beneficial hormone. Balding does not lead to the death of an individual, but if testosterone can inhibit hair growth, for example, what else might it be doing to the organism? Posponement of the appearance of such hormones in time was probably necessary to achieve a physiologically uniform increase of longevity. One effect of castration, such as seen in the eunuch, is a lack of balding and a longer life span of about 6 to 10 years.[116]
3. Age-dependent decrease in hormone receptors. A substantial number of cells have now been shown to undergo a quantitative loss of specific hormone receptors.[117-121] Because response to hormones play an important role in determining a cell's differentiated state, this decrease in receptor number is likely to lead to slight changes in the cell's differentiated state, such as its response to hormone stimuli. In addition to hormone receptors at the cell membrane and within the cytoplasm, they also exist as part of the chromatin structure and consequently may be importantly involved in governing the differentiated state of cells. Age-dependent changes in the chromatin thyroid receptor were measured for this reason, and preliminary data suggest that a decrease with age may be occurring.[122] It is also important to note that most of the age-related changes found for the hormone receptors are quantitative in nature; that is, a change in number of receptors per cell occurs most frequently with age, not a qualitative alteration in the structure of the receptors, as would be evidenced by a change in binding

affinities. This is consistent with the concept that no errors in protein synthesis or altered proteins underlie the change, but rather a change in the expression of genes involved in determining the differentiated state of the cells.

4. Age-dependent increase in cancer. Many properties of cancer cells are consistent with a dysdifferentiated-state condition.[82,84,94,95,96,123-125] This is evidenced by the appearance of new cell functions, such as the synthesis of foreign proteins, ectopic hormone producing tumors,[126] the loss in sensitivity to normal controlling elements of cell division, altered patterns of isoenzymes,[127-129] and changes in properties of the cell membrane.[130-134] It is also well known that the probability of cancer cells appearing as a function of time increases with an individual's age. What is not as well known is that the probability of cancer cells appearing as a function of time also increases with a species' aging rate; that is, longer-lived species are able to live longer before the probability of cancer appearance is equal to that of shorter-lived species.[125,135,136] These data lead to the prediction that the same processes governing the aging rate of a mammalian species are also likely to govern the time-dependent probability of cells transforming to cancer cells. The link between cancer and aging being proposed is that both are the result of dysdifferentiation processes and the probability of cancer and aging are both governed by differentiation-state stabilizing processes, the LDPs. The cancer cell is postulated to be a special type of aged cell and, as such, is part of and not separate from the general aging process that is occurring in all cells with time. What makes cancer cells special is that their particular type of dysdifferentiation becomes amplified by their nonrestricted proliferation properties. Other aged cells remain normal in this respect when they drift from the proper state of differentiation. Thus, the same processes governing aging rate, the proposed differentiation stability processes, act also to reduce the probability of cell transformation to cancer.[137] If this is the case, most types of cancer will not likely be preventable to a significant degree without also altering the processes governing aging rate.
5. Age-dependent increase of metaplasias. With increasing age, there is found an increased number of metaplasias, the presence of abnormal cells in tissues.[138-142] An example is intestinal-like cells appearing in the lining of the stomach. These cells do not have the intrinsic protection they need in this environment and appear to have a higher frequency of being transformed to a cancerous state.
6. The age-dependent frequency of autoimmune disease. Some types of autoimmune disease may have a dysdifferentiative basis if, for example, genes are expressed in the adult that were repressed during the period of the immune system development.[7] The synthesis of embryonic proteins, for example, in adult would then appear foreign and induce an autoimmune reaction. Immune reactions associated with the cellular change in senile dementia could be another example, such as the appearance of senile plaques and perhaps neurofibrillary tangles.
7. The age-dependent expression of endogenous viruses. The origin of slow virus diseases could be due to a slow age-dependent relaxation of the repression of endogenous viral genes.[147-151] Many viruses are endogenous in nature[152-154] and are known to be involved in age-like diseases.[155-159] A significant age-dependent increase of mouse leukemia virus (MuLV) and mouse mammary tumor virus (MMTV)-related RNA in liver and brain tissues of C57BL/6J male mice has been shown.[160-162] The type of increase is qualitative in that more of the viral genome appears to be represented in the cell. Most but not all of the viral RNA sequences appear to be restricted to the nuclei and are not transported to the cytoplasm.[7,161]

An interesting aspect of these viral studies is that agents known to enhance viral expression are usually toxic in nature, such as carcinogens and/or mutagens. Studies on the mechanism of phage induction indicate that mutagenic processes of the DNA are not necessarily involved. For example, the induction of the λ-phage by UV light has been shown to occur by alteration of a repressor protein.[163]

These data also suggest that the dysdifferentiation process might not only involve an alteration of control of expression of genes required for normal differentiation and development to occur but also the alteration and control of endogenous viral and perhaps other DNA sequences that never play a functional role in the development or survival of the organism.[1] For example, there may be a great number of defective viral sequences, evolutionary-like DNA,[164] nonfunctional or junk DNA,[98] and even the so-called selfish DNA sequences[66-68] that are normally repressed but could become expressed with increasing age. It is of interest that mutagens not only alter given states of differentiation but also can induce cancer. Important evidence in this regard is that cancer can be induced by carcinogenic agents[94,95,165] without causing any apparent mutations. Moreover, the work of Fahmy and Fahmy[94,95] has indicated that alteration of the state of differentiation is much more likely to occur by epigenetic-like mechanisms than by mutations when low levels of mutagens are used.

It is also interesting that amino acid analogues such as ethionine can induce activation of embryonic genes[166] and that carcinogens have been shown to induce embryonic hemoglobin in adult tissue.[167] Also, activation of nonviral-related genes has been observed when tumor viruses are activated.[168] Protein synthesis is known to be required to maintain the transformed state of cells,[169] and in this regard a positive energy-requiring effort must be made by the cell to maintain this particular state of differentiation. Also, evidence has been found that the extent chromatin is packaged, in terms of repeat lengths of the nucleosomes, may be involved in maintaining a given differentiated state.[170] These results are all consistent with normal toxic by-products of metabolism and/or development being able to alter the dysdifferentiated state of cells.

8. The age-dependent appearance of foreign-like proteins associated with age and senile dementia. The appearance of neurofibrillary tangles could be a result of improper gene expression and as such reflects a normal characteristic of neuron aging.[171-174] Thus, the type of dysdifferentiation processes occurring with age are likely to be highly dependent on the normal differentiated state of the cell.
9. Age-dependent changes in cell morphology. Gross changes in cell morphology[175] like the degeneration of dendrites in neurons[176,177] or changes in cell membrane composition could be reflective of changes occurring in the cell's differentiated state. The loss of dendrites is usually thought of as being the result of some damaging process. However, it could just as well be the result of a repression of the genes necessary to produce dendrite structures.
10. The age-dependent decrease in the rate of RNA and protein synthesis. It appears clear that most evidence for mice and rats indicates an age-dependent decrease in the rate of RNA and protein synthesis.[178] Such changes are likely to be adaptive in nature and not to be the result of intrinsic cell impairments. A large number of different enzymes vary in their activity with increasing age, with about equal number increasing and decreasing in activity.[179] These changes are also likely to reflect either adaptive or dysdifferentiational processes occurring.
11. The age-dependent changes in gene expression. Evidence that changes in gene expression, particularly of a qualitative nature, occurring with increasing age would support the dysdifferentiation hypothesis. Recent models of gene control during development and differentiation processes[180,181] suggest that differences in the genes being transcribed would be expected in cells with different states of differentiation. The Davidson and Britten model[181] of gene control in eukaryotic cells suggests that, although some gene control is at the transcriptional level,

there is also control at the posttranscriptional level. In addition, most genes would be expected to be "leaky", that is, genes not necessary for the function of the cell would nevertheless be turned on to a small degree. Support for this concept is the presence of embryonic mRNA in the adult tissues of the sea urchin,[182] ovalbumin RNA synthesis in response to estrogen in nontarget tissue,[183] and globin RNA in adult brain and liver.[7]

There is also considerable evidence that gene repression occurs normally with development.[184] Gene control mechanisms which could operate during development are extracellular modification factors[185] and DNA modification mechanisms[186] such as DNA methylation.[187]

Our early studies on the possible qualitative changes in RNA with age indicated a general decrease with increasing age,[1,188] which is consistent with the work reported by Hill[189] and the model proposed by Caplan and Ordahl.[184] Such a repression was also consistent with a number of other studies on the age-dependent changes occurring in chromatin and RNA sequence complexity changes.[5,190] Furthermore, recent studies have indicated posttranslational modification of RNA[191] and an age-dependent decrease in the relative concentration of 5-methylcytosine in rat liver DNA.[192] More recent studies, however, on possible age-dependent changes in the sequence complexity of RNA have been negative.[193-197] The reason for the differences between the early and later findings is not clear, but with the new techniques now being employed, it appears that the early studies may have been in error.

It was for these reasons (the lack of sensitive techniques and the difficulty in interpreting the results) that we turned to the assay of specific genes. These studies showed about a twofold increase with age in liver and brain tissues for $\alpha$ and $\beta$ hemoglobin but no change with casein.[7,198] A qualitative increase in the expression of c-type virus MMTV and MuLV was found with increasing age.[7,198] Thus, it appears that age-dependent changes in genes do occur in terms of changes in the presence of different types of RNA in a cell. As yet no studies on loss of expression of specific genes have been reported.

Also, it is likely that substantial changes can occur in the differentiated state of cells without changes in the type of RNA present in the cell. In this case, differences in gene expression would occur by posttranscriptional types of modulations. Thus, the data so far on changes in RNA synthesis with age is consistent with the dysdifferentiation hypothesis, and the present data basis provides no good evidence for an absence of intrinsic cell aging processes, as proposed by Finch.[196,199] It should be pointed out that much of the data Finch has used to argue against intrinsic cell age changes is in fact highly consistent with dysdifferentiational processes occurring, where many of the changes in cell function would be caused by humoral effects.[199]

12. Age-dependent alteration of membranes. The qualitative characteristics of membrane composition is known to play an important role in determining the differentiated state of cells. Similarly, membrane changes are known to be associated with the occurrence of cancer[130-133] and with aging.[134,200] Some of these changes involve specific proteins, such as the sulfated proteoglycans[201] and other lipid fluidity changes.[201,202] This latter observation may be quite important, for the age-dependent decrease in fluidity (increase in viscosity) has been shown to modulate the binding of serotonin. Thus, changes in this type of membrane property could change a cell's response to specific hormones by altering receptor binding site availability. This might be what is occurring when a loss of hormone receptor is found. Also, such changes would be consistent with dysdifferentiation occurring in these cells. Changes in membrane fluidity could be a result of a change

in the relative amount of its constituents. However, there is evidence that oxidative damage also increases as a function of age in rat adipocytes, which may reflect a loss of protection and/or a decrease in repair (turnover) of the membrane.[203]

*3. Testing the Hypothesis*

The major prediction of the dysdifferentiation hypothesis of aging is that cells from older animals will be found that have properties different in terms of their differentiated state than corresponding cells from a young animal. These changes are predicted to be sufficient in degree and scope, involving critical function of an organism, to account for the aging of the organism. It is unlikely that serious decreases in vital cellular function will take place as the result of the accumulation of errors according to the error catastrophe hypothesis or the appearance of a large number of nonfunctional abnormal proteins. It is possible that a relaxation of fidelity of DNA replication, transcription, or translation could occur, resulting in the appearance of mutations and abnormal proteins that would then further lead to the decline of the cells. In fact, one could almost explain almost every type of cell change with age as being caused by a change in the differentiated state of a cell. But a fundamental point of the dysdifferentiation hypothesis is that the changes in cell properties that mainly contribute to the aging process are those properties that created the organism. For example, the cellular properties that distinguish a neuron from a liver cell, that are involved in organizing cells into tissues and organs — and these into an organism are the differentiated states most likely to drift and not the basic vital processes of a cell. Thus, the prediction is to look for high-order changes in the differentiated state of cells in the state of tissues, and in the communication between tissues with increasing age. Homeostasis control processes are also necessary to maintain a high-ordered differentiated state of the organism, and its loss with age may form an important component of aging without affecting intrinsic properties of cells.[134,204-207] Finally, a time-dependent increase in dysdifferentiation is predicted, the rate being inversely related to MLP.

The following methods and techniques are suggested to test the hypothesis that dysdifferentiation of cells are occurring with increasing age.

1. Investigate the possible age-dependent increase in expression of specific genes in tissues where their expression would not normally be expected. The use of complementary DNA probes (cDNA) to specific genes has proven to be a sensitive technique for detecting specific RNA sequences. Some structural proteins where cDNA probes are now available (a) $\alpha$ and $\beta$ hemoglobin (mouse and human), (b) casein (human), (c) $\alpha$-fetoprotein (mouse, rat), (d) insulin (mouse, human), (e) growth hormone (mouse, human), and (f) albumin (rat). Endogenous viruses where cDNA probes are available are (a) mouse leukemia virus (MuLV), (b) mouse mammary tumor virus (MMTV), and (c) a number of different primate-related viruses.
2. Investigate the possible age-dependent changes in the expression of isoenzymes in tissues where such changes would not be expected. In this regards, the same techniques and method used by other investigators to identify cancer cells and how they differ from normal cells could be employed. One technique is high-resolution two-dimensional polyacrylamide gel electrophoresis. Another technique is isoelectric focusing. Over 20 different isoenzymes have shown changes in their isoelectric profiles as a function of different states of differentiation and/or normal vs. cancerous tissues.[128]
3. Investigate the possible age-dependent changes that occur in cell morphology and membrane proteins that characterize its differentiated state. Examples are the

metaplasias and cancerous-like cells.[138-142] This includes nodules, benign foci, lesions, or precursor lesions appearing in normal tissue. A systemic search and classification of abnormal-appearing cells with age has not yet been done to my knowledge. Also, alteration of HLA histocompatibility antigens would be an indication of altered states of differentiation.[208-210]

### C. Developmentally Linked Biosenescent Processes

#### *1. Experimental Support*

What aspects of development might contribute most to the dysdifferentiation of cells is not clear. It is clear, however, that hormones involved in differentiation and development do have aging effects. For example, the adrenocortical hormones are known to accelerate the senescence of the Pacific coast salmon, trout,[211-219] and the octopus.[220] There is also evidence that these effects might involve a change in the methylation of DNA.[221] Steroid metabolism is also associated with toxic effects, as demonstrated by Hornsby.[222-225] This is a particularly interesting example, in that antioxidants appear to protect the cells in terms of stabilizing the cell's differentiated state. These data also imply that steroid metabolism produces free radicals. Relevant to this observation is that the pituitary, the hypothalamus and the adrenocorticoid tissues have unusually high levels of antioxidants such as vitamin C, vitamin E, and glutathione.

Postponement of aging by hypophysectomy, as reported by Everitt[226-228] and Denckla,[229-233] support the toxic effects of hormones. The compensation-threshhold concept of Dilman[74-79] is also supportive of the open-ended nature of the genetic program of development and the long-term toxic effects of hormones. Recent studies by Landfield and co-workers[234-239] are based on the concept that hormones such as the glucocorticoids may play a role as a cause of aging. Thus, the possibility of a long-term accumulatory effect of hormones causing dysdifferentiation is gathering support.

Other supporting data is the good correlation of the rate of development and aging rate. This correlation is an important part of the argument that postponement of the appearance of DLBPs is an important longevity determinant process.[6,12] Evidence indicating that nontoxic methods which reduce developmental rate also increase longevity lends support to this proposal.[12,240] Thus, a straight-forward prediction is that any nontoxic process that reduces rate of development would also be expected to lengthen life span. The increased life span achieved by dietary restriction could operate by this mechanism.

Other LDPs that evolved to counteract the DLBPs could be the high concentration of antioxidants in the neuroendocrine tissues associated with the control of development and sexual maturation. In this case, it would be of value to determine if neuroendocrine tissues such as pituitary, hypothalamus, and adrenal of longer-lived species have higher levels of antioxidants.

The androgen, dehydroepiandrosterone (DHEA), has been implicated recently as a possible longevity enhancement agent and to be able to inhibit the increase of certain types of cancers, as well as to protect cells from carcinogenic agents.[241,242] In primates and other mammalian species, the plasma and tissue levels of DHEA are very low shortly after birth and up to sexual maturity.[243] During sexual maturation, DHEA levels dramatically increase, and shortly afterwards show a slow but progressive age-dependent decline.[244] One mechanism of action of DHEA may be its inhibitory effects on glucose-6-phosphate dehydrogenase. By inhibiting this enzyme, DHEA could act to reduce detoxification processes, DNA replication, cell division, and a number of other functions.[245] Another possibility is that DHEA increases during sexual maturation because it is required as a protective agent against the pleiotropic effects of the hormones and other growth factors that are also increasing in levels at this time. Support for this possibility is that DHEA does appear to have antioxidant properties, as do a number of other steroids.[246,247]

*2. Testing the Hypothesis*

Some tests for the hypothesis of the existence of DLBPs are the following:

1. Determine how strong the linkage is between developmental rate and aging rate. The positive correlation found by Goodrick and co-workers[240] between developmental rate and aging rate using calorie-restricted and fasted animals is consistent with the hypothesis, but this correlation could be coincidental. Experiments designed to uncouple the rate of growth and development to the aging rate should be undertaken using for example specific growth-stimulating or retarding factors.
2. Accelerate aging by increasing the plasma concentration of the glucocorticoid hormones.[238]
3. Extend life span by removing and/or decreasing the concentration of hormone products of the pituitary or adrenal glands before and after sexual maturation.[237] The increase in longevity obtained by Everitt,[226-228] Denckla,[229-233] and Dilman,[74-79] using such methods, are representative of this approach.
4. Use in vitro cell culture to determine the possible toxic effects hormones, growth factors, or growth inhibitors have on target as well as nontarget cells and if long-term exposure of cells in culture to these agents acts to stimulate the appearance of dysdifferentiation-like processes.[222-225]

**D. Continuously Acting Biosenescent Processes**

*1. Overview*

The major difference between the DLBPs and the CABPs is that the latter does not change in qualitative aspects as a function of development. The major contributor to the CABPs is believed to be processes associated with energy and heat generation. These and a number of other metabolic reactions are known to produce free radicals, such as the superoxide free radical $O_2^-$ and the more toxic hydroxyl free radical $\cdot OH^-$.[103-110] In fact, a substantial number of products associated with normal metabolic reactions could act to destabilize the differentiated state of cells.

In support of the postulated connection between metabolic rate, aging rate, and the incidence rate of cancer is the impressive argument by Totter,[137] based on cancer incidence studies in the U.S. These studies suggest that the univalent reduction of oxygen in normal metabolism to $O_2^-$ and the resultant production of more harmful radicals can account for the rate of spontaneous cancer. Other arguments have also been presented, suggesting a relationship between free radical damage, aging, and the incidence of cancer.[248]

To reduce the harmful effects of these toxic agents, the cell has evolved repair and protective processes.[1,5,6,12] Some of these processes are (1) the detoxification reactions,[249] (2) the DNA repair processes,[250-252] (3) the naturally occurring antioxidants,[253] (4) free radical scavenger enzymes,[247,254-256] and (5) random and selective protein degradation.[257-259] Not all of the repair and protective processes are expected to have played a role in mammalian or primate evolution of longevity. To determine if such a role was played by a certain class of protective or repair process, it is necessary to determine if a correlation exists between its intensity of action and the longevity of the species.

*2. Experimental Support*

***a. Redundancy of Genes***

After the formulation of the working hypothesis in 1972, this laboratory began screening for potential LDPs. Our first effort was to look at the possible role of gene redundancy.[260] The essential concept here is that, if accumulation of mutations were important to aging, and if most mutations either resulted in the synthesis of inactive protein or no protein, then extra genes should enhance the survival of a species. From studies of reassociation rate analysis of DNA from different species as well as using similar data from other laboratories, it was concluded that longevity in mammals does not appear to be related to gross differences in redundancy levels of DNA sequences. This analysis included the highly reiterated and the intermediate DNA sequence classes.

A study of the redundancy level of specific genes followed, which included the ribosomal RNA and transfer RNA genes.[260] Similarly, no correlation was found in the degree these genes were repeated and the maximum life span of the mammalian species investigated. There was, however, the possibility that a few critical genes having a redundancy frequency of only a few copies (like the hemoglobin and histone genes) existed which played a longevity determinant role. To study this possibility, the reiterated frequency of messenger RNA populations was compared in different mammalian species using a DNA·RNA reassociation rate analysis. These results did show a positive correlation, but because a number of assumptions were required in analyzing the data, the results cannot be highly convincing.

Another possibility is that redundancy may not be related directly to MLP but rather to a reserve capacity effect.[260] To determine this, a ratio called the genetic reserve capacity (GRC) was calculated. This is defined as follows.

$$\text{GRC} = \frac{\text{Maximum transcription capacity possible per genome}}{\text{Actual transcription rate occurring per genome}} \quad (1)$$

Another method was to calculate a ratio called the genetic environmental hazard (GEH). This is defined as follows.

$$\text{GEH} = \frac{\text{Basal specific metabolic rate}}{\text{Number of specific genes per genome}} \quad (2)$$

The GRC and the GEH values for the rRNAs and tRNAs did not increase significantly with the MLP of the species studied, but some correlation was evident. Most of the data was derived from tissue culture studies, and more accurate in vivo data might indicate a better correlation.

### *b. DNA Repair*

The possible correlation of DNA repair levels with MLP was predicted in 1972,[1] and this prediction was confirmed in 1975 when Hart and Setlow published their findings of a correlation of UV light repair levels with longevity for several mammalian species.[261] Their report represents the first experimental evidence that supported the special hypothesis.

In analyzing the Hart and Setlow paper, it is important to note that the correlation is not linear, but exponential.[6] Species showing a life span of 4 to 8 years (an increase of 4 years) had the same increment of increase of DNA repair as species from 50 to 100 years (an increase of 50 years). Thus, either increases of DNA repair was reaching a point of diminishing effectiveness in the evolution of longer-lived species or smaller increases in DNA repair were being more effective in longer-lived species. There was also the need for a number of controls which were needed to clearly interpret if the unscheduled DNA synthesis being measured was really reflecting DNA repair and, if so, how much.[262] These controls include measuring thymine pool size, the species-related patch-size repair areas, and the relative number of thymine dimers produced by a given amount of radiation.

Most importantly, it was not clear nor was it pointed out if a correlation existed with the species used in this study of DNA repair levels with their sensitivity to UV light (in terms of killing effects). In fact, it appears as if such a correlation may not exist.[263-266] X-ray and $\gamma$-ray sensitivities of normal human cells in culture appear to vary over a wide range (from 100 to 160 rads, $D_o$).[264,267,268] The inactivation of cells, on the other hand, has been found to be similar, in spite of differences in radiation response for human diploid cells.[269] No significant differences were found in unscheduled DNA synthesis for two murine mammary tumor cell lines with substantial differences in radiosensitivities.[270] Finally, there exists a wide variation in the ability to transform clones of a given mouse strain by UV light, but with no difference shown in their sensitivity to UV light.[271]

In short, mouse cells appear equally sensitive to the killing effect of UV light as human cells. Unfortunately, it was assumed by many not in the field that more unscheduled DNA repair implied an increased resistance and enhanced survival. It is also not known if higher levels of DNA repair reflect constitutive levels of the DNA repair enzymes, induction of DNA repair enzymes, or differences in chromatin structure such as the degree of the helical state in determining accessibility of a constant level of DNA repair enzymes.[262]

Most consistent with the special hypothesis is that DNA repair enzyme levels would be higher in longer-lived species. Implication of differences in chromatin structure to account for the different DNA repair levels appears more complicated and implies that fundamental differences in chromatin structure change as a function of MLP in primates. Of course, such differences might indeed exist as a result of different enzyme levels of gyrase.[272] These chromatin structure changes may have other advantages for longevity than an enhancement of DNA repair levels, such as the stabilization of the differentiated state of cells.

A similar correlation of UV-DNA repair was found as a function of MLP by Regan's group[273] and Walford's group.[274] Both of these studies also reported an exponential type of correlation of DNA repair to MLP. Regan's group reported no significant correlation of the UV repair levels between the few primate species used, but Walford's group, using only primate lymphocytes, reported an excellent correlation. This latter study is of particular interest in that freshly-prepared lymphocytes were used from the different primate species. A major difficulty using the skin fibroblast cells is that DNA repair levels are known to decrease dramatically on early passage number.[275] Thus, depending on the passage number, the cells can be found in a wide range of DNA repair states. The use of lymphocytes would appear to eliminate this problem and to represent a more normal situation. In this regard, it would be of value to determine if the lymphocytes from the different species had a corresponding difference in their sensitivities to UV light, and if the differences in UV-DNA repair levels were actually reflecting DNA repair enzyme level differences ($\beta$-polymerase) and not differences in chromatin structure, thymine pool levels, or response to mitogen. In this latter case, the ability of lymphocytes to perform repair sythesis following UV damage is highly dependent on its state of DNA replication.[276]

Hart et al.[277] have also found that UV-DNA repair levels of cells in tissue culture from *Peromyscus leucopus* were higher than similar cells from *Mus musculus*. These two rodent species have MLPs of about 3 and 8 years, respectively.

Two studies have been reported which did not find a correlation of UV-DNA repair with MLP. The first was by Kato's group,[278] where cells from 19 different species were examined. For the three different primate species that were used in this study, no differences were observed in relative DNA repair levels, although MLP ranged from about 10 to 100 years. Also, no correlations with MLP were found for the other species examined. The second study was by Woodhead and Setlow[279] on UV-DNA repair levels in three species of cold-blooded vertebrates. No differences were found, in spite of life spans ranging from 3 to 118 years. The difficulty in this study is the use of species that are not closely related to another evolutionarily. Also, it should be emphasized that DNA repair levels could be correlated with MCC (total metabolic potential) and not MLP. Clearly, what needs to be developed are in vivo methods where DNA repair levels can be measured in postmitotic cells of closely related mammalian species under normal circumstances. Such techniques are now available and should be employed.[280-282] Finally, it is interesting that, on exposing 27 different mouse strains to whole body x-irradiation over their life span, the longer-lived strains were found to be more resistant to low levels of radiation.[283]

### *c. Detoxification Processes*

Mammalian species with a higher MLP have been found by Schwartz and co-workers[284,285] to be less sensitive to the mutagenic action of hydrocarbon precarcinogens such as 7,12-dimethylbenz(*a*)anthracene (DMBA) and benz(*a*)anthracene (BA).[285,286] Longer-lived mammalian species do not appear to activate these hydrocarbons to mutagens as readily and/or as effectively as shorter-lived species. A clear implication of these results would be that longer-lived species are more resistant to environmental toxins, as well as to endogenously produced toxins. Because a number of different enzymes are involved in the activation of precarcinogens, some of them might be changing their relative levels of activity with MLP. One important difficulty in interpreting Schwartz's data as reflecting a LDP is that the intensity of activation of precarcinogens is usually proportional to the species' intensity of detoxifying other toxins. Thus, one appears to gain in terms of less activation of precarcinogens but to lose in terms that many other toxins would not be expected to be detoxified as readily in longer-lived species.

A key question then is, do humans have less ability to detoxify endogenous and exogenous compounds as compared to shorter-lived species or is general detoxification ability maintained or even enhanced — and at the same time activation of precarcinogens reduced? It is also important to note that a comparison of activation of DMBA and BA has not been made between different primate species, so these results might not be relevant for human's recent evolution of longevity. Finally, the molecular basis for the differences in the activation of the precarcinogens between the different species has not yet been accounted for, such as in terms of differences in the levels of specific enzymes.

### *d. Superoxide Dismutase*

Our laboratory has recently found a correlation of superoxide dismutase (SOD) activity levels (the Cu/Zn type) with MLP in primate species[11] (see Figure 1). Ten different primates plus two rodent species were used in the study, and SOD levels were determined in liver, brain, and heart tissues. The assay did not measure the enzyme level directly, but the activity of the enzyme to remove the superoxide free radical $O_2^{\cdot-}$. However, because the amino acid sequence and structure of the enzyme appears to be remarkably conserved in all mammalian species, a reasonable assumption is that the different activity levels measured reflect different enzyme concentration levels. The correlations found can be described by the equation.

$$\text{SOD} = k\ \text{SMR}\cdot\text{MLP} = k\ \text{MCC} \tag{3}$$

where SOD is superoxide dismutase (units of activity per mg protein), SMR is specific metabolic rate (calories/g) of the whole organism or tissue, MLP is maximum life span potential (years), and MCC is the maximum life span potential calorie consumption.

For most mammalian species it is known that:

$$(\text{MLP})\cdot(\text{SMR}) = \text{MCC} \cong \text{constant} \cong 200{,}000 \text{ calories/g} \tag{4}$$

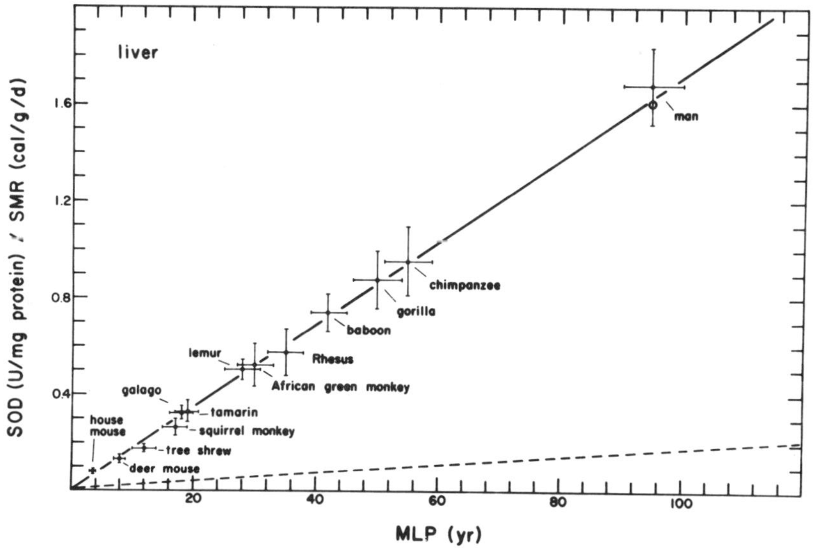


FIGURE 1. Correlation of maximum life span potential (MLP) of mammalian species with the ratio of Cu/Zn Mn superoxide dismutase (SOD) activity to specific metabolic rate (SMR). Dashed line represents the ratio of SMR if liver is used in the calculation rather than whole body.[11]

For example, mouse, elephant, and a number of primate species have the same MCC values. On this basis, it could be predicted that they would also have the same SOD values. This is essentially what we found. However, human and a few other primate species, mainly the tamarins, lemurs, and chimpanzee, have unusually high MCC values, running from about 600,000 calories/g for the nonhuman primates to 800,000 calories/g for human. It has been a puzzle for many years why humans are able to utilize such a great amount of energy (up to fourfold over most mammals) per unit body weight over their life span.[41] One answer this study has provided is that humans have a much higher tissue level of SOD, and this is likely to provide better protection to the cells against harmful by-products of energy metabolism.

Preliminary studies with these same primate species have shown a similar correlation with the Mn-SOD type, and studies underway in our laboratory are determining the relative amount of Cu/Zn and Mn-SODs in primates as a function of their MLP.

This SOD correlation represents the first time an enzyme level (or activity) has been correlated with MLP (or MCC). Moreover, the quantitative rather than a qualitative change observed is right in line with the prediction of the special hypothesis as being a regulatory type of change. Also, the correlation with MCC is linear, not exponential, suggesting that the SOD increase may have played a more important role in the evolution of longevity in the hominids than increased DNA repair levels. It should be pointed out that high confidence in the SOD studies should await until a larger number of different species are studied using several different SOD assays. For example, a puzzling result of our findings was that SOD levels of heart and brain were found to be equal to that of liver. We would have expected SOD levels of heart and brain to be much less.

### *e. Guanylate Cyclase*

The activity of guanylate cyclase is known to be increased by its interactions with free radicals and a number of mutagenic agents.[287,288] Cigarette smoke is found to activate guanylate cyclase and to result in an increase of guanosine 3′,5′-monophosphate in tissue, the active component of the smoke being nitric oxide.[289] Estrogens and progesterone increase guanylate cyclase activity, and this may be related to their possible promoter effect for cancer.[290] In fact, there is substantial data linking an increase of cyclic GMP to cell injury and to the detoxification of chemical carcinogens as well as natural toxins.[291]

Interestingly, adenylate cyclase is activated in rat brain tissue by lipid peroxidation reactions,[292] so perhaps both adenylate and guanylate play a role in detecting cell injury. Also of interest is the observation that plasma levels of insulin and glucagon are correlated with hepatocyte levels of guanylate cyclase, suggesting some type of regulatory linkage.[293] This may be important in view that the $\beta$ cells of the islets of Langerhans appear to be unusually sensitive to the toxic effects of free radicals.[294] The concept that changes in the oxidation/reduction state of a cell may be linked to guanylate cyclase activity in the cell, and thus cGMP levels, is supported by the reversible inactivation of guanylate cyclase by disulfides.[295] It has been observed that, when the nematode *Caenorhabditis elegans* was exposed to cGMP in the growth media, a significant increase in longevity was observed (33 to 42 days).[296] The levels of cGMP used appeared to be nontoxic and not to alter normal development. Possibly related to the effects of cGMP is the evidence that addition of cAMP to cell culture or injecting into mice enhances their radiation resistance by a yet undiscovered mechanism.[297-301] Guanylate cyclase activity has also been found to increase with age in the skeletal muscle of the Rhesus monkey.[302]

We were interested in seeing if guanylate cyclase might play an important role in the detection and genetic regulation of LDPs in the cell. Our initial investigation was to determine if the activity of soluble guanylate cyclase correlated with MLP in primate species. We found a reasonably good inverse correlation, the opposite of what was found for SOD.[11,80,81] Typical results for guanylate cyclase activity in brain are shown in Figure 2. These results are consistent with the following derivations.

$$(O_2^-) \alpha \, (GS)_A = \text{constant} \tag{5}$$

where $(GS)_A$ represents the activated levels of guanylate cyclase (GS) and $(O_2^-)$ is the concentration of the superoxide free radical, other free radicals, or normal endogenous agents that activate (GS).

$(O_2^-)$ is constant at equilibrium, where:

$(O_2^-)$ is constant at equilibrium, where:

$$(SOD)\,(O_2^-) \, \alpha \text{ rate of removal of } O_2^- = \text{constant} \tag{6}$$

giving:

$$(SOD)\,(GS)_A \, \alpha \text{ constant} \tag{7}$$

or, more general:

$$(\text{level of antioxidants})\,(GS)_A = \text{constant} = k_1 \tag{8}$$

From these results, it is proposed that guanylate cyclase may act as a free radical detector and thus as a regulatory enzyme in a system governing the intracellular reductive/oxidative potential of a cell by regulating the intracellular levels of antioxidants and free radical scavengers. A simple schematic drawing of this control is shown in the following diagram.

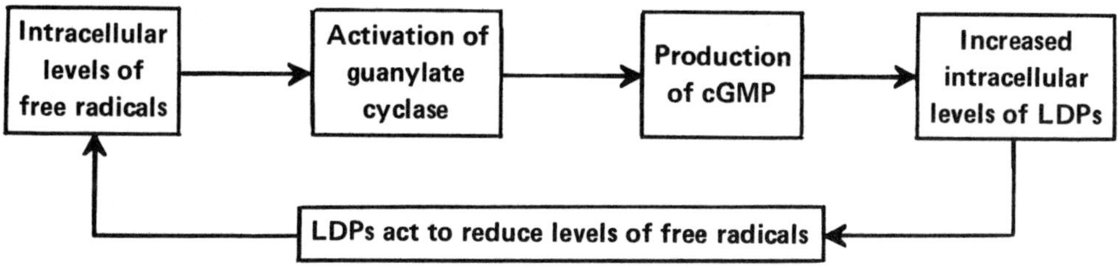


Sensitivity of the feedback loop is predicted to determine the constitutive intracellular levels of free radicals. An increased sensitivity of the feedback loop would be predicted for longer-lived species (a higher $k_1$ value; see Equation 8), resulting in higher levels of LDPs and lower levels of free radicals. An age-dependent change of the ratio cAMP/cGMP, which has been found in some cells,[304] would be consistent with a change in the level of mutagens and free radicals in the cell. This could also imply an age-dependent increase of damage now being accumulated. Consistent with this prediction is the age-dependent increase in guanylate cyclase in Rhesus muscle[301] and in SOD found in houseflys.[304] However, SOD appears to remain constant throughout the life span of the mouse and a number of primate species, including human.[11] Thus, $(GS)_A$ in most tissues would be expected to be constant with age.

### *f. Urate and Ascorbate*

Urate is the terminal product of purine metabolism in human and a few other species and is generally thought to be a waste product with no function.[305-307] In most other mammalian species, urate is further converted to allatoin by uricase. This additional step presumably aids in the removal of urate. Thus, the loss of the ability to convert urate to allatoin in the human is thought to be a metabolic defect.[308] Urate is removed from the plasma by the kidneys, only to be replaced again. The result of this recycling, plus the lack of uricase, gives human one of the highest plasma and tissue levels of urate of all mammals. In fact, the concentration in plasma is close to saturation in normal individuals, and this high level may play a role in the frequent incidence of gout in humans.

Recently, Ames and co-workers[309] have found that urate is an excellent free radical scavenger, which at physiological levels can protect membranes of red blood cells from lipid peroxidation reactions. They have proposed that urate may be an important protective agent against normal membrane peroxidation processes. In addition, because urate is much higher in humans than in other mammalian species,[310] it might be a LDP and have played an important role in the recent evolution of longevity in the hominids.

On examining the literature on urate plasma concentrations in primates, a good correlation with MLP was found. This preliminary data are presented below. A better correlation might be obtained if all the assays for urate were done by the same laboratory using the same procedure (see Figure 3).

Ames and co-workers have also suggested the possibility that the loss of the higher-evolved primate species' ability to synthesize ascorbic acid through the loss of the enzyme L-gulonolactone oxidase may have occurred at about the same time as the loss of uricase. This is suggested because less harmful side effects may have resulted than if ascorbate was further increased. Like the absence of uricase in human, the absence of L-gulonolactone oxidase in human has previously been considered to be a genetic defect.[312,313]

Both urate and ascorbate are antioxidants, but ascorbate is also involved in a number of other biochemical reactions, such as in the synthesis of collagen.[314] Moreover, ascorbate can convert spontaneously to a free radical form which might prove hazard-

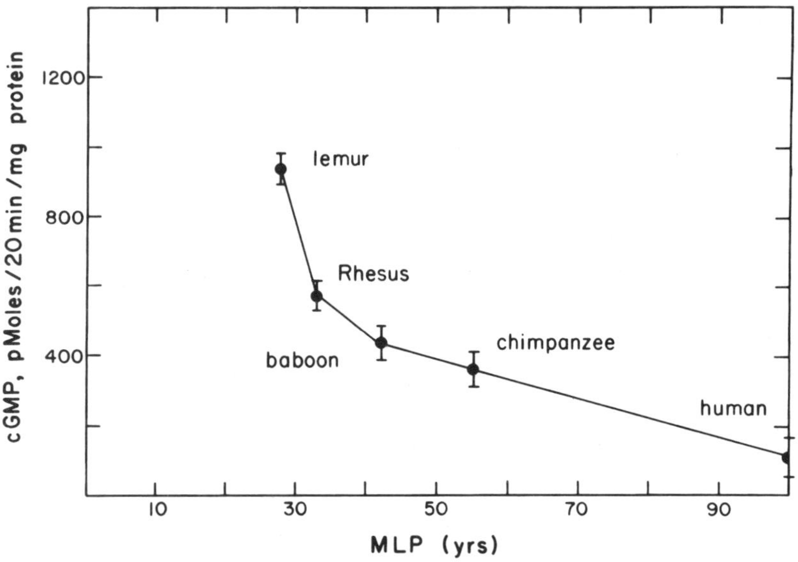


FIGURE 2. Soluble guanylate cyclase activity levels in cerebral cortex brain tissues or primate species as a function of maximum life span potential (MLP).

ous if at high concentrations.[316,317] Urate, on the other hand, does not appear to be involved with any biochemical reactions, and so its further increase in concentration as an antioxidant would be expected to have less complicating effects.

The evolution of ascorbate synthesis has been studied in a number of different species. The biosynthesis of ascorbate appeared in the kidneys of amphibians, remained in reptiles, and in mammals was transferred to the liver. Ascorbate synthesis ability was then lost in the guinea pig, flying mammals (bats), and a number of primates, including human.[317] On examining whether a correlation exists with ascorbate plasma levels with longevity in primates, using what limited data was available, it was found that only a slight increase occurs with increased MLP with the shorter-lived species. Past the 30-year MLP point, ascorbate plasma levels appear to be constant up to human, but urate plasma levels appear to begin to increase with MLP more sharply. Thus, the Ames prediction appears correct.

Also, of considerable interest is the correlation of high plasma urate levels and intelligence.[318-320] Thus, the increase of urate in plasma and tissue levels may have played a role in increased intellectual capacity as well as increasing longevity.

The digestion of yeast RNA is known to be highly effective in increasing plasma levels of urate. Adding RNA to tissue culture cells was found to increase protection against X-rays and $\gamma$ irradiation.[321] Also, the addition of yeast RNA to the diet of rats has shown a dramatic enhancement of MLP. For example, Odens[322] has reported an increase from 800 to 900 days (control) to 2750 days. An increase in life span has been observed by other investigators, but to a lesser degree (about 10 to 20%).[323] Diabetics also tend to have low urate levels,[324] which might enhance this disease if urate protects the $\beta$ cells as an antioxidant. Another interesting finding is that low DHEA levels have been found to be associated with high levels of urate in patients with gout.[325,326] This may be the result of some type of compensational process by urate. Alterations in the purine metabolism pathways have been associated with a number of human inherited diseases,[307] one of which involves the overproduction of adenosine deaminase. This results in impaired immunological function and also in an inbalance affecting urate, cAMP, and cGMP, among other metabolites.[327] Thus, as Walford has suggested, aging could be the result of such metabolic inbalances.[303]

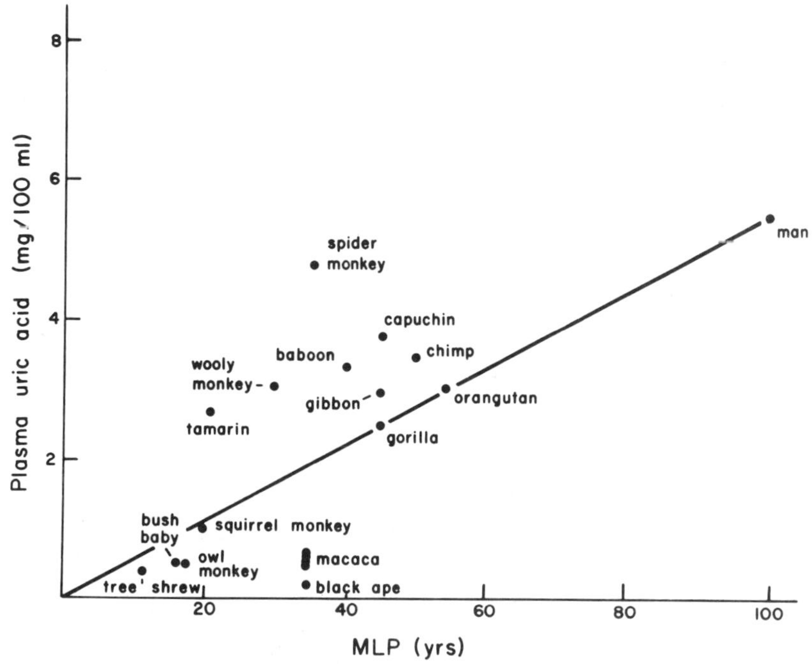


FIGURE 3. Blood plasma concentration of uric acid as a function of maximum life span potential (MLP) in primate species. Uric acid values taken from Ref. 311.

These data imply that the recent loss of the ability to synthesize uricase and L-gulonolactone oxidase during the evolution of the higher primate species may not have been a genetic defect, as has been formerly proposed, but are essential for the evolution of longevity. This suggestion, if proven correct, would serve as a good example that basic genetic and biochemical characteristics of human and other species cannot be explained correctly if the mechanisms determining the basis of aging and longevity processes are ignored.

### *g. Dehydroepiandrosterone*

Schwartz and co-workers have found that the steroid dehydroepiandrosterone (DHEA), when given orally to mice or rats, increases resistance to induction of cancer by precarcinogenic agents, increases fat utilization, and extends life span.[241,242] Many of the characteristics observed in animals given DHEA appear to be remarkably similar to animals placed on a calorie-restricted diet. Thus, the age-dependent decline in DHEA level may be a causative factor in aging. Another interesting point is that, as with urate, humans appear to have the highest plasma levels of all mammalian species, and as yet the biological role of DHEA has not been explained satisfactorily.

It has been proposed by Schwartz and co-workers, as well as by others, that one mechanism of how DHEA may produce its anticarcinogenic effects and calorie restriction-like effects is by its rather specific inhibition of the enzyme glucose-6-phosphate dehydrogenase. DHEA may also be important because of its alleged antioxidant properties. Support for the latter concept is that the metabolism of some steroids appears to produce free radicals, and the adrenal glands are known to have unusually high levels of vitamin C, vitamin E, and DHEA-sulfate.

For DHEA to be a LDP, it would be expected to be at higher plasma levels in longer-lived species. It is not sufficient for it simply to decrease in age. A correlation was therefore sought between the plasma levels of DHEA and DHEA-S in primates as a function of MLP. Results shown in Figure 4 indicate that the DHEA and DHEA-S

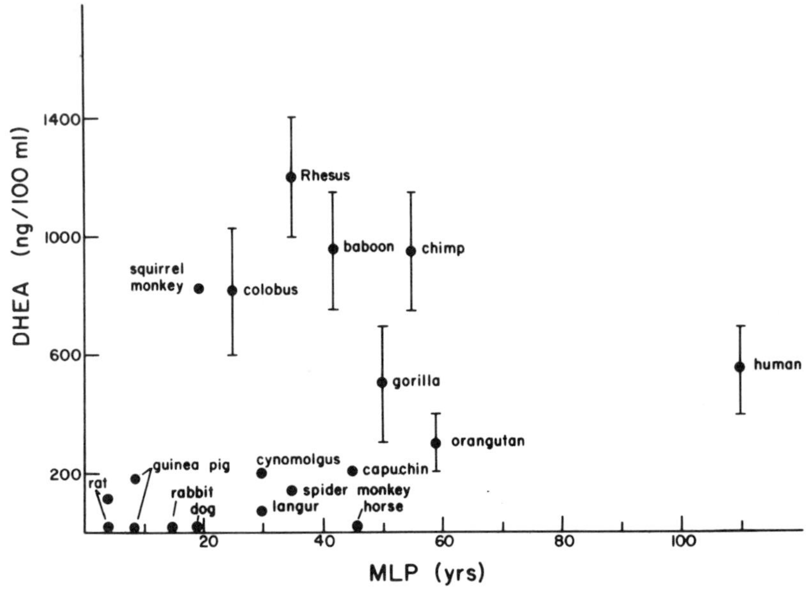


A

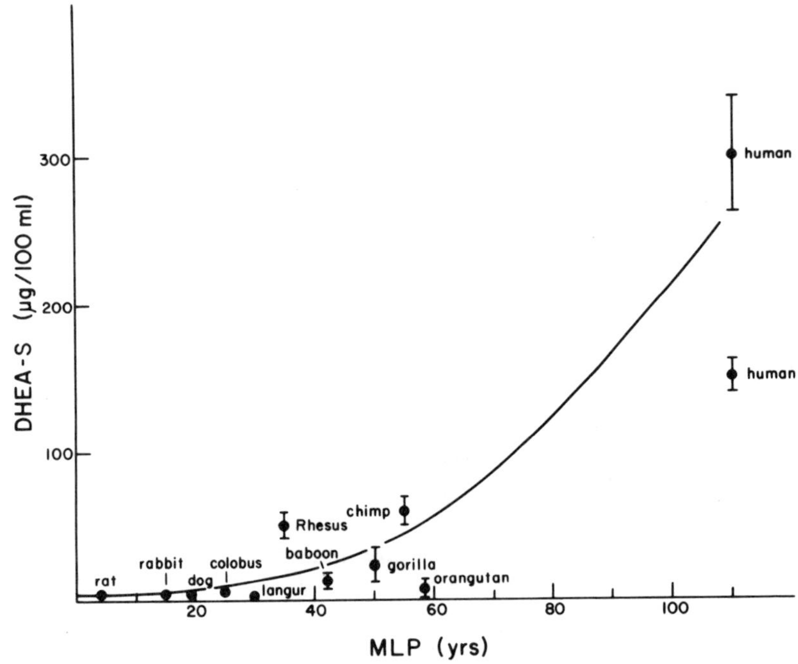


B

FIGURE 4. Dehydroepiandrosterone (DHEA). (A) Dehydroepiandrosterone sulfate (DHEA-S). (B) A function of maximum life span potential (MLP) in primate species. DHEA and DHEA-S values taken from Refs. 242, 328, 329.

levels in the nonprimate species are generally very low, are somewhat higher for primates other than human and the great apes, and are highest in human and the great apes. Overall, DHEA-S shows the best correlation with MLP.

Table 1
VITAMIN A (AS β-CAROTENE)

| Species | MLP (yrs) | Level/mℓ plasma (μg)[a] | Level/100 mℓ blood (μg)[a] |
|---|---|---|---|
| Human | ∼110 | 220 | 120 |
| Horse | ∼49 | 100 | 65 |
| Cow | ∼30 | 70 | 40 |
| Sheep | ∼20 | 10 | 7 |

[a] Taken from Altman and Dittmer.[331]

Table 2
TOTAL CHOLINE

| Species | MLP (yrs) | Level/100 mℓ plasma (mg)[a] |
|---|---|---|
| Human | ∼110 | 26—35 |
| Horse | ∼49 | 12—15 |
| Cow | ∼30 | 16.5 |
| Sheep | ∼20 | 10.0 |

[a] Taken from Altman and Dittmer.[331]

### *h. Vitamins and Minerals*

There is little data in the literature on what could be defined as normal tissue or plasma levels of vitamins and minerals in primates or other mammalian species. For example, there are very few published values of vitamin C levels in plasma of the great apes. Similarly, very little data exists for trace minerals. These points are noted here to emphasize that, beyond the need to know these values for a screening test for potential LDPs, such data would also be of value for more general biological purposes, even if the MLP correlation were negative.

Vitamin A and its related derivatives such as the retinoids and carotenoids have been implicated as effective anticancer agents.[330] A search in the literature for a possible correlation of plasma values of retinoids with increased life span potentials shows a positive correlation with β-carotene, as far as the biochemical data was available (Table 1). Positive correlations were also found for choline (Table 2) and vitamin E (Table 3). In this screening, it is important to emphasize that no MLP correlations were evident for the following vitamins: vitamin A, vitamin $B_{12}$, biotin, vitamin D, nicotinic acid, pantothenic acid, pyridoxine, riboflavin, and thiamin.

These correlations of urate, vitamin C, DHEA-S, β-carotene, choline, and vitamin E with MLP, as obtained from literature values, represent a very rough evaluation of these agents as LDPs. Proper controlled studies using the primate species clearly need to be undertaken with both tissue and plasma levels. Also, key tissues should be studied. For example, the pituitary, hypothalamus, and the adrenal glands have unusually high concentrations of antioxidants, and the concentrations of a given antioxidant or other LDP in these critical tissues could be uniquely correlated to MLP, while other tissues would not show a correlation.

### *i. Turnover Rate of Protein*

The degradion and removal of enzymes within a cell has usually been thought to be necessary only for purposes of enzyme level adaptation.[257-259] However, high turnover

**Table 3**
**VITAMIN E**

| Species | MLP (yrs) | Level/100 mℓ plasma (mg)[a] |
|---|---|---|
| Human | ~110 | 1.2 |
| Cow | ~30 | 0.4 |
| Pig | ~25 | 0.1 |
| Sheep | ~20 | 0.02 |

[a] Taken from Altman and Dittmer.[331]

**Table 4**
**TURNOVER OF PROTEIN AS A FUNCTION OF MLP**

| Species | MLP (yrs) | Albumin half-life (d)[a] | γ-Globulin half-life (d)[a] |
|---|---|---|---|
| Human | ~110 | 15 | 13.1 |
| Rhesus | ~35 | — | 6.6 |
| Cow | ~20 | 20.7 | 21.2 |
| Dog | ~18 | 8.2 | 6.6 |
| Rabbit | ~12 | 5.7 | 8.0 |
| Guinea pig | ~6 | — | 4.6 |
| Mouse | ~3 | 1.2 | 1.9 |

[a] Adapted from Spector.[332]

rates of structural and enzymatic proteins are known to occur in tissues (such as liver) that apparently are not required to adapt to any enzymatic change very rapidly. For example, in mouse, the average half life of the protein in liver is about 5 to 7 days. This represents a substantial energy expenditure for degradation and resynthesis. Another reason for such high rates of protein turnover may be the need to produce heat for maintenance of body temperature. For small animals, we would therefore expect to see high rates of turnover and for larger animals, a corresponding lower rate of protein turnover. Such a correlation does indeed appear to exist, but this mechanism appears rather crude for heat production. A more direct conversion of ATP to heat has been proposed, which is the hydrolysis of ATP by ATPase within the mitochondria.

If cellular components do have a finite functional life span due to interactions with proteolytic enzymes and oxidizing or reducing agents, it may well be of value to a cell, particularly the slowly dividing and postmitotic cells, to turn over the composition of the cell as a renewing process. In this manner, defective proteins and other cellular components could be eliminated, a process that would similate the effects of division. One means to test this concept would be to determine if longer-lived species have higher rates of protein turnover than shorter-lived species. Unfortunately, this author has not yet been able to obtain sufficient data of the turnover rate of protein in tissues other than in blood as a function of MLP. For proteins found in the blood, an excellent correlation does exist,[332] as shown in Table 4. But this correlation is in the opposite direction as predicted; that is, longer-lived species have a lower rate of protein degradation. Moreover, the correlation appears best as a function of body weight rather than with maximum life span potential. Thus, overall protein degradation does not appear at first glance to be an important LDP for the recent evolution of human longevity and may indeed exist primarily for heat generation. It is of course also possible that a decrease in rate of protein degradation results mainly from a scaling factor and as such is a neutral or even negative carry-along characteristic. The lower degradation rates in longer-lived species may not be too serious because of their lower SMRs plus higher levels of LDPs serving to protect the proteins. Thus, proteins in longer-lived species may turn over slower with no serious posttranslational changes occurring.

On the other hand, impressive evidence supporting the scavenger role for protein degradation has been provided by Goldberg,[257-259] showing that abnormal proteins are selectively degraded at higher rates than normal proteins. In a collaborative study with Sacher, we measured selective protein of two rodent species having different MLPs.[333] The two species were *Mus musculus* (house mouse) having a life span of 3 years and *Peromyscus leucopus* with a life span of about 8 years. The basic experiment was similar in design to those measuring in vivo protein turnover rates in specific tissues using radioactive amino acids. The major difference in our studies was labeling two groups of proteins in the animals, one with a normal amino acid (such as $^{14}$C-leucine) and the other with an amino acid analogue (such as L-canavaline). Our results indicated a substantially higher ability (about twofold) for the longer-lived *Peromyscus* to recognize and degrade abnormal proteins as compared to normal proteins. A technical difficulty with these studies is that it is not yet known if the proteins labeled in the two rodent species incorporate the same amount of amino acid analogues. Higher rates of degradation do appear to be related to the degree of abnormality in protein tertiary structure. However, a higher level of incorporation of the amino acid analogue in the protein of the longer-lived species would not be expected (if anything, it should be the other way). In any case, this study indicates that specific types of protein degradation may act as LDPs and clearly indicates that types of studies need to be undertaken to determine if, for example, human has a superior ability to remove abnormal proteins once they occur.

#### *j. Life Span of Red Blood Cells*

Many of the cells in a mammalian species such as skin cells and intestinal mucosa cells normally divide throughout the life span of an animal. This cell turnover is usually explained as a means to eliminate damaged cells that have served their purpose and to replace them with nondamaged cells. In fact, the process is frequently called cell renewal. In addition, cell renewal may also have important protective functions by eliminating dysdifferentiated cells such as cancer cells. Cells exposed to gastric-derived carcinogens, for example, would be sloughed off before they are transformed or can metastasize. The lack of significant turnover of cells in lung tissue of primates and other mammals which are now being exposed to toxic compounds from the air may contribute significantly to the now ever-increasing incidence of lung cancer. Because such air-born toxins were not present in the atmosphere when the species evolved, turnover in lung tissues would not have the evolutionary pressure to evolve.

Sufficient data from the literature have not yet been found to determine if a correlation exists between the turnover rate of specific types of nonblood cells and MLP. However, there is extensive data on the life span of red blood cells in different species.[334-336] The red blood cells have a finite life span, which decreases slightly with increasing age. The reasons for the finite life span of the red blood cell appears to be related to an accumulation of membrane damage through physical utilization and oxidative reactions, as well as possible biochemical changes in the membrane composition. Thus, a longer life span for red blood cells would likely reflect higher levels of protection, both inside and outside the cells. Also, longer life span of red blood cells in a given species might reflect superior protective processes present for other types of blood cells such as the lymphocytes and for the cells of other tissues.

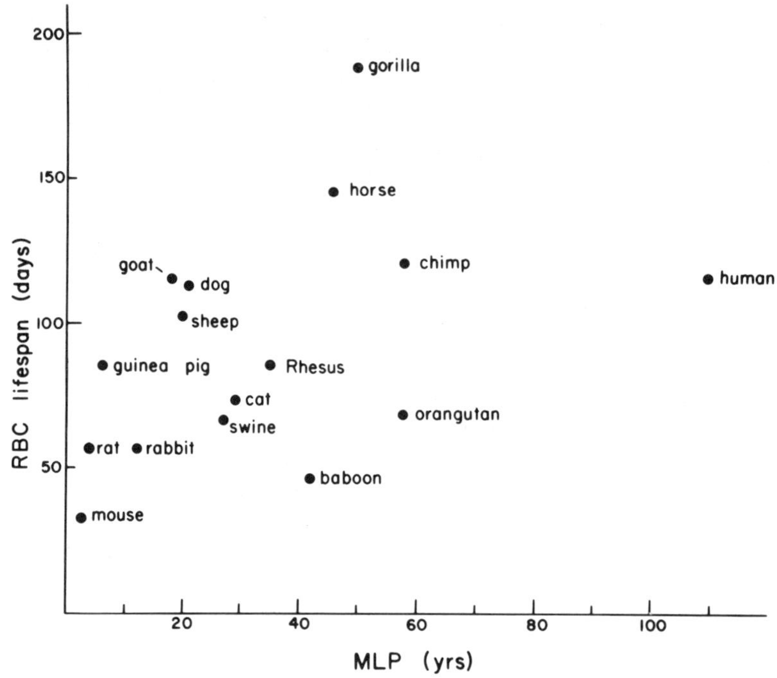


FIGURE 5. Life span of red blood cells (RBC) as a function of maximum life span potential (MLP) in mammalian species. Life span of RBC taken from Refs. 336—338. Note that high correlation is not found when primate data is included with other mammals.

A comparison of 10 nonprimate and 6 primate species shows a weak but positive correlation of halflife of red blood cells in young adult with MLP, again in the opposite direction of what would be expected (Figure 5). Other data, mainly from nonprimate species have shown that halflife of red blood cells is inversely correlated with specific metabolic rate. Better data is necessary to determine if this holds true for primate species having different specific metabolic rates.

An important point in seeking MLP correlations is that a great number of parameters in mammals appear to correlate amazingly well with body weight. Not only do we have SMR and MLP, but also the rate of protein turnover, life span of red blood cells, halflife of drugs, plasma clearance of inulin, respiratory cycle, and the cardiac cycle.[73] These correlations could be viewed as neutral carry-along consequences of scaling; that is, they are interrelated by a highly-coordinated program of development, where one change caused the other — and so forth. Such a genetic linkage of development could place extraordinary restriction on what can or is most likely to evolve.

### *3. Regulatory Linkage Between Antioxidants and Detoxification*

Since the formulation of the free radical hypothesis of aging by Harman,[59-61] there have been many attempts to increase the life span of experimental animals by feeding them synthetic non-natural free radical scavengers. In most of these studies with mammals, MLP was not extended to any significant degree, but in some cases, mean life span was extended significantly.[339-345] However, with the nematode and diptera, both mean and maximum life span was extended significantly. These results were interpreted as supporting the free radical hypothesis of aging, although free radicals were not shown to be present and the feeding experiments to reduce their levels.

An interesting aspect of the antioxidant studies using different mouse strains is that the antioxidant therapy appeared most effective in those animals having unusually short life spans, particularly those strains frequently dying of various types of cancer or under high stress or adverse living conditions.[346] Thus, life span appears in many cases to have been extended by reducing cancer frequency or particular dysfunctions rather than by reducing overall aging rate. In fact, most all inbred mouse strains do have some sort of unusual pathology that results in shortening their normal life span and have a general aging rate similar to that of the wild-type mouse.

On considering these data, it appears that the life span extension effects of antioxidants found for the mouse strains and perhaps for other species as well is not due to a decrease in free radicals of tissues but rather to a selective enhancement of endogenous detoxification processes. This suggestion derives support from the extensive studies of L. W. Wattenburg and others on the inhibitory effect of antioxidants on the activation of precarcinogens.[347] Butylated hydroxyanisole and ethoxyquin have been found to induce quinone reductase, glutathione S-transferase and epoxide hydratase in liver and digestive tissues of mice.[348] Similarly, toxic compounds like tetrachlorodibenzo-*p*-dioxin (TCDD) also induce higher levels of epoxide hydratase, glutathione S-transferase, as well as aryl hydrocarbon hydroxylase (AHH) and UDPglucoronyl transferase. Also, animals fed antioxidants have a reduced rate of growth and body weight and an increased rate of ascorbic acid secretion.[349]

Some of the most effective protective agents against the precarcinogens were found to be the same chemicals found to be the most effective in enhancing life span: for example, butylated hydroxyanisole (BHA), butylated hydroxytoluene (GHT), ethoxyquin, and cystamine.[13] Thus, the life span extension effect of these chemicals might not be by a reduction in free radicals but rather due to a decrease in the unusually high rate of cancer and related diseases whose incidence is related to precarcinogen activation and detoxification. It is likely that these short-lived mouse strains have a deficient level of detoxification enzymes, some are perhaps $Ah^-$,[350] and that the antioxidant aids in bringing these levels back to normal. In this case, antioxidant therapy would be expected to be less effective in wild-type mice because they normally have sufficient levels of these detoxification enzymes.

An interesting aspect of the protective effect of antioxidants against precarcinogens is their possible mechanism of action. Wattenberg has proposed three general mechanisms:[347] (1) a direct blocking of enzymatic activation of the carcinogen to its reactive ultimate carcinogenic form, (2) direct scavenging of reactive carcinogenic species by the inhibitor, and (3) the stimulation of a coordinated detoxification response resulting in increased activity of detoxifying enzymes in the microsomes and the cytosol.

This latter mechanism implies that the relative concentrations of the various enzymes in the detoxification system which frequently activates compounds to a carcinogenic form can be shifted by the presence of antioxidants such that detoxification rather than activation is the predominant reaction. The possibility that these enzymes can vary their concentration in a coordinate manner to enhance detoxification is of considerable interest because this is what may have occurred naturally during the evolution of longevity. Perhaps this is the mechanism behind the decrease in activation of precarcinogens with MLP found by Schwartz et al.[284-286] It is also of interest that an antioxidant stimulates the coordinated enhancement of detoxification. If antioxidants are also involved as determinants of longevity, this result suggests some type of feedback control process where higher tissue levels of antioxidants are coupled by a regulatory linkage to enhance higher levels of enzymes related to detoxification.

Wattenberg has proposed the existence of a receptor for detecting antioxidants, which in turn governs the levels of detoxifying enzymes.[347] The antioxidants are suggested to mimic (as an analog) the carcinogens, which is what the receptor normally evolved to recognize. However, it could be that this receptor (like the guanylate cyclase model previously proposed) recognizes the antioxidant level of cells, which in turn controls the effectiveness of the detoxification process. A model like the following could be possible, where the detoxification enzyme levels would be regulated by the postulated regulatory protein.

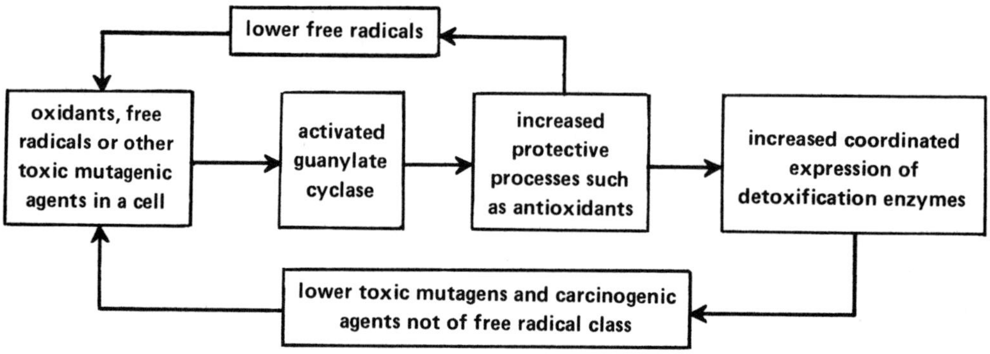


The above model could be tested by determining if (1) an increase of cellular levels of free radicals or mutagens results in an increase of guanylate cyclase, DNA repair, antioxidant levels and detoxification enzymes, and (2) an increase of cell levels of antioxidants increases detoxification enzymes, DNA repair, or affects cAMP/cGMP intracellular levels. There appears to be a similarity in the effects of antioxidants and DHEA. Both reduce cancer induction by chemical mutagens, reduce the rate of growth, and mimic the effects of calorie-restricted diet life span extension. Could DHEA be acting as an antioxidant, as was earlier suggested in this paper, and thereby be increasing the levels of detoxification and simultaneously decreasing the levels of precarcinogen-activating enzymes?

*4. Theoretical Basis of Maximum Life Span Correlations*

The following equations are used to develop a rationale of what type of functions we might expect relating endogenous levels of potential LDPs with MLP of different species. Seeking only a linear or an exponential relation may be an error. For example, it was found that a normalization of the SOD data with SMR was necessary to obtain the correlation with MLP, such that:

$$\text{SOD} = k(\text{SMR})(\text{MLP}) \tag{9}$$

On the other hand, the correlation of UV light DNA repair levels, as well as the activation of precarcinogens with MLP was found to be an exponential function, such that:

$$\ln(\text{MLP}) = k\,(\text{DNA repair level}) \tag{10}$$

Normalization of these data with SMR (such as the DNA repair per SMR) had the effect of removing elephant from the MLP correlation. A theoretical basis would therefore be of value in screening potential LDPs in providing what type of mathematical function might be expected according to the hypothesis being tested, as well as provide a theoretical basis for their mechanism of action.

At the cellular level it appears reasonable to assume that:

$$\left.\frac{d(O_2)}{dt}\right|_{organism} = k_1 \left.\frac{d(O_2)}{dt}\right|_{cell} = k_2 \left.\frac{d(O_2^-)}{dt}\right|_{cell} \tag{11}$$

where $O_2$ is amount of oxygen utilized by the organism or cell and $O_2^-$ is concentration of superoxide free radical. The above relation simply states that the rate of oxygen consumed per body weight by an organism is proportional to the rate of oxygen consumed at the cellular level, which is in turn proportional to the rate of superoxide free radical produced by the cell. The rate of removal of $O_2^-$ is then assumed to be governed by:

$$(SOD)\,(O_2^-) = k_3 \left.\frac{d(O_2^-)}{dt}\right|_{cell} \tag{12}$$

or the rate of removal of $O_2^-$ from within the cell is equal to the product of the cellular concentration of SOD and $O_2^-$.

On rearranging Equation 12 we have:

$$\left.(O_2^-)\right|_{cell} = \frac{1}{SOD} \cdot k_3 \left.\frac{d(O_2^-)}{dt}\right|_{cell} \tag{13}$$

But, it is also reasonable to assume that:

$$\left.\frac{d(O_2^-)}{dt}\right|_{cell} \propto \left.\frac{d(O_2)}{dt}\right|_{organ} \propto \left.SMR\right|_{organisms} \tag{14}$$

where SMR is specific metabolic rate, as measured by the oxygen consumption of an organism per unit body weight. This relation, when inserted into Equation 14, gives the equation:

$$\left.(O_2)\right|_{cell} = k_4 \frac{\left.SMR\right|_{organism}}{\left.SOD\right|_{cell}} \tag{15}$$

Now, let us also assume that at equilibrium within a cell we have:

$$\left.\frac{dD}{dt}\right|_{produced} = \left.\frac{dD}{dt}\right|_{repaired} \tag{16}$$

where dD/dt is rate of damage produced or repaired within a cell. Here we make the important assumption that damage does not accumulate within the cell with increasing age. It is also considered reasonable to assume that the rate of damage being produced in a cell is proportional to the concentration in the cell of ($O_2^-$), so we have:

$$\left.\frac{dD}{dt}\right|_{\text{produced}} \alpha \left.(O_2^-)\right|_{\text{cell}} = k_4 \frac{SMR}{SOD} \tag{17}$$

Now, the rate of how fast damage is removed by DNA repair processes at a given time (t) is also assumed to be proportional to how much damage exists at that time-point, or:

$$\left.\frac{dD}{dt}\right|_{\text{repaired}} = k_5 \left.(D)\right|_{\text{cell}} \tag{18}$$

where D is the level of damage at a given time. If equilibrium is assumed between rate of damage produced and rate of repair, then D is a constant. Thus, on equating Equation 17 to Equation 18, we have:

$$k_4 \frac{SMR}{SOD} = \left.\frac{dD}{dt}\right|_{\text{repair}} = k_5 (D) \tag{19}$$

We now assume that the rate a cell will drift from its proper state of differentiation is proportional to the equilibrium mutational level (D) being carried in its genetic apparatus. The rate of this drift is in turn assumed to be proportional to the aging rate of the organism. And where we have:

$$\left.\text{aging rate}\right|_{\text{cell}} \alpha \left.\text{aging rate}\right|_{\text{organism}} \alpha \left.\frac{1}{MLP}\right|_{\text{organism}} \tag{20}$$

Then:

$$\left.(D)\right|_{\text{cell}} = k_6 \text{ (aging rate)} = k_7 \left(\frac{1}{MLP}\right) \tag{21}$$

giving:

$$k_4 \frac{SMR}{SOD} = k_5 \cdot k_7 \left(\frac{1}{MLP}\right) \tag{22}$$

or:

$$\frac{SMR}{SOD} = \frac{k_5 \cdot k_7}{k_4} \frac{1}{MLP} \tag{23}$$

and on rearrangement, we have:

$$\left.SOD\right|_{\text{cell}} = \frac{k_4}{k_5 \cdot k_7} \left.(SMR)(MLP) = K\,(MCC)\right|_{\text{organism}} \tag{24}$$

where MCC is maximum calorie consumption. This is the same Equation 9 found experimentally to fit the data best for the tissue levels of SOD and organ or total body SMR with MLP. Thus, the assumption made in deriving this equation appears consistent with the data. It is also consistent with the concept that an equilibrium mutational load of damage exists in typical cells of an organism, the magnitude of which is characteristic of the species innate longevity potential.

It is important to note in the derivation of these equations that DNA repair processes were defined in Equation 18, which can be rearranged as:

$$k_5 = \frac{\left.\frac{dD}{dt}\right|_{\text{DNA repair}}}{D} = \text{SDR} \tag{25}$$

where SDR is defined as specific DNA repair levels. If cells are given an acute dose of the same amount of damage (a constant level of D), say by UV light irradiation, then the amount of DNA repair seen per unit of damage induced over a given time-period would be equal to specific DNA repair, as defined by this equation.

Taking this definition of DNA repair and inserting it into Equation 24 gives us the equation:

$$\text{SOD} = k_6 \frac{(\text{SMR})\,(\text{MLP})}{(\text{SDR})} \tag{26}$$

Equation 26 predicts that, for the primate species used in the SOD studies, specific DNA repair levels would be expected to be unchanged. This prediction is consistent with Regan's[273] and Kato's[278] published reports but is inconsistent with Walford's.[274]

The general equation for MLP, as it is related to SOD and DNA repair, is found by rearranging Equation 26, giving:

$$\text{MLP} = k_7 \frac{(\text{SOD})\,(\text{SDR})}{(\text{SMR})} \tag{27}$$

If SOD is taken to reflect the kinetics of other free radical scavenging enzymes, antioxidants and SDR levels to all types of DNA and protein repair processes, a general equation would be:

$$\text{MLP} = K \frac{(\text{protective level})\,(\text{repair level})}{(\text{specific metabolic rate})} \tag{28}$$

A similar approach can be taken to derive more complicated relations, where for example an equilibrium is not assumed and a net accumulation of damage in cells occurs. Here, we would have:

$$\left.\frac{dD}{dt}\right|_{\text{net}} = \left.\frac{dD}{dt}\right|_{\text{protective}} - \left.\frac{dD}{dt}\right|_{\text{repaired}} \tag{29}$$

In this case we find:

$$\left.\frac{dD}{dt}\right|_{net} = k_1 \frac{SMR}{SOD} - k_2 D = k_3 \frac{1}{MLP} \tag{30}$$

and assuming that:

$$D \, \alpha \, \frac{\text{chronological age}}{MLP} \tag{31}$$

Then we have:

$$k_3 \frac{1}{MLP} = k_1 \frac{SMR}{SOD} - k_2 \frac{Age}{MLP} \tag{32}$$

and where $k_2$ = SDR levels, then:

$$k_3 \frac{1}{MLP} = k_1 \frac{SMR}{SOD} - \frac{(SDR)\,(Age)}{MLP} \tag{33}$$

or:

$$MLP = K_1 \frac{SOD}{SMR} (K_2 + SDR \cdot Age) \tag{34}$$

In this case, then where we assume:

$$(SOD) \, \alpha \, (MLP)\,(SMR) = \text{constant}, \tag{35}$$

then:

$$K_2 + (SDR \cdot Age) = \text{constant} \tag{36}$$

Here, DNA repair levels would be predicted to be an inverse function of age but not MLP. Another possibility is that, instead of the aging rate of the organism being proportional to the aging rate of its cells, the total number of cells in the organism under risk needs to be considered. That is:

$$(\text{aging rate/cell})\,(\text{number of cells/organism}) \, \alpha \, (\text{aging rate of organism}) \tag{37}$$

In this case, we find the relation:

$$MLP = K \frac{(\text{DNA repair level})\,(\text{protective level})}{(SMR)\,(\text{body weight})} \tag{38}$$

Giving the prediction that, if:

$$SOD = K(SMR)\,(MLP) \tag{39}$$

then:

$$(\text{DNA repair}) \, \alpha \, (\text{body weight}) \tag{40}$$

which, according to most of the data of Regan's paper,[273] appears to roughly hold true.

The above equations clearly represent a rough attempt to derive a theoretical basis for the type of correlation one would expect to find between LDPs, MLP, SMR, and body weight. The rationale in presenting these derivations is to formulate at least some theoretical basis which would serve as another means to help test the special hypothesis and to stimulate more sophisticated approaches.

*5. Testing the Hypothesis*

The experimental method used to screen LDPs of the continuously acting type has been to determine the relative levels of enzymes or functions that are involved in detoxification, DNA repair, and protective processes in species as a function of MLP. A correlation with MLP would be considered as evidence that it may have played a causative role in the evolution of longevity of the species used in the comparison. Of course, such a correlation is not proof that it did indeed play a causative role, and further experimentation would need to be carried out after such a correlation is obtained. The correlation with MLP is thus only one of the first of a number of other screening tests that need to be conducted to finally identify a LDP. To date, of course, no LDP has definitely been identified.

It is to be expected that most LDPs essential for determining MLP were not involved in the recent evolution of longevity in mammals. Also, the LDPs that were important for short-lived species might not be important any longer for longer-lived species. Thus, to obtain an understanding of the biological mechanisms involved in the evolution of longevity in the hominids, it is considered to be of particular importance that comparative studies be conducted using primate species.

Potential LDPs of the continuously acting type which could be screened by determining the intensity of their function in mammalian species as a function of MLP are as follows:

1. Immunological system: (a) sensitivity and specificity of immunological reactions, (b) inducibility (rate of response) of immunological reactions.
2. Interferon: (a) sensitivity and specificity of the various types of interferon, (b) inducibility (rate of response) of interferon production.
3. Gene control systems: Intracellular mechanisms may act to stabilize the differentiated state of cells, such as: (a) critical gene control elements may be redundant, (b) genetic reprogramming during each cell division cycle may be more complete in longer-lived species,[1] (c) eukaryotic cells having no operons and the structural genes in a given pathway are frequently dispersed. Lack of operons could act as a protective process against one mutation inactivating whole clusters of genes. Genes and their controlling element may be arranged in the chromosomes in a special manner in longer-lived species to further decrease the probability of such mutations affecting the differentiated state.
4. Detoxification processes: a noncomprehensive list of enzymes known to be involved in the detoxification reaction that could be screened is[249] (a) mixed function oxidases: cytochrome P-450 reductase, microsomal flavin-containing monoxygenases, (b) oxidative-reduction enzymes: alcohol dehydrogenases, aldehyde reductase, aldehyde-oxidizing enzymes, ketone reductase, xanthine oxidase, aldehyde oxidase, SOD, glutathione peroxidase, monoamine oxidase, quinone reductase, (c) conjugation and hydrolic processes, glucuronidases, *N*- and *O*-methylases, glutathione, glutathione S-transferases, (d) peptide bond and mercapturic acid formation, cystein conjugate $\beta$-lyase, thiol S-methyltransferase, acetylase, arylhydroxamic acid actyltransferase, sulfotransferase, glyoxalase, epoxide hydrolase, carboxylesterases, and amidases. Also, levels of gastric mucoproteins that may play protective roles against gastric carcinogens could be investigated.[139]

5. DNA repair processes: many of these processes are likely to involve common enzymes: (a) enzymes involved in X-ray repair, (b) enzymes involved in UV light repair, (c) enzymes involved in repair of damage due to different types of chemical mutagens, (d) enzymes involved in repair of endogenous damage of a spontaneous nature, such as in depurination.
6. Sensitivity and survival of cells: mutagenic, carcinogenic, and other toxic agents could be used to test the sensitivity, survival, and transformation frequency of cells in tissue culture taken from species of different MLPs. Use of agents known to produce endogenous free radicals such as dinitrophenol or paraquat might also be used. In these tests, it may be important to use near physiological levels of these toxic agents.
7. Natural antioxidants, free radical scavengers, and heavy metal chelators: (a) SOD (CuZn and Mn types and relative amounts of their isoenzymes), (b) glutathione peroxidase (Se and Se-independent types), (c) catalase, (d) glutathione, (e) cysteine, methionine, histidine, tyrosine, (f) ascorbic acid, (g) $\alpha$-tocopherol, (h) cytochrome peroxidase, (i) ascorbate free radical reductase, (j) glutathione reductase, (k) dehydroascorbate reductase, (l) ceruloplasmin, (m) unsaturated-to-saturated fatty acid ratios in membranes, (n) polyamines, (o) urate and related derivatives, (p) vitamin A, retinoids, carotene, and related derivatives, (q) metallothionine (r) ubiquinone (coenzyme $Q_{10}$).

   A particular good organ to study in regards to relative levels of natural antioxidants and free radical scavengers is the eye.[351,352] It is obvious that the function of the eye, including the lens, last for a much longer period in longer-lived species. It is also well known that proper maintenance of the eye requires comparatively high levels of antioxidants such as ascorbate, $\alpha$-tocopherol, and glutathione. In addition, SOD and glutathione peroxidase are likely to play important protective roles. Oxidative damage to a number of structural proteins is known to occur, such as to aldolase and pyruvate kinase.[353] Also, there appears to be a relation between incidence of diabetes and formation of cataracts. Thus, a correlation of the amount of antioxidants and free radical scavengers in the various tissues of the eye with MLP would be expected.
8. Cellular renewal processes: (a) rates of nonselective protein and lipid degradation (nonselective implies equal rate of removal of abnormal protein as normal protein), (b) rate and specificity of selective protein degradation (abnormal proteins selected for degradation), (c) organelle replacement, such as mitochondria, peroxisomes and lysosomes, (d) whole cell turnover rates (mitotic rate), (f) protein repair processes. The level of methionine sulfoxide reductase may be involved in the removal of methionine sulfoxide in proteins.[354,355]
9. Redundancy process: (1) molecular level: tetraploid cells as a protective process, redundant levels of critical structural genes, overlap functions and compensation processes, (b) cellular level: cellular structures and organelles, cell number in a given tissue, (c) organ level; overlap of functions between different tissues, number of separate organs for same function.
10. Specific metabolic rate. Efficiency of energy utilization: (a) relative efficiency of ATP production in terms of $O_2^-$ and $\cdot OH$ radicals produced, role of increased body size in decreasing SMR, (c) biochemical pathway of heat energy production and its possible role as a high source of free radical production in comparison to the production of kinetic energy, (d) the role of daily sleep in primates as a LDP by reducing energy requirements and body temperature, and consequently the mean free radical production over a life span.[1,6]

Some potential LDPs of the continuously-acting type that may also be related to developmentally-linked changes are as follows:

1. Developmental rate. Experiments would focus on the role the decrease in rate of development and differentiation might play in the evolution of longevity, such as (a) postponement in time of the appearance of growth inhibitors which control organ size and finite overall size of a given species, (b) postponement in time of appearance of some steroid hormones and the hormones associated with sexual maturation processes, (c) possible protective role of DHEA and DHEA-S and related derivatives against the long-term harmful effects of hormones related to cessation of growth and sexual maturation.
2. Homeostasis control processes. Experiments would determine if (a) an increase in the precision of homeostatic control processes occurred with increased MLP, (b) what role does the increase of brain size play in governing longevity, and (c) is pH, temperature and maintenance of steady-state levels of nutrients and other factors in blood plasma under more precise control in longer-lived species.
3. Relative enzyme levels. Shifts in the relative levels of enzymes in metabolic pathways may have been involved to increase the efficiency of pathways and to reduce toxic by-products: (a) change in the ratio of the isoenzyme of lactate dehydrogenase. Preliminary results have indicated a good correlation of the a/b types to longevity in primates, particularly in different tissues of the brain.[6] What does such a correlation mean and are there other isoenzyme correlations with longevity, (b) alteration in the levels of enzymes in the mixed function oxidase system. Many alterations in the levels between different species are known, but the reasons are not understood. Antioxidants appear to alter these ratios towards greater efficiencies of detoxification, (c) alterations in the levels of enzymes in the mitochondria to reduce possible leakage of $O_2^-$ and $\cdot OH$ radicals. Is the structure of mitochondria in longer-lived species such that leakage of free radicals is reduced?
4. Structural components of a cell: (a) change in the ratio of saturated-to-unsaturated fatty acids or other constituents of the membrane, providing it with more resistance to lipid peroxidation reactions, (b) mechanism underlying the age-dependent increase in membrane viscosity (decrease in membrane fluidity). Is this age-dependent change related to species aging rate and, if so, what mechanisms govern the rate of change, (c) changes in the amino acid content of proteins, making them less susceptible to oxidation reactions.[351,353] A decrease in the methionine and other amino acids might decrease the sensitivity of proteins to oxidation or racemization types of alterations.

## IV. GENETIC LINKAGE OF LONGEVITY DETERMINANT GENES

### A. General Implications and Evidence

There may be advantages for the many different LDPs to be linked such that many different LDPs could be modulated in a coordinated fashion by a few regulatory genes. One reason for such a linkage is that, if a proper distribution of expression of the longevity determinant genes is required for each cell type within an organism, which might also change with development, then a mechanism for the coordinated control of the expression of these genes might be essential. For example, an increase of SOD activity without a corresponding increase of catalase or glutathione peroxidase to remove the $H_2O_2$ produced in the removal of the superoxide free radical would not be beneficial. Another reason might be to provide a mechanism for the rapid evolution of longevity or an adaptive-like where either an increase or a decrease in longevity might prove beneficial.[356] It is also of practical interest to determine if linkage of LDPs exist for, if so, the problem of learning how to manipulate their expression would be considerably reduced. Thus, if linkage of LDPs did exist, the problem of uniform enhancement of the expression of the LDPs would be reduced to identifying the key regulatory genes and determining how they might be manipulated.

The expression of genes can be linked in two ways. One is by their physical linkage, such as found in a prokaryotic operon. The other is an indirect linkage through regulatory gene products. In this latter case, the genes being controlled, as well as the regulatory genes, can be dispersed throughout the genome. In fact, because an operon has yet to be discovered in the mammalian cells, it is likely that physical linkage of the LDPs might be restricted to prokaryotic and primitive eukaryotic cells. However, one possible example of a physical linkage of genes having a common function in higher organisms is the histocompatibility complex. Also, it appears that specific sets of genes have remained together over long periods of evolution in higher eukaryotic organisms.[357]

What evidence do we have of genetic or regulatory linkage of LDPs in prokaryotic and primative eukaryotic cells? One suggestive finding was when *E. coli* was exposed to DNA-damaging agents, a stimulation of specific genes occurred at a number of different specific loci (DIN genes).[163] This supports the coordinated expression of LDPs due to regulatory rather than physical linkages. However, at each stimulated loci, a gene cluster could be involved. Also, apparently a single-point mutation in *E. coli* has resulted in a coordinated decrease in SOD, glutathione peroxidase and catalase.[358] This strongly suggests the existence of either a genetic or a regulatory linkage being involved in determining their cellular levels.

However, the most convincing evidence so far that LDGs at least in part are clustered together as a genetic linkage is from the work of Munkres and co-workers.[359-361] They have studied the biochemistry and genetics of the processes involved in determining the longevity of conidia of *Neurospora*. In studying a large number of mutations affecting the longevity of the conidia, they found that there are at least 16 different genes clustered together at the termini of the right arm of chromosome 1. This cluster is called the Age-1 complex.

Mutations occurring in this region affecting longevity are dominant in nature, and an outstanding feature of this region is its extremely high mutability. Two other gene clusters located have also been identified and are called Age-2 and Age-3 complexes. The enzymes which appear to be affected by mutation occurring in the Age complex regions are SOD, ascorbate free radical reductase, glutathione peroxidase, catalase, glutathione reductase, and cytochrome peroxidase. The SOD, glutathione peroxidase and catalase were found to be highly correlated with the life span of the conidia. A model was proposed by Munkres, suggesting that the genes located in the Age-1 complex are functioning and spatially redundant and may consist of seven contiguous genes, a regulatory loci, and at least five structural genes. Not only are these potential LDGs close together, but also they are highly redundant. Thus, species' levels of LDPs may be determined simply in many cases by gene dosage, and regulatory genes are not involved. The genes that appear to determine the longevity of the conidia are protective against the toxic effects of oxygen, thus supporting the harmful pleiotropic nature of oxygen utilization.

Munkres and Cutler have recently investigated the genetic maps of *Neurospora, Drosophila,* mouse and human to determine if there exists similar clustering of genes that could be LDGs. They set up a list of a number of different enzymes or compounds known to be antioxidants, free radical scavengers, recombination/repair processes, pigmentation, detoxification, development and growth, susceptibility to virus induction, and immunological parameters. Their major source of data was recently published genetic maps.[362] Their preliminary results suggest that the genes for these functions are not randomly distributed over the chromosome and suggest the possibility that clustering of LDPs may indeed exist in these organisms. However, much more data is required to confirm this possibility.

Their findings with mouse were of particular interest, in showing that a number of these potential LDGs appeared to be located close to the various histocompatibility regions. Examples are the Aox-1 (aldehyde oxidase) gene by the H(ln,fz) region on chromosome 1, the Cs-1 (catalase) gene near the H-3 region and the Ir-2 (immune response) region on chromosome 2, and the Hao-1(hydroxyacid oxidase-1) and a (non-agouti) genes near H-13 on chromosome 2. On chromosome 4, the b (brown gene) and H-21 regions are near one another (brown is associated with high cancer incidence), and the db (diabetic) gene loci is near H-15 and H-16 histocompatibility regions. Also, on chromosome 4, pgk-1 (phosphoglycerate kinase-1), Fv-1 (Friend virus susceptibility-1) Gpd-1 (glucose-6-phosphate dehydrogenase-1) and ecl (epistatic circling, C57L/J) all map close to the H-2 histocompatibility region. On chromosome 5, rd (retinal degeneration) is near H-27, and on chromosome 7, the Coh (coumarin hydroxylase) gene loci and the H-24 regions are close. Ldh-1 (lactate dehydrogenase-1) and p (pink-eyed) are close to H-4. Eh (hairy ears) is close to H(Eh) on chromosome 15. Chromosome 16 contains the close linkage of If-Rec (interferon receptor) and SOD-1 (superoxide dismutase, Cu/Zn).

One of the most interesting potential linkages of LDG is found on chromosome 17, near the NO end. Here, the T loci, involved with a wide number of developmental defects, are close to the H-39, H-33 and H-2 regions. Near the H-2 region is also the Ce-2 gene for kidney catalase.

There does not appear to be a clustering of the oxygen-related defense enzymes in mouse or human, as is found in *Neurospora.* The SOD-1 and If-Rec genes are both mapped together on chromosome 16 in the mouse and 21 in human. For the mouse, Ce-2 (kidney catalase) is on chromosome 17, Cs-1 (catalase) on chromosome 2, Gr-1 (glutathione reductase) on chromosome 8, SOD-1 (superoxide dismutase, Cu/Zn) on chromosome 16, and DNA repair (UV) genes on chromosome 4.[363]

Other points of interest are that Ce-2 (kidney catalase) activity varies with H-2 type in the mouse,[364] and genes that affect the susceptibility of cortisone-induced cleft palate are closely linked to the lr genes on chromosomes 2 and 17.[365] Also, some of the Ah loci involved with regulation of metabolism of detoxification reactions may reside on chromosome 17.[366]

Genetic analyses of mouse have shown that the genes for pancreatic and salivary amylase isoenzymes are tightly linked and may involve up to 20 tandemly-structured genes. Only one of the 20 isoenzymes are produced in a given mouse. Expression of β-glucoronidase is affected by several regulatory loci, and these map at or near the structural gene.[367] Thus, regulatory genes do appear to exist in mammalian cells and may indeed map close to the genes they control. A number of human inherited diseases, including senile dementia, are associated with neuraminidase deficiency. It is of interest then that the gene for this enzyme (New-1) maps on the mouse chromosome 17 near the H-2 region.[368]

In the rat, a gene region termed the growth and reproductive complex has been identified which may be similar to the T complex in mouse.[369] This complex also resides near the major histocompatibility complex in the rat.

In human, the major histocompatibility complex (MHC) is on chromosome 6. Mapping close to this region are the enzymes P6M3 (phosphoglucomutase-3), GLO-1 (glyoxylase-1) and the ME-1 (malic enzyme), which might be related to LDPs. SOD-2 (superoxide dismutase, Mn type) is mapped in the upper q section of the chromosome arm, which is still quite close to the major histocompatibility region.

Developmentally related genes that may be linked to the human MHC region are the ASD2 (atrical septal defect), ASH (asymmetric septal hypertrophy) and DMJ (juvenile diabetes mellitus). The hemochromatosis (HCh) is not likely to be an immune dysfunction and may be linked to HLA, as is hereditary hypercholesterolemia (CHOL), which in turn could be related to a deficiency in antioxidants.

Also, on chromosome 6 is the gene for adrenal hyperplasia (21-hydroxylase deficiency, AH3), which may be related to a deficiency in antioxidants, since free radicals have been shown to inactivate this enzyme when the cells are deficient in levels of antioxidants. Also, located near this site is the gene related to baboon M7 virus infection (BEVI). On chromosome 21, within the region frequently identified with Down's syndrome, are the linkage groups, glutathione peroxidase (GPX-1), superoxide dismutase (SOD-1, Cu/Zn) and interferon receptor (If-Rec). Because many of the characteristics of Down's syndrome appear as accelerated aging processes,[370] the linkage of these three enzymes is highly suggestive of a functional relationship to aging. However, other interferon genes are located elsewhere, such as on chromosome 5. Also, glutathione peroxidase (GPX-1) is on chromosome 3, glutathione reductase on chromosome 8, and aryl hydrocarbon hydroxylase (Ah) on chromosome 2. In addition, all Down's syndrome patients do not have an extra chromosome 21 segment (21q22) and many patients that do, do not have Down's syndrome.[371] In Down's syndrome patients, there is not only an increase of SOD-1 Cu/Zn levels in the cells (presumably due to gene dosage effects) but also a decrease in SOD-2, Mn. This decrease would be consistent with some type of regulatory linkage between the two enzymes.[371] Of interest is the conservation of autosomal gene synteny groups in mouse and human.[372] This conservation, in spite of numerous chromosome rearrangments which have occurred during the divergene evolution of primates and rodents, is consistent with the concept that, during vertebrate evolution, certain gene clusters were presevered in that they determine the relative gene expression occurring during differentiation and development.[372] The conservation of LDG clusters could perhaps represent other ancestral synteny groups. Finally, the increase of glutathione peroxidase in Down's syndrome might not be a gene dosage effect but a compensatory effect perhaps caused by unusual production of oxidation-types of damage.[373]

### B. Histocompatibility Linkage with Longevity Determinant Processes

For some time, and previous to these mapping studies, Walford and co-workers have been emphasizing the importance of the MHC as being involved in some manner in the aging process.[374] Some of their evidence has been that (1) the immune system can, as a function of age, give rise to many types of physiological dysfunctions, resembling normal aging processes, and (2) congenic H-2 mouse strains have different life spans, where the only genetic difference between these strains is an allele located within the H-2 region.[375] However, the fact that immunological dysfunctions can alter life span is not surprising and the differences in MLP of the congenic strains was not great. This data by itself lends little support to the concept that the H-2 region is involved somehow in governing aging by the same mechanism that aging rate is governed in different mammalian species. But substantial support for the H-2 involvement in aging was gained on learning that DNA repair levels in mouse lymphocytes appeared to be associated with the H-2 congenic type.[376,377] Again, however, this correlation by itself could most easily be explained as processes modulating the DNA repair assays such as by a difference in membrane surfaces of the lymphocytes affecting penetration of radioactive precursors or mitogenic effects known to affect DNA repair which are controlled by the alleles of the H-2 regions. Further experiments are necessary, demonstrating that DNA repair was truly enhanced by measuring relative DNA repair enzyme levels and that sensitivity of the lymphocytes to the killing action of the radiation and/or mutagen is correlated to H-2. It is also not known if the allele in the H-2 region affects DNA repair similarly for cells other than lymphocytes.

However, recent evidence has been published indicating that SOD levels in liver of mice are related to the allelic changes in the H-2 region.[378] These results, along with the results of Walford's group, now indicate much more strongly the possibility that

## Table 5
## CORRELATION BETWEEN EXPRESSION OF POTENTIAL LONGEVITY DETERMINANTS AND MAJOR HISTOCOMPATIBILITY GENES IN CONGENIC MOUSE STRAINS

| Mouse strain | H-2 Allele | Life span[a] | SOD[b] | cAMP[c] | Ultraviolet DNA repair[d] | Bleomycin DNA repair[d] |
|---|---|---|---|---|---|---|
| B10Br/Sg | k | 149 ± 1.1 | 23 ± 2 | 0.95 ± 0.2 | 2.0 ± 0.18 | 72 |
| C57BL/10 | b | 155 ± 4.0 | 46 ± 2 | 1.29 ± 0.18 | 3.7 ± 0.28 | 120 |
| B10A/2R | h2 | — | 46 ± 2 | 1.76 ± 0.32 | — | — |
| B10A/4R | h4 | — | 48 ± 2 | 1.76 ± 0.32 | — | — |
| A.BY | b | 114 ± 3.5 | 45 ± 1 | 1.39 ± 0.16 | — | — |
| A.CA | f | 127 ± 3.0 | 48 ± 2 | 1.48 ± 0.13 | — | — |
| C3H/HeDi | k | 138 ± 0.7 | 18 ± 1 | 0.99 ± 0.28 | 1.7 ± 0.15 | 90 |
| C3H.SW | b | 150 ± 1.2 | 58 ± 1 | 1.25 ± 0.37 | 2.1 ± 0.23 | 125 |

[a] Tenth decile, male.[374]
[b] Units SOD/mg protein in liver.[378]
[c] Picomoles cAMP/mg liver wet weight.[380]
[d] Expressed as amount of unscheduled DNA replication in treated lymphocytes at a given dose divided by amount of DNA replication of untreated cells.[377]

the H-2 and perhaps other histocompatibility regions might indeed represent genetic regions where regulatory and/or structural LDGs might reside. The genetic and biochemical mechanisms determining the levels of DNA repair, free radical scavengers, and antioxidant processes in a cell are not known, and so the possibility that these processes might be related somehow to the mechanisms also involved in determining immunological properties is very intriguing. An investigation into the literature showed that levels of cAMP in liver are also altered by the H-2 region.[379-382] The effect appears not to be a variation of the enzymatic levels involved with cAMP synthesis but rather a modification of the membrane and thus an alteration of the availability of hormone receptors that are involved in controlling the synthesis of cAMP. In relation to these findings is the observation that addition of cAMP to cell cultures or injection of cAMP into mice enhances radiation resistance.[297-301] Interestingly, a number of radioprotectors have also been found to increase intracellular levels of cAMP.[383] Thus, perhaps addition of antioxidants not only directly removes free radicals but also acts to enhance detoxification and other LDPs through a mechanism involving cAMP induction. This possibility may also help explain the radioprotective effect of antioxidants, which is still not clearly understood.[384]

On comparing the life spans, DNA repair, SOD, catalase, and cAMP levels for the different congenic H-2 mouse strains, this author found a fairly good correlation existed; that is, higher levels of DNA repair, SOD, catalase, and cAMP correlated with longer life span in the H-2 strains. However, a few exceptions did exist. This correlation is shown in Table 5.

A summary of these data and other evidence suggesting a role for the histocompatibility gene loci in LDPs are as follows:

1. Mutations occurring within the H-2 loci of mice appear to coordinately change the levels of liver SOD,[378] kidney catalase,[364] lymphocyte DNA repair,[374,375] liver cAMP,[379-382] and life span of mice in the expected direction; that is, higher levels are found with a greater life span. High levels of cAMP may reflect lower levels of cGMP and in turn lower guanylate cyclase activity.
2. Similar coordinated effects of potential LDPs have been found in other organisms. These are: (a) *E. coli:* catalase, peroxidase, SOD, and DIN genes,[163,358] (b)

*Neurospora:* catalase, glutathione peroxidase, glutathione reductase, nonspecific peroxidase, ascorbate free radical reductase, life span.[359-361] (c) *Drosophila* (vestigial mutant): SOD, DNA repair, sensitivity to chemical mutagens, life span.[385-387]

3. Age-dependent derepression of endogenous virus is affected by H-2 loci alleles.[162]
4. A number of potential LDPs are not randomly scattered along the chromosomes of *Neurospora, Drosophila,* mouse and human but appear to be asymmetrically distributed, with many clustering near the histocompatibility loci.
5. Aryl hydrocarbon hydroxylase (Ah) levels appear to be correlated frequently with the life span of mice and genetic mapping is consistent with the possibility that some regulatory genes of Ah level may be near the H-2 loci.[366] An interesting similarity exists between the detoxification system and the immune system in many of their functions.[388]
6. A large number of different human diseases and dysfunctions have been associated with specific types of histocompatibility antigens.[389,390] Moreover, many of these diseases do not clearly involve immunological dysfunctions.[391,392] In some of these MHC-linked diseases, potential LDPs appear to be involved; for example, (a) systemic lupus erythematosis: MHC-linked and low level of DNA repair,[393] (b) rheumatoid arthritis: MHC-linked and low level of SOD,[394] (c) diabetes mellitus: MHC-linked and altered levels of cyclic nucleotides similar to those found in normal older persons,[395] (d) multiple sclerosis: MHC-linked, low glutathione peroxidase activity,[396,397] and abnormal proteins.[398]
7. A number of potential LDPs not yet linked to MHC but associated with diseases and other dysfunctions have been identified: (a) human disorders which show an increased sensitivity of cells to the induction of genetic damage by various means are xeroderma pigmentosum, ataxia telangectasia, Fanconi's anemia, Bloom's syndrome, and Cockayne's syndrome.[399] Many of these diseases show developmental effects and physiological disorders similar to that of accelerated aging,[400] (b) Down's syndrome is of special interest, having higher than normal levels of Cu/Zn SOD and interferon receptors and lower than normal levels of Mn SOD.[371,401] There is also the interesting correlation of low erythrocyte glutathione reductase levels in Down's syndrome patients. These patients are known to have abnormalities in their central nervous system, show accelerated aging, such as an accumulation of neurofibrillary tangles, which mimic aspects of Alzheimer's dementia.[370] The extra gene dosage of the DNA segment of chromosome 21 associated with Down's syndrome may produce a regulatory imbalance of LDPs and improper nervous system development by cells being less stable in their differentiated state. Thus, accelerated aging in Down's syndrome may be reflecting accelerated dysdifferentiation, during embryonic development and thereafter, (c) Parkinson's disease: low levels of glutathione peroxidase and catalase, (d) Fanconi's anemia; low levels of SOD,[402] (e) granulomatous disease: low levels of glutathione peroxidase,[403] (f) $\beta$-thalassemia: unusually high levels of SOD, catalase and glutathione peroxidase in the red blood cells, probably due to high oxygen tension due to this inherited disease,[404] (g) diabetes: Note is taken here both of the MHC linkage of diabetes and also that the $\beta$ cells in human islets of Langerhans are rich in SOD activity.[405] Agents known to be toxic to pancreatic $\beta$ cells such as streptozocin or alloxan are also known to inactivate SOD.[294] Thus, the genetic proneness of an individual towards diabetes (which also reflects accelerated aging in many respects) may be related to the antioxidant protection level of this tissue, which in turn may be reflected by the patient's HLA spectrum.

Additional support for the regulatory linkage of SOD, catalase, and glutathione peroxidase is found when the activity of these three enzymes were all increased in the red blood cells of subjects with β-thalassemia minor and chronic hypoxaemia.[406] This is likely to be in response to hemoglobin autooxidation, and it would be of interest if plasma urate is also increased. Rats fed a diet deficient in vitamin E and selenium show an increase of glutathione S-transferase[407] and plasma urate levels. The similar genetic organization of the chromosomes carrying the MHC in human and other primates support the concept that qualitative differences in primate immune function and in the function of the MHC are minimal.[408]

There is also considerable evidence that the histocompatibility antigens are involved with embryonic cell recognition events,[409,410] cytoskeletal elements,[411] and cell-to-cell recognition.[412] That the expression of the histocompatibility complex may be importantly involved in dysdifferentiation is supported more directly by the relation of the major histocompatibility antigens to the carcinoembryonic antigens on human cells.[413]

The genetic linkage of the interferon receptor to SOD may be of functional significance. It could be that interferon serves two roles as a LDP, one as an agent to reduce viral infection and the other more primitive in origin as a continuously-acting LDP to stabilize the differentiated state of cells. For example, a wide variety of infectious agents and chemicals are capable of inducing synthesis of interferon. Most of these inducers act to disturb the cell surface.[414] The possibility has been raised that interferon is normally produced in cells that are not infected or injured.[415] More impressive, however, is that interferon enhances guanylate cyclase activity[416] and has protective effects to mice previously exposed to lethal irradiation.[417] Also, interferon becomes induced when detoxification systems are inhibited,[418] is known to inhibit cell division[419] and at high levels can inhibit the expression of specific genes such as the rRNA gene.[420] Finally, there is evidence that SOD along with interferon may be necessary for the establishment of the antiviral state,[421] which suggests a mechanism of why these two genes are syntenic in both mouse and human.

The evolutionary rationale suggesting that the histocompatibility complex may be involved in the coding and/or regulating of levels of LDPs is as follows.

The function of the immune system is the maintenance of proper self through self- and nonself recognition processes acting as the cellular level against abnormal cells or organisms coming from the external as well as perhaps from the internal environment of the organism.[422,423] The functions of the LDPs are also the maintenance of proper self, which is the maintenance of the proper differentiated state of cells and thus of the whole organism. In addition, the mechanism of action of the LDPs is related to self and nonself recognition processes such as DNA repair and selective protein degradation. For example, vitamin E, urate, SOD, and glutathione peroxidase are involved in maintenance of proper self through the protection of cell membranes and the genetic apparatus of the cell. The protection of a cell's outer membrane may be even more essential than genetic protection, for its integrity is necessary for maintaining normal sensitivity to humoral and other regulatory factors and cell-to-cell interactions essential for the cell to be able to maintain its proper state of differentiation. Thus, the immune system and all its complex functions may have evolved as part of the more general LDPs of an organism, having a common purpose or function and acting through common mechanisms.

In this sense, the immune system may have had a similar evolutionary history, being a more recently appearing LDP, as compared to SOD or DNA repair processes. Support for this concept is the similar tertiary structure of SOD and the γ globulins[424] and the common functions shared by the immune system with the cell's detoxification system.[388] In fact, an early function of the immune system may have been of an endogenous nature, such as to eliminate cells which have drifted too far from their proper state of differentiation during the period when multicellular organisms were first appearing. Later evolved functions of the immune system would be the protection of the organism from external hazards such as foreign organisms, viruses and bacteria. It should also be remembered that the maintenance of the immune system itself required the presence of other LDPs, such as SOD, glutathione peroxidase, and DNA repair. Finally, the suggestion that the genes involved in control of rates of development, neoteny processes, reproduction, and morphology may be linked or part of the LDPs gains support on finding that genes affecting these processes are often located near the histocompatibility complex region. Thus, the clustering of the LDP's near the histocompatibility gene region may have both a common evolutionary history as well as a common functional significance. The coordinate control of the LDPs with immune-related and developmental processes by a few key regulatory genes would clearly provide advantages during evolutionary processes of increased longevity.

In summary of the data presented in this paper suggesting possible linkage of LDPs, the following processes appear to be associated with one another in their expression: developmental rate, fertility, differentiation and development processes, detoxification and activation of precarcinogens, purine metabolism (salvage pathway/urate), free radical scavengers/antioxidants, DHEA/adrenocorticoids, DNA repair, turnover rate of proteins, interferon, guanylate cyclase, adenylate cyclase, cGMP/cAMP levels, and metabolic rate. These processes frequently appear to affect sensitivity to radiation, chemical mutagens, lipid peroxidation, the incidence of diseases, and MLP. Furthermore, a number of these are associated with the histocompatibility complex, including DNA repair, cAMP, kidney catalase, possibly SOD, possibly detoxification, fertility, developmental rate, differentiation and developmental processes, a broad spectrum of immune-related functions, a broad spectrum of human diseases including diabetes, free radical pathology, and MLP.

### C. Humoral Modulation of Intracellular Longevity Determinant Genes

A mechanism of how the alleles in and near the histocompatibility regions may control cellular LDPs could be by governing the number or sensitivity of membrane receptors to humoral factors. This model is similar to that proposed by Edidin and co-workers for the regulation of cAMP levels.[379-382] The histocompatibility region so far is only known to alter membrane composition and structural changes.[425] Because membrane modifications are also known to be importantly involved in differentiation, such changes could also govern intracellular levels of LDPs such as SOD and DNA repair. It is therefore proposed that the number and/or sensitivity of specific types of cell membrane receptors to humoral factors may govern the intracellular levels of many LDPs, which in turn act to stabilize a cell's differentiated state.

It is usually assumed that DNA repair and SOD levels are intrinsically controlled; that is, DNA repair and SOD levels in mammalian cells have not yet been considered, to be affected by humoral or extracellular factors. It appears that these processes are usually thought to be controlled by intracellular processes, such as appears to be the case in *E. coli.* DNA repair and SOD levels,[426] as well as many of the other potential LDPs are known to be inducible. Their induction methods, however, all involve production of intracellular damage to a cell such as UV light or X-ray irradiation. In the study of DNA repair processes, the use of tissue techniques are frequently employed, where the growth media for the cells does not have the same composition as in vivo conditions. Thus, human cells grown in tissue culture using calf serum might only express LDPs at the level between human and calf. Perhaps the wide variation seen in DNA repair levels between different tissue culture strains and the highly random and sometimes negative results of studies seeking a correlation of DNA repair levels with MLP using tissue culture cells derived from different primate strains can be explained in part by not culturing these cells in serum from the same species that the cells were derived from. This author has been unable to find any studies of DNA repair levels using tissue culture cells grown in serum of their own species. Also, the doubling potential of normal diploid cells is usually determined in media supplemented with calf serum, and the possible effect of growing such cells in homologous serum has not been extensively studied. Skin fibroblast cells grown in vitro undergo a progressive decrease in DNA repair level with increasing passage number and also lose many of the normal histocompatibility antigens, as noted previously. In fact, an early loss of histocompatibility antigens on aging cells in tissue culture is correlated with loss of proper differentiated state of the cells.

It may be that each type of differentiated cell has a characteristic sensitivity to a complex of circulating longevity determinant humoral factors which determine each cell's unique intracellular level of LDPs and, in turn, the life span of the organism. Thus, a simple increase in concentration of such humoral factors may effect a uniform and coordinated increase in a number of LDPs throughout the entire organism. To test this possibility, the following suggestions are made: (1) determine the sensitivity and DNA repair levels of mouse and human cells to various mutagens (UV light and chemical mutagens) when grown in tissue culture using serum taken from different species, and (2) determine the levels of SOD, cAMP, and DNA repair in parabiotic H-2 congenic mouse pairs having different individual levels of these constituents.

## V. ENHANCEMENT OF LONGEVITY DETERMINANT GENE EXPRESSION

### A. A Direct Test of the Special Hypothesis

The basic postulates of the special hypothesis to test are (1) Specific longevity determinant genes exist, (2) all mammalian species have a common set of these LDGs, and (3) life span or aging rate is determined by their timing during development and degree of expression. One method proposed to test these postulates has been to chose a potential LDP and to measure its relative level as a function of MLP in different mammalian species. A common relative age would be used for all species, such as young sexually mature adults, and data from primate species is considered to be more relevant if we are interested in the mechanism of aging and longevity in human.

A second method to test these postulates is to take potential LDPs such as DNA repair or SOD and to determine if deficiencies in tissue concentration of these LDPs would result in accelerated aging. Such appears to be the case for SOD in *Neurospora* and *Drosophila* and for DNA repair processes in a number of human genetic diseases.

A third method would be to increase the production rate of the developmentally-linked or continuously-acting biosenescent processes. Evidence that increased metabolic rate, as produced by raising animals below ambient temperature, accelerates aging is consistent with the by-products of metabolism accelerating aging.[427-429] To be more conclusive, these studies would have to take into consideration that the normal levels of continuously-acting LDPs remained the same and were not increased when metabolic rate increased (the metabolic rate per amount of LDP needs to be measured). Overnutrition (*ad libitum* feeding), where developmental rate is accelerated over normal, would be another example.

A fourth method is to study the many different inherited diseases which mimic many age-like functions. Most of the human inherited diseases (the so-called segmental progeria) are not likely to be associated with a normal aging process.[190,430] However, it should be pointed out that the fact that any point mutation or other small genetic abnormality causes broad time-dependent changes similar to aging processes strongly supports the concept that small but different disorders in metabolism or states of differentiation can lead to a broad and common spectra of symptoms. The potential value of segmental progeria diseases to testing the special hypothesis lies in the possibility that these diseases may represent alterations in the LDGs or in the regulatory genes governing their expression.[431] Thus, experiments screening such inherited diseases for abnormal levels in potential LDPs may prove extremely valuable. Down's syndrome would be a good candidate, as are a number of other human inherited diseases already listed.[430] If some segmental progeria diseases are indeed a result of improper LDG expression, then it would be possible to estimate the total number of genes involved in LDPs by estimating the ratio of how many of these types of segmental progeria diseases exist to the number of diseases not of the segmental progeria type. Such an estimate was made by Martin.[432] However, it is likely that very few of the segmental progeria diseases he used in this calculation had LDP alterations, and until experimental evidence is available to demonstrate this, then this method to estimate total number of genes involved in aging has little scientific basis.

A fifth method would be to devise a means where a number of potential LDPs would be enhanced in their expression, resulting in a clear extension in time of good health and vigor and a longer MLP. This method would provide the most direct test of the special hypothesis. To achieve this objective, several areas need to be investigated. One is that it is not known which of the two biosenescent processes (CABPs or DLBPs) might contribute the most to aging or which of the two corresponding LDPs contribute the most to longevity. To date, on reviewing papers on life span extension experiments in nonmammals and mammals, this author is not convinced that life span, as measured by the time an organism spends in maximum vigor and good health or total energy consumed over its life span per unit body weight (MCC), has ever been significantly increased[13] (see Section IV). Calorie restriction and/or intermittent fasting does lengthen MLP and perhaps MCC with reference to *ad libitum*-fed control. This lengthening of MLP and MCC appears to be caused primarily by a decrease in rate of development[6,8,12] and a decrease in the toxicity of foods due to overnutrition. Thus, the increase in MLP and MCC might have been even greater if both a decrease in developmental rate and an increase in the expression of other LDPs was achieved.

**B. Compensational Nature of Longevity Determinant Processes**

This brings us to a major problem in all life span extension studies, and that is the possibility of compensatory processes. Vitamins E and C and other antioxidants have been fed to animals to test the free radical hypothesis of aging.[13,433-435] No significant life span effects were found, and the experiments were interpreted as not supporting the free radical hypothesis. But, if there exists a number of antioxidants and/or free radical scavenger mechanisms in the cell, where their protective effects are overlapping, and whose levels of expressions are governed by a central regulatory process, then an excess of vitamin E level in the cell might result in a corresponding decrease of vitamin C, for example, such that the net result is no effect of total life span. Knowledge that vitamin E lowers the rate of accumulation of lipofuscin does not provide proof that compensation is not occurring elsewhere in the cell.[436] Even if vitamin E reduces the specific metabolic rate of the animal as well, life span extension would be seen in terms of chronological time, but not likely measured by metabolic time (MCC) or total vigor.

Coordinate compensational processes in the expression of the LDPs, both for the CABPs and the DLBPs, is to be expected, particularly if the LDPs are genetically linked and under common regulatory factors. Simply feeding an animal an antioxidant without measuring the effect it might have on the levels of other antioxidants within the cell or on completely different LDPs such as DNA repair will not yield conclusive results of the effectiveness of feeding that antioxidant to lengthen life span, regardless of what the effects on life span might have been.

There is experimental data suggesting that potential LDPs are inducible. SOD (Mn type) has been induced to higher levels by a number of agents increasing intracellular levels of $O_2^-$. These are paraquat, menadione, juglone, streptonigrin, nalidixic acid, and pyocyanide.[437] The uncoupling agent, 2,4-dinitrophenol has been shown to enhance repair of mammalian cells to X-ray.[438-440] UV repair in *E. coli* is inducible,[441] and exposure of *E. coli* to low levels of chemical mutagens has been shown to induce a new type of DNA repair system.[442-445] Carcinogens have been shown to enhance the survival of UV-irradiated SV-40 in treated monkey kidney cells, which may be inducing DNA repair,[446] and the pretreatment of Chinese hamster cells with a low nontoxic dose of a chemical mutagen gives more resistance to a following larger dose of the mutagen.[447] These latter effects were proposed to result perhaps more from an enhancement of the cells ability to recover from cellular damage rather than from just an increase of DNA repair.

There is also evidence for the enhancement of a DNA repair process in Chinese hamster cells and human skin fibroblast cells on giving them low doses of a chemical mutagen.[448] SOD has been enhanced in brown adipose tissue and liver of rats by noradrenaline administration,[449] and alcoholics have elevated SOD activity in their red blood cells, presumably in response to the toxic by-products of alcohol metabolites.[450] Levels of catalase are increased by feeding high levels of cholesterol[451] or ethyl-$\alpha$-$\varrho$-chlorophenoxisobutyrate.[452] On the other hand, prolonged treatment with X-rays did not increase levels of SOD in *Drosophila* or mice.[453]

As pointed out, SOD can be induced, but so far it can only be induced by toxic agents such as increasing oxygen tension[454] or feeding an animal free radical-generating compounds such as paraquat or dinitrophenol.[426] Longevity is not enhanced in these cases, possibly because the damage produced is not overcompensated by the protective processes induced. Usually the animal has an even shorter than normal life span. Similarly, as noted previously, human diseases such as $\alpha$-thalassemia result in higher cellular levels of SOD, catalase, and glutathione peroxidase, but longer life span is not seen, presumably because the oxidative level is greater than the enhanced protection.[404] Vitamin E-deficient animals have excess levels of urate in the plasma and tissue, indicating a compensatory process occurring. Similarly, higher tissue levels of metal poisons also appear to enhance higher levels of urate.[309] The higher levels of the Cu/Zn SOD in Down's syndrome cells are accompanied by lower levels of the Mn SOD type, which may be a compensatory process.[371,401]

Relative to the argument that compensation is likely to occur among the LDPs that govern life span, is the criticism that, if indeed few genes exist that govern life span, why do we not see at least a few people living an unusually long time, such as 150 to 200 years? Two answers have been given in the past to answer this criticism: (1) the number of genes governing aging rate are likely to be more than one or two but probably less than 600, the point here being that the number of LDGs may be quite large but is still substantially less than that involved with the total operation of the organism, and (2) if such mutations did indeed occur in one individual such as to give that person a MLP of say 150 years, the probability of this person living out this potential plus this event being recorded would be very small. Death by accident or disease would probably occur before the individual reached 100 years of age, and before death an appearance of being 33% younger than normal at say the age of 75 is not likely to be noticed and/or taken seriously.

But if compensatory processes occur in the relative expression of LDGs, it is much easier to explain both the remarkable constant length of life span between different individuals of a given mammalian species and why exceptionally long-lived individuals have never been seen. Basically, the idea is that too much or too little in the expression of one type of LDP would be counteracted by corresponding compensations occurring in other LDPs, resulting in MLPs being held constant. By this mechanism, aging rate would be governed much like body temperature, where the factor to be kept constant is likely to be MCC and not MLP.

### C. Direct and Indirect Longevity Determinant Methods

Taking these considerations in mind, experiments in our laboratory have been taking a different approach in the development of life span extension techniques over the past 3 years. This has been the investigation of methods to enhance the expression of a complex spectrum of LDPs by attempting to interfere directly or indirectly with the mechanisms which control their level of expression. For example, the levels of DNA repair and antioxidants might be determined (in addition to the humoral factors) by the degree genetic damage exists in a cell (the mutational equilibrium load). This could be the level of excised DNA damaged regions or chromatin damage diffusing back to the cytoplasm or the level of damage present in membrane structures.

The basic rationale is to try to trick the cell's LDG regulatory processes into thinking that the cell has too much damage when it really does not and to consequently stimulate it to produce more DNA repair enzymes and/or protective antioxidant agents. This technique to increase innate resistance to aging is similar in principle to developing a vaccine to increase resistance to polio. For example, defective polio virus is used to stimulate the organism into making antibodies, this protecting the organism when exposed to the real virus. The mechanism of how the virus causes paralysis is not known nor how the defective virus stimulates antibody production. Yet, substantially increased resistance to the disease can be enhanced.

So far, we have been testing the possible effects of thymidine dimers, DNA protective adducts, and other DNA and cell organelle-damaged products produced by UV light, X-rays and oxidative agents for their ability to enhance resistance to these toxic agents. Our preliminary results indicate that survival of tissue culture cells and mice can be enhanced by these methods, but much more testing is required to determine how reproducible this enhancement is and if it is due to changes in levels of LDPs. This new approach is only noted here to illustrate another means to test the special hypothesis and what possible pitfalls to avoid.

While we were undertaking these studies, the success of a similar approach was reported, showing that the population doubling potential of *Paramecium* could be enhanced by first exposing the cell to UV light, followed by exposure to photo-reactivating light.[455] The limited proliferation potential of *Paramecium* appears in many respects to be the result of an accumulation of damage primarily of a genetic nature.[456,457] The UV light exposure would produce thymine dimers and, if left intact, the cells would undergo fewer doublings. However, photoreactivating light exposure would remove most of the thymine dimers, and the cell would presumably be left with excess repair and thus be able to proliferate for a greater number of rounds. Later, it was reported that exposure to photoreactivating light was not necessary if the intensity of the UV light was reduced sufficiently.

The major problem with this interesting study is that it has not yet been shown directly that any type of DNA repair, free radical scavenger, antioxidant or other potential LDP has been enhanced in the *Paramecium*. The possibility is being explored, however, that DNA repair enzyme levels are not increased but instead the accessibility of the DNA to repair enzymes is increased by a change in the DNA helical content.[272]

Even before these results, it has been known that small doses of irradiation can lengthen life span of mice, insects and other animals.[458,459] A number of interpretations for the mechanism can be given, but one was, as Smith-Sonneborn has suggested, an enhancement of DNA repair processes occurs. Sohal and co-workers[460] have found, however, that low radiation exposure of houseflies reduces their mean specific metabolic rate (they do not fly as much) and as a result they live longer.

Supporting this result are studies by Miquel and co-workers,[461] showing that many chemicals as well as X-ray and UV light irradiation which lower metabolic rate in *Drosophila* also result in a lengthening of life span but not total oxygen consumption over the life span. Chemical agents tested were thiazolidine, carboxylic acid, 2,4-dinitrophenol, nordihydroguairetic acid and vitamin E. Thus, the compensation process of the LDPs may be operating by keeping total energy consumption (MCC) over the life span at a constant level, not chronological time. Could it be that the extension of proliferation doubling potential in *Paramecium* achieved with UV light works by a similar process, that the total energy consumption per unit metabolic mass of the culture has remained unchanged? If total number of doublings increased, this could mean slower division rate and/or smaller cells. From these considerations, it appears important for all longevity-enhancing studies to measure total energy consumption over the life span of the animal (MCC), as well as to measure chronological life span (MLP), to evaluate the possibility that compensation processes involving the LDPs may be occurring.

It is also essential in experiments designed to enhance life span by attempting to enhance LDPs or by any other means, that the type of organism used be carefully considered. For example, the nematode and diptera organisms have essentially no cell turnover and no turnover of mitochondria. Such turnover may be essential for significantly longer life span, regardless of how high the levels of LDPs can be raised. Thus, a number of organisms may represent a dead end evolutionary genotype that precludes further enhancement of longevity by the processes that normally evolved in other species.

Similarly, a key point of the method to enhance individual LDPs is the concept of further increasing levels of *natural* processes involved in determining longevity and health maintenance. Synthetic antioxidants or other drugs commonly being used in life span extension studies[462] may have long-term detrimental side effects. For example, if vitamin E or vitamin C did not normally increase with increased longevity during primate evolution, then there may be a good reason for this, and artificially enhancing their levels may prove to have harmful long-term effects.

Finally, it should be emphasized that the LDPs are likely to be able to handle only normal physiological levels of harmful by-products of metabolism. This may be an important consideration in designing experiments to test if a potential LDP has been enhanced. For example, if a method used to induce a cell's normal antioxidant capacity is to be evaluated, one might test a change in a cell's resistance to a chemical producing high intracellular levels of free radicals. If the levels of free radicals produced, however, are much larger than normally exist, an increased protection may not be seen. This is well illustrated by the kinetics of SOD removal of $O_2^-$.[463] SOD has been found to be only effective in reducing $O_2^-$ levels that are already at low levels. This action is analogous to a second-stage oil vapor vacuum pump, where the pump will not reduce air pressure from atmospheric pressure but works only if the air pressure is already substantially reduced. Thus, cells with very high levels of SOD, as compared to cells with normal SOD levels, would be expected to show the same sensitivity to high levels of superoxide free radicals. The difference in sensitivity would only become evident when the level of the superoxide radical is reduced to levels of the same order of magnitude normally found in the cell.

These results indicate that longer-lived species may not be more resistant to higher doses of free radicals or other damaging agents but would be expected to be more resistant to long-term low dosage levels of these agents. Similar values for the LD50/30 survival for acute X-ray exposure of animals[464-467] and the sensitivity of cells in culture to the killing effects of X-rays and UV light, independent of the species MLP, support this concept.[399] Thus, the most effective means to determine if an enhanced potential LDP really is effective in lengthening life span appears simply to be to measure its effect on longevity.

## VI. CALORIE RESTRICTION AND INTERMITTENT FASTING

### A. Life Span Extension Interpretation

Calorie restriction and/or intermittent fasting is often cited as the only means found that significantly extends the life span of animals.[468-470] The well-known studies of McCay,[471,472] Carlson,[473,474] Berg and Simms,[475,476] Barrows,[477] and Ross,[478] clearly demonstrate the life span extension effects of reduced calorie intake and/or intermittent fasting. Recent results also demonstrate the reduction in the age-related loss of a specific function such as the immune system[470,479,480] or of hormone receptors[481] in calorie-restricted/intermittent-fasted animals. Consequently, a rationale of current studies of calorie restriction have been to learn of the mechanisms of how calorie restriction lengthens life span in order to gain insight into the genetic and biochemical processes governing the life span of mammalian species. Work from this laboratory a few years ago, however, seriously questioned this rationale, and this study will be reviewed and an alternative viewpoint presented.

### B. Life Span Shortening Interpretation

The possible accumulation of altered proteins with age, namely glucose-6-phosphate dehydrogenase, was studied and was successful in showing a substantial age-dependent increase in the amount of temperature sensitive enzyme in mouse liver.[482] To determine if the rate of accumulation of the altered protein was coupled with aging rate, the age-dependent levels of the altered protein were assayed in mice that were intermittently fasted (1 day without food but with water and 2 days with food *ad libitum*). It was found that fasting, even for 1 day, almost completely removed the altered component of this enzyme. The conclusions were that calorie-restriction and fasting may extend life span by two different processes, one by reducing rate of development and the other by stimulating degradation processes, thus accelerating the selective degradation of altered cellular constituents.

However, it was also proposed that calorie-restricted diet and intermittent fasting are not likely to result in a species living a life span beyond its normal genetic potential. Instead, this diet acts to bring the animal back to the aging rate it would normally have if living in its natural ecological niche. The reasoning behind this suggestion is that most animals living in their natural habitat are usually in a feast or famine condition and also normally exercising more than animals in captivity. Seldom if ever do animals in the wild go throughout their entire life spans eating *ad libitum* or having all they want to eat all the time. However, it was generally thought, particularly during the period the McCay experiments were carried out, that animals given food under *ad libitum* conditions, where maximum rate of growth is achieved, should be the most healthy. What has been learned since is that there is no positive correlation between the rate of growth and the extent of general good health, vigor, and longevity. In fact, a negative correlation is usually found. Also, animals in a calorie-restricted diet or intermittent fasting schedule are much more active than their *ad libitum*-fed controls.

From this viewpoint, studies of the effects of calorie restriction and intermittent fasting on lengthening life span appear to be studies on the effects of over-nutrition and under-exercise on shortening life span. In other words, the control animals (the *ad libitum*-fed animals) are actually the experimental animals.

One of the most significant features of calorie-restricted animals, as compared to their *ad libitum*-fed counterparts, is the remarkable postponement of many types of cancers.[483] Indeed, most of the extension of life span appears to be derived from a reduction in cancer. It is also important to note that similar beneficial effects have been recorded for human populations on a reduced intake of calories. These natural experiments occurred during war or famine and such populations have been observed to be remarkably free of cancer and other types of diseases seen frequently in the older population.[484] When this same population returned to an *ad libitum* type of diet, the onset frequency of diseases were found to return to normal high frequency.

But how can over-eating accelerate aging? One mechanism is that it accelerates growth and development and shortens the time when the DLBPs will be expressed. Why this occurs may be related to a population regulatory process where, in time of plenty, it would be advantageous to reach sexual maturity earlier, thereby increasing reproduction rate; whereas in times of food scarcity, reproduction rate would decrease accordingly. Another possible reason is that an organism simply may not be designed to handle all the food it wants to eat all the time because such a situation rarely occurred during its evolution. Thus, a safeguard mechanism to prevent overeating did not evolve and, most importantly, means to prevent the harmful side effects of overeating in terms of accelerated aging did not evolve. Thus, when food does become plentiful, as is with most laboratory animals and for most humans in the developed nations, overeating and accelerated aging occurs.

According to this viewpoint, over-nutrition results in long-term detrimental effects that act to accelerate a number of aging processes, including an increase in the rate of cancer incidence. The toxic effects of high levels of some types of amino acids is well known, particularly on the nervous system, but there are likely to be other possible adverse effects.

A means to determine how much food animals should eat was approached by Young in a study of amino acid constituents in the blood plasma as a function of increased food intake.[485] Starting from a low intake of protein and increasing the amount fed to an animal, little change in the level of amino acids in the blood plasma was found, indicating that almost complete cell utilization was taking place. However, when food intake passed a certain level, further cell uptake quickly stopped, and plasma levels of the amino acids began to rise. The point of where cell utilization of food constituents in the plasma no longer occurs may be near an adequate dietary intake.

Since most humans do eat *ad libitum,* this viewpoint would predict that, if humans would also return to the feast/famine conditions which would ideally also include the same types of food we evolved to digest and to detoxify, the same degree of exercise we evolved to undertake, and the same level of stress we evolved to handle, then according to the mouse and rat studies, we should live perhaps 20 to 30 years longer than the present mean or maximum life span potential. This extension of life span would, of course, occur by taking advantage of our present biological potential, and we would in effect be living a more normal life span.

Also, if this viewpoint of the calorie-restriction/intermittent-fasting life span extension data is correct, an understanding of the long-term effects of overeating and how it enhances disease frequency and shortens life span may be of less value than commonly thought in learning of the genetic and biochemical mechanisms of aging and longevity. For example, if both human and chimpanzee were on the calorie-restricted diet and exercised sufficiently, the twofold difference in their aging rate or MLP would still exist. Thus, calorie restriction and intermittent fasting, as well as exercise, may only modify the effectiveness of the LDPs but not their levels. When we do finally learn of the mechanisms of how life span is affected by lowering calories or fasting, we may learn nothing of the basic genetic and biochemical processes governing aging rate. Thus, the term life span extension used in describing the calorie-restricted and intermittent-fasting studies should be clearly defined as to what is meant to avoid confusion. Life span extension is most frequently thought to be a process that prolongs life beyond what is the normal genetic potential for the animal. Calorie restriction and/or intermittent fasting does not appear to be such a process.

It may be advantageous in future life span extension experiments to use, as controls, animals having a truly normal aging rate as it would exist in their normal ecological niche. Such control animals could be those placed on a calorie-restricted and/or intermittent-fasting diet with adequate exercise. Clearly, a treatment resulting in an increase of MLP and/or MCC over these controls would be impressive. This would enable the detection of life span extension beyond the normal genetic potential of the species. No method has succeeded in increasing life span in any animal according to this definition.

### C. Thrifty and Obese Gene Effects

Some adaptive evolution to *ad libitum* feeding may be occurring in the human population and other mammals not now living in their normal ecological niche. This idea gains support from studies using the obese and diabetic mouse mutant strains. These mouse strains appear to be able to derive more calories and deposit more fat, as compared to so-called normal control mouse strains.[486] Because of this phenomena, the genes affected in these mouse strains have been called "thrifty genes". It could be that such genes may be closer to the normal genotype, where in feast and famine conditions, the mice would not become obese or diabetic but would likely survive better than the less thrifty inbred mouse strains. Under *ad libitum* feeding the obese mouse strain has a very short life span, but under calorie-restriction, Harrison has found that their life span can be increased over twofold, to a value equal to or slightly more than calorie-restricted nonobese long-lived mice.[487] These results suggest that by-products of inefficient metabolism may play a role in accelerating aging. Perhaps overnutrition operates in the same manner; that is, *ad libitum* feeding induces inefficient utilization of food, producing high levels of toxic by-products which act to accelerate aging. A mouse strain not now expressing the thrifty gene phenotype might have an advantage which evolved since the mice were placed in captivity under *ad libitum* feeding conditions. Thus, perhaps the best control animals for longevity studies in mice would be to use the thrifty wild-type strains under calorie-restriction and/or intermittent fasting with adequate exercise.

### D. Short-Lived Mouse Strains

Most of the inbred mouse strains have life spans shorter than the wild type, and many of the causes of their death are related to immunologically-related dysfunctions or to cancer. These diseases are frequently described as a result of genetic changes involved directly with the tissue or systems they affect. Examples are the NZB strain with high frequency of autoimmune disease or the AKR strain with high frequency of mammary cancer. It is now clear that calorie-restriction and/or intermittent fasting can significantly reduce the age-dependent frequency of these diseases and lengthen the life span of the short-lived strains. These results are often interpreted as evidence for the life span extension effects of calorie restriction.[13,479]

This author would like to offer a different interpretation as to the biological nature of some of the short-lived mouse strains and how calorie-restriction operates to increase their life span. It is proposed that the mutations these mice carry increase the sensitivity of particular tissues or systems to the toxicity or life-shortening effects of *ad libitum* feeding. Such mutations would not be nearly as effective in shortening life span in calorie-restricted and/or intermittent-fasted animals. Life span of normal mice fed *ad libitum* is considered to be shortened by an accelerated rate of development and an increased rate of toxic by-products of metabolism. The short-lived mutant mouse strains may have mutations in the LDGs of both the DLBS and CABS types. Thus, *ad libitum* feeding would amplify the effects of this class of mutations, allowing their adverse effects to be detected by calorie-restriction and/or intermittent-fasting. A prediction of this model is that many of the shorter-lived mouse strains whose life span can be lengthened by calorie-restriction and/or intermittent-fasting would be found deficient in LDPs. If this proves to be correct, these mouse strains would be valuable in studying these LDGs and how they function. There also exists the possibility that many human inherited diseases operate in a similar manner by making an individual more sensitive than normal to *ad libitum* feeding.

## VII. BIOMARKERS OF AGING AND LONGEVITY

### A. Biomarkers of Aging

Biomarkers of aging are considered essential in life span intervention experiments in order to ascertain as quickly as possible whether a certain treatment is having any effect. A second need for biomarkers of aging is to be able to measure a person's physiological or functional age equivalent. This is important in view of the remarkable differences which exist in aging rates in human populations and the necessity to arrive at a rational retirement age (mandatory retirement for airline pilots is 60 years).

In developing biomarker assays, it is essential to realize that changes which simply correlate with age do not necessarily mean that they are importantly involved with the aging process. This has been a common error. For example, in rats, it has been shown that the time required to induce a number of specific enzymes increases with age.[488] A remarkable linear correlation has been found between the age of the animal and the lag-time of enzyme induction. Such an increased lag time in induction kinetics has been termed a "biochemical defect", implying that if it did not occur, the animal would presumably live much longer. Accordingly, it is reasoned that if the mechanism underlying this lag is found, we would be able to understand at least one aspect of aging processes at the molecular level. However, it is equally probable that this age-dependent lag is a compensatory process required to maintain overall homeostasis in the animal and is not related to any manner as a causative element in aging. Thus, an insight to the biochemical mechanism related to the increased lag-time may not result in new insight of the mechanisms of aging but instead of the mechanisms of compensation of other types of aging processes occurring. Consequently, enzyme induction lag-time may not be a direct measure of the aged state of the animal, and as such it may not be a very good biomarker.

Similarly, other changes frequently termed as defects or dysfunctions are the age-dependent decline in protein and RNA synthesis rates and changes in enzyme levels (some increase and others decrease). These changes could also be compensatory processes. In fact, the changes may not even be compensatory in nature but instead may have no effect, simply being part of a feedback control, reflecting other types of age-dependent processes occurring in the organism. Still other age-dependent changes that may be compensatory in nature are the decrease in specific metabolic rate,[230] the decrease in plasma levels of DHEA/DHEA-S,[241] and the decline in function of the immune system.[489] A dramatic reduction in metabolism occurs in early life (on a total body weight basis), and it has been suggested that this may be an important cause of aging.[70] Similarly, a dramatic decrease in plasma levels of DHEA/DHEA-S occurs, which has usually been described as a possible cause of aging. However, it may be that, if SMR or DHEA/DHEA-S levels did not decrease, the animal would have a much shorter life span; consequently it may be quite harmful to return the SMR or plasma DHEA/DHEA-S levels in an older person to that of a young adult. The same could be said for the immune system, for it may be beneficial for the immune system to decrease its function with age in order to reduce the possibly more serious consequences of increased autoantibody production. The decline and cessation of reproduction is another example,[490] where reduction of reproductive potential may be a positive result of a genetic program and not related at all to normal aging processes. Here, a decrease in reproduction may have species survival value by decreasing the incidence of birth defects and other genetic abnormalities that occur with increasing age.

In terms of searching for biomarkers of aging, ideally the marker should measure primary aging processes or their effects as directly as possible, the critical objective being that if aging rate is really being slowed down, this fact should not be missed by the use of indirect or irrelevant biomarkers. One method of determining if a given age-dependent change is playing an important role in determining aging rate is to investigate its rate of change as a function of MLP in different species. In other words, the correlation should be found to be dependent on aging rate, not just on the rate of passage of time. For example, there is evidence that collagen cross-linkage increases with age, and accordingly, there is a collagen cross-linkage hypothesis of aging and the suggestion that it should be a good biomarker of aging.[491] However, there has been other data indicating that the rate of change in collagen structure is more dependent on temperature[492] and hormones,[493,494] not on MLP of a species.[495,496] In our experience, collagen from old humans appears to be highly cross-linked, while collagen from the same organs from old mice is more like that of a 2 to 3-year-old human's tissues.

The age-dependent rate of collagen cross-linkage with MLP has recently been reported for a few mammalian species, and in these studies the rate was slower in longer-lived species.[497,498] However, more work of this nature needs to be completed, particularly for different primate species, before we should seriously consider a collagen hypothesis of aging to be relevant for humans or suggest collagen cross-linkage as a biomarker of aging. This problem is much clearer for the rate of racemization of amino acids.[499] The rate of racemization is not a function of MLP (body temperature of mammals is almost equal) but is simply a function of chronological time.

Potential biomarkers related to the postulated dysdifferentiative nature of aging may prove to be of value. Any assays that would be able to detect a small drift of cells from their proper state of differentiation could be used. This would include changes in membrane characteristics of cells such as hormone receptor proteins or HLA antigen patterns and changes in the amount and types of proteins and RNA.

Possible noninvasive techniques that may be useful as biomarkers of aging are those currently being used as biomarkers of cancer in humans. Because it has been postulated that, a cancer cell is a specific type of aging cell (a specific type of dysdifferentiated cell), many of the biomarkers of cancer may be biomarkers of aging. A list of such markers that may be of value in this regard are (1) alpha-fetoprotein, (2) β-glucuronidase, (3) breast-cyst fluid protein, (4) calcitonin, (5) carcinoembryonic antigen, (6) colon mucoprotein antigen, (7) colon-specific antigen, (8) fetal sulfoglycoprotein, (9) galactosyl transferase isoenzyme-11, (10) human chorionic gonadotropin, (11) lactic acid dehydrogenase, (12) pancreatic oncofetal antigen, (13) prostatic acid phosphatase, (14) prostate-specific antigen, (15) Tennessee antigen, and (16) zinc glycinate marker. In addition, the interesting observation has been made that most cancerous cells have a deficiency of the Mn-SOD type.[500] Perhaps such a decrease is involved in the normal process of age-dependent dysdifferentiation. Other possibilities are the measurement of by-products of lipid peroxidation and other oxidative reactions related to cellular damage by determining levels of pentane in the breath.[501]

Of course, before any of these methods could be used, it must first be shown that aging is a dysdifferentiative process and that such measurements are effective in measuring this state. Therefore, the first step would be to determine if age-dependent increases in the low background level of these markers occur in noncancerous patients.

## B. Biomarkers of Longevity

### *1. Theoretical Basis*

Biomarkers of aging are considered useful to determine both physiological age and aging rate when measured over a given time interval. A prediction of an individual's life-long characteristic aging rate could be determined early in life by measuring their biomarkers of longevity. This method comes from the predictions of the special hypothesis that aging rate is governed by a special set of genes called the LDGs. Thus, if the degree of expression of these genes can be determined, the characteristic aging rate of an individual could theoretically be estimated at a very early age without having to take measurements over a long period of time. Furthermore, since techniques of life span intervention may involve the enhancement of the expression of these LDPs, then these same biomarkers measuring their effectiveness in enhancing levels of LDPs could be used as biomarkers of longevity.

Of course, the major difficulty with this suggestion is that the basic concept of LDPs is far from proven. Nevertheless, there is sufficient evidence that individuals with unusually low levels of known potential LDPs are likely to be at greater risk to physiological dysfunctions. Examples are individuals with abnormally low levels of DNA repair, SOD, glutathione peroxidase, and detoxification. A set of such measurements could be made using a single plasma sample or a tissue culture of cells taken from a skin sample. Another possibility is that an individual's characteristic lymphocyte HLA antigen pattern might reflect not only his innate immunological capacity but also endogenous levels of some of these LDPs (see Section IV). Thus, a combination of both biomarkers of aging and longevity might be the most effective means of monitoring the effects of life span intervention techniques.

*2. Population and Physiological Markers of Aging Rate*

Not too long ago, considerable interest was placed on the analysis of survival curves in the development of models and hypotheses of aging.[61,502] An important criteria for a successful model of aging was its ability to predict the nonlinear Gompertz function from the linear decline in physiological functions. The Gompertz function is derived from the equation:

$$\frac{dN}{dt} = a_o e^{\alpha_o t} N \tag{41}$$

where N is number of individuals in the population at any time, t, and $a_o$ and $\alpha$ are constants.

The Gompertz function is the normalized rate of death and is frequently called the mortality rate. It is written as:

$$\frac{1}{N}\frac{dN}{dt} = a_o e^{\alpha_o t} \tag{42}$$

This relation holds good only after sexual maturation and to about 80% of a species' MLP. The theoretical basis of this equation can be explained if it is considered that survival is determined by two components, a random component based on the intensity of external environmental hazards and an aging component based on how the processes of aging effectively increase this random probability of death as a function of time. For example, if a population was immortal, where no aging processes occurred, $\alpha_o$ would be zero and the Gompertz function would be expressed as:

$$\frac{dN}{dt}\frac{1}{N} = a_o \tag{43}$$

This function describes what is frequently seen for animals living in their natural ecological niche. Under these circumstances, death by accident or predators occurs largely independent of the age of the individual and is completely random. On the average, death usually occurs before senescence reduces the animal's vigor to the point that the probability of death is significantly increased. However, for animals in captivity and removed from their natural environmental hazards (and as it is for most humans today), a nonexponential survival curve is found, where senescence clearly plays a role in determining probability of death in later life. Here, $\alpha_o$ is not zero. Thus, a straight-forward interpretation of the Gompertz function is that the constant $a_o$ represents the random death component and $\alpha_o$, the aging component of the population being followed as a function of age.

According to the special hypothesis, longer-lived species would live under less hazardous conditions, allowing them to benefit from their innate longevity potential. Thus, $a_o$ would be expected to decrease as MLP increased. The value of $a_o$ would be related to the species' innate LDP levels and its external environmental hazards. Different species in captivity living under the same environmental hazards would accordingly have relative $a_o$ values determined largely by their innate differences of LDPs, as reflected by their characteristic MLP.

A theoretical question of long standing has been how $a_o$ and $\alpha_o$ constants describing the survival curve might be related to the biological aging or longevity characteristics of the individuals making up the population.[61] Some insight to this question might be gained by determining the $a_o$ and $\alpha_o$ values for different species raised under similar external environmental hazard conditions whose life spans have been shortened or lengthened by various genetic, dietary, or biochemical means.[459] Under these conditions, acute radiation of mice was found only to reduce $a_o$ but not $\alpha_o$, but chronic radiation exposure over the life span decreased $\alpha_o$ and not $a_o$. Increase of life span by calorie restriction was also found to increase $a_o$ and to decrease $\alpha_o$. Antioxidants appear to decrease $a_o$ and to leave $\alpha_o$ relatively unaffected.

These type of data led Sacher to postulate a different interpretation of what the $a_o$ and $\alpha_o$ constituents implied than has just been presented.[459] He has suggested that the shape of the survival curve is determined by two parameters, one controlling initial vulnerability to disease and death ($a_o$) and the other controlling the rate this vulnerability increases with age, or $\alpha_o$. It was concluded that most life span intervention techniques have only altered the vulnerability parameters ($a_o$) and have not truly altered innate aging rate. Only a decrease in body temperature and calorie restriction alteration appear to have altered the aging rate parameter, $\alpha_o$.

This interpretation of the biological meaning of the $a_o$ and $\alpha_o$ constituents appears to have been widely accepted without question, but a number of difficulties are evident.[503] The most fundamental is the attempt to derive information on the biological basis of aging of individuals within a population from an equation used to describe the age-dependent frequency of death of individuals. There is no data or mathematical derivation I am aware of that supports the postulate that $\alpha_o$ is related to the biological aging rate of an individual and is accordingly inversely related to MLP. Moreover, in terms of practical matters, the shape of survival curves can easily be altered for a given species by simple changes in diet and/or environmental housing conditions, thus dramatically changing $a_o$ and $\alpha_o$ values. Yet, under such changes, little or no changes are seen in the innate MLP, as shown by the survival curve. The best example supporting this conclusion is the shape of human survival curves in different countries, where large differences in mean survival are evident with no change in MLP. It is generally accepted that the differences in mean survival represent environmental differences affecting the death of the population, not innate differences in the aging rate of the individuals. Indeed, it is not known what genetic or biochemical factors actually do determine the characteristic shapes of survival curves. For example, are the deaths of individuals near the 50% mean survival value occurring because they have aged faster than the individuals still alive or because they were killed by random effects, where the aging rates of the population are all similar? In other words, how homogeneous is aging rate in a population? The interpretation given by Sacher for the Gompertz function assumes innate biological aging rate among the different individuals to be identical, but this has never been proven.

The shape of survival curves of inbred mice also appears to be similar to outbred mice and does not have a more squared shape, as would be expected if aging rate were more homogeneous between the individuals. Also, the shape of survival curves of humans in developed countries appears like that of an inbred mouse; but on estimates based on identical twin studies of humans, the human survival curve would be more squared if all humans were inbred. These observations question how genetically and physiologically homogeneous are inbred mice. No one has actually shown that inbred mice are indeed homogeneous in genetic composition. Perhaps the random migration of transposon elements during development produce a distribution of genotypes in the inbred mice which result in a distribution of aging rates in the population. For example, slightly different genotypes would affect a cell's drift rate towards dysdifferentiation.

A second difficulty in attempting to derive biological parameters of aging for individuals from population death frequency data centers on the suggestion by Sacher that two independent biological parameters define the survival curve: (1) vulnerability and (2) innate aging rate which acts to increase vulnerability. This is essentially saying that longer-lived species are less likely to be killed at all ages, which instinctively must be the case. But why are the longer-lived species less vulnerable? At the peak of health and vigor are longer-lived species healthier or more vigorous? This author thinks not. Instead, they have less of a probability to die throughout their life span because they are living in a less hazardous environment and are aging less rapidly.

To emphasize the importance of the issue here, Sacher has suggested that longevity intervention techniques could be developed where only vulnerability would be increased and aging rate would be left unchanged.[503] In this manner, he predicts that a longer more vigorous life span would result, but MLP would remain unchanged. This author believes this is impossible. It appears more plausible that vulnerability of individuals to death and their innate aging rates are the result of the *same* LDPs and, as such, cannot be controlled independently. Thus, a decrease in $\alpha_o$ would be predicted to result in a corresponding decrease in $a_o$ if changes in LDPs are involved. A comparison of $a_o$ and $\alpha_o$ as a function of MLP in the different mammalian species supports this prediction.

An illustration of how MLP is related to $a_o$ and $\alpha_o$ is illustrated in Figure 6.

$$\ln \left| \frac{\frac{dN}{dt}}{N} \right| = \ln (a_o) + \alpha_o t \tag{44}$$

and typical curves for two species having different MLPs are illustrated where species 1 has a lower MLP than species 2.

MLP is the life span where all individuals of a given population have died. This point can be defined when the probability of death or mortality rate reaches a certain value over a given length of time. This value would be expected to be equal for all species, and $a_o$ and $\alpha_o$ would determine the time necessary to reach a given mortality rate. Using this concept to define MLP, we have:

$$\text{MLP} = \frac{\ln \left| \frac{\frac{dN}{dt}}{N} \right| - \ln(a_o)}{\alpha_o} \tag{45}$$

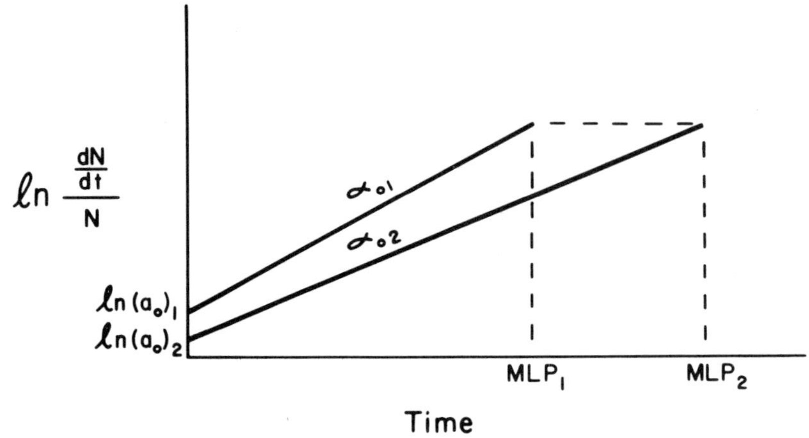


FIGURE 6. A plot of the Gompertz function for two hypothetical species having maximum life span potentials of $MLP_1$ and $MLP_2$, which correspond to the slope of the lines $\alpha_{01}$ and $\alpha_{02}$, respectively. MLP or equivalent physiological age of the population at any time would be defined here as the time when the probabilities of death dN/dt/N are equal.

where for practical purposes $\ln\left|\frac{\frac{dN}{dt}}{N}\right|_{MLP}$ would be defined as a value that results in about 10% remaining survivors of a given population.

But then how can the biological aging rate be measured for an individual if it cannot be derived from survival curve data? The only means would be from physiological data on individuals from a longitudinal study. The age-dependent decline of a large number of physiological functions are known, both for mouse and human, and these occur in approximately a linear manner for both longitudinal and cross-sectional populations.[504]

The slopes of these various curves measuring physiological functions with increasing age however are different, suggesting at first sight that different physiological functions age at different rates. A more likely possibility is that the fraction of loss of all physiological functions per unit time of an individual is a constant. For example, if P represents the magnitude of a given physiological function at a time, t, then:

$$\frac{\frac{dP}{dt}}{P_{MLP}} = K = \text{constant} \tag{46}$$

Integrating this function over an individual's lifespan (t = 0 to t = MLP), we have:

$$\int_{P_o}^{P_{MLP}} dP = KP_{MLP} \int_{o}^{t=MLP} dt \tag{47}$$

or

$$P_{MLP} - P_o = KP_{MLP}\,(MLP) \tag{48}$$

giving

$$MLP = \frac{P_{MLP} - P_o}{KP_{MLP}} = \frac{1}{K}\left[1 - \frac{P_o}{P_{MLP}}\right] \qquad (49)$$

By this definition, K would represent the physiological aging rate of the species and MLP would be defined by the ratio of $P_o/P_{MLP}$ of any physiological function.

The major assumption of this derivation is that the relative rate of decline of all physiological functions is equal. This has yet to be tested experimentally, but instinctively it is difficult to see how natural selection would favor the maintenance of a given physiological function in excess over another function, particularly in view of the concept that longevity evolved. This author believes it is more reasonable to assume that longevity of the organism evolved uniformly by reducing the relative aging rate of each physiological function uniformly.

## VIII. DYSDIFFERENTIATION OF NORMAL DIPLOID CELLS IN CULTURE

### A. Finite Division Potential: Biological Relevance

An interesting phenomena of normal diploid cells grown in tissue culture is that they apparently have a finite doubling potential.[505-507] Whether or not this effect is a result of inadequate growth media or other artifacts does not diminish the fact that, under defined conditions, such cells in culture do undergo a number of biochemical, genetic and morphological changes and finally end as a nondividing population.

The question of why cells stop dividing is clearly an interesting one, and it is obvious that this phenomena can be used as a useful model system to study mechanisms of control processes governing mitosis in cells.[508] Furthermore, since transformed cells and cells from cancerous tissue appear to have unlimited proliferation capacity grown under the same conditions, there is the possibility that a knowledge of why normal diploid cells stop dividing or why cancer cells do not stop dividing might lead to new insights on how cancer cells are different and to means of how their proliferation can be stopped in vivo.

Vaccines for human are now being produced using normal human diploid cells, which requires of course a very detailed study of their growth characteristics and other relevant biological parameters of the particular strain of cell being used for this purpose. Unfortunately, because such normal diploid cell strains have finite proliferation capacity, and of course transformed cells would not be used for the purpose of vaccine production, this limitation has been a serious handicap for their use in this regard. Thus, an understanding of how doubling potential might be extended would have considerable economic benefits.

In addition to the above reasons for studying the mechanisms of limited proliferation capacity of normal diploid cells in culture, it has also been proposed that the proliferation limit may be reflecting or is actually an aging process identical to that occurring in cells in vivo.[507,508] To emphasize this point, advocates of the use of normal diploid cells for aging studies describe the culturing of these cells as "aging cells" and the cells in phase three as "senescent" or "old" cells.[505] In support of its validity as a model for aging, it has been implied that shortly after cell division ceases in phase three, death occurs and the culture dies out.

As a result of the apparent attractiveness of this in vitro system a substantial effort over the past 10 years or so has been made on a worldwide scale in characterizing this so-called aging phenomena in tissue culture to gain insight on in vivo cellular aging processes. Most of the past work on the tissue culture aging model has been of a descriptive nature, and today a substantial list can be compiled of what changes with population doublings and what does not.[507] The tissue culture aging model has also been popular in testing a number of aging hypotheses, such as the error catastrophe hypothesis[53,54] and the altered protein hypothesis of aging,[509] but the mechanism is still not known why these cells stop dividing and finally die.

### B. Indefinite Life Span Potential: Biological Relevance

Early studies by Alexis Carrel had indicated that normal cells in culture did not stop dividing and consequently did not die. Later studies indicated that Carrell's conclusions were incorrect on both accounts; normal diploid cells have a finite doubling potential and they do die.[506] However, it now appears that these cells may not die, at least shortly after they stop dividing. There is surprisingly little data on this important point, but the relatively recent results of Bell and co-workers[510,511] have indicated that, although cell division does stop, cell viability can nevertheless be maintained in the nondividing state for up to 2 or more years if the media is changed on a frequent and regular basis. Personal communication with several researchers in this field has confirmed this result.[512-515] It appears that it is not known just how long the cells can be maintained in the viable nondividing state, but it is at least 2 or more years. In this light, certainly the terms "senescence", "aging", "death", and "proliferation death" are misleading and scientifically incorrect if it is not known if the culture does die out at some stage. Of course, it can be argued that loss of cell division potential is a loss of a critical function and is equivalent to death, but postmitotic cells in young animals (neurons for example) are certainly not dead. Before the loss of proliferation potential can be termed an aging phenomena, it appears necessary to demonstrate that loss of proliferation increases at least the probability of death in the culture. This is the standard definition of aging and to my knowledge this has not yet been demonstrated.

This is not an argument of sematics. The seriousness of this situation can be demonstrated by the use of the tissue culture aging model for testing aging hypotheses that were proposed to account for aging in vivo. For example, most experiments testing the Orgel error catastrophe hypothesis have used the tissue culture aging model. One of the methods used was to test the ability of viruses to replicate in phase three cultures.[516-518] If the cells were undergoing an error catastrophe and nearing death because of an increasing load of abnormal proteins, then low titers and defective viruses would be expected to be produced. The results indicated that viral replication does not decrease significantly as a function of population doubling. These data were therefore interpreted as not supporting the error catastrophe hypothesis of aging.

However, Orgel's hypothesis or other error hypotheses are hypotheses of senescence and death, not hypotheses of how division might cease. Moreover, these results could have been easily predicted on prior knowledge that these cells in culture did not die at least for 2 or more years. If fact, just on this basis one could rule out the error catastrophe model of aging playing any role in the cessation of cell division. It is therefore not surprising that no accumulation of errors[519] or altered proteins[520] or the production of defective viruses[516-518] have been found in phase three cells. Thus, the conclusions drawn from using the in vitro cell culture model of aging to test these hypotheses appear to be in serious error as to their implications to normal cell aging processes in vivo. On the other hand, it would be interesting to learn how long the nondividing cells can be maintained and if they would begin to undergo aging processes leading to their death. A study of such cells may indeed show an accumulation of errors.

### C. Normal Diploid Cells in Culture as a Model of Dysdifferentiation

Still, the cessation of division, even if cell death does not immediately follow, could reflect some normal type of cellular aging process. It has been suggested that the changes seen during phase two before cell division stops are more indicative of normal in vivo cellular aging processes.[505,507] But it can also be argued that these changes reflect the alteration most cells normally undergo when division is being genetically programmed to stop through nonsenescent processes. Cells taken from older individuals have been shown to have a shorter doubling potential, which is supportive that doubling potential is related somehow to physiological age.[505,507] But a close examination of this data indicates its scattered nature. For example, one can find the doubling potential of cells from an elderly individual being similar to the doubling potential of cells from a young individual. Of course, physiological parameters, particularly as age increases, are also increasingly scattered, but in this case the suggestion is not made that a decline in a given physiological function is causing aging. Instead, it is generally accepted as reflecting more fundamental aging changes.

The doubling potential of normal diploid cells has been shown to correlate with MLP of different species, and this data is frequently given as support that the finite doubling potential of cells in culture does reflect in some way the MLP of different species.[505,507] This comparative approach appears at first sight to be a good method to determine the validity of the in vitro cell culture model to aging, but this author is unaware of any data showing a positive correlation of doubling potential of cells in vivo with MLP. Instead, doubling potential in vivo appears to be more related to body size or SMR if the life span of red blood cells are any indication of other dividing cells of an organism.

Unfortunately, very little effort appears to have been placed on testing the validity of the tissue culture aging model by using the comparative method or any other method. The comparative data usually cited is a collection of results from different laboratories of widely different types of species such as human, Galapagos tortoise, mink, chicken, and mouse. Such studies would be more meaningful if the same type of cells from different primate species were used and the experiments carried out by the same laboratory. One study was carried out in the same laboratory using cells from a number of different species. No correlation of doubling potential with MLP was found.[521] On the other hand, another recent study indicates that cells from longer-lived species do have greater doubling potential.[522] A puzzle in this latter study is the reported high number of cells found with abnormal genotypes as population doubling increased. Similar results have been reported,[523] but if this indeed occurs, then why not postulate loss of genes or a gene dosage effect as a possible cause of loss of doubling potential as the simplest model rather than speculate on more sophisticated models such as genetic-programmed aging processes which imply an intact genome? Also, if such genetic alteration from the normal diploid state occurs, then the loss of reiterated sequences, as reported by Shmookler and Goldstein,[524] could be reinterpreted simply as due to a different chromosome distribution. Clearly, much more work needs to be done before we can consider the normal diploid cell in vitro culture system as an unquestioned model for in vivo cellular aging.

On considering the history of development of in vitro tissue culture techniques, the most impressive fact is that mammalian cells can be grown in vitro.[525-527] Most differentiated cell types cannot be grown in vitro, and those that can grow, usually always change to some degree from their proper state of differentiation. Thus, the question of why normal cells change their state of differentiation when taken from an organism and placed in tissue culture has attracted interest in the tissue culture technique, for this phenomenon may prove to be important in understanding the processes leading to the proposed dysdifferentiation processes which have been proposed to occur in vivo.

On considering the number of processes which are thought to be involved in determining the proper state of differentiation, it is not surprising that such changes in these processes may occur in vitro. For example, when cells are placed in culture, normal cell-to-cell contact is lost and the cells have lost their normal exposure to a wide number of growth factors, hormones and other regulatory agents (most of which are probably still unknown) that determine differentiated states of cells.[525,527] In addition, potential LDPs such as vitamin C, vitamin E, choline, urate, DHEA-S, and β-carotene are likely to be altered from their optimum concentrations, particularly when growing human cells in calf serum for instance. Most data appears to be consistent with the interpretation that the closer the normal in vivo environment of cells can be similated in culture, the greater the stability of the differentiated state of cells in culture. This fact then already leads to the concept that the various factors now required to grow cells in defined media, for example, act to stabilize the differentiated state of cells, and that changes with age could act to promote cellular aging in terms of dysdifferentiation.

Thus, the limited proliferation capacity of cells in culture along with the initial and progressive changes taking place in the cells when placed in culture may be the result of dysdifferentiation processes. Such dysdifferentiation processes would reflect a cell's normal response to being placed in an artificial and/or improper environment where this in vitro environment would be similar to what occurs naturally with aging in vivo. This interpretation implies that aging can be caused or enhanced by a deterioration of a cell's normal environment. Growth of normal diploid cells in culture as it is presently being conducted may then accelerate dysdifferentiation processes. Dysdifferentiation, as it has been defined here, should be understood as being different from terminal differentiation, which implies the normal continuation of a genetic program.[510,511,528]

Further support for the dysdifferentiation nature of proliferating cells in culture is that renewing cells in vivo show many features of nonrenewing cells in vivo as a function of age.[529] It has also been demonstrated that small changes in the growth conditions of cells can lead to modification of their phenotypic expression.[530] Since division is highly complicated and is a differentiation process, then a change from a dividing to a nondividing state represents a change in the differentiated state. All the other morphological and biochemical changes known to occur as a function of doubling potential could also be reflecting dysdifferentiation. Cells taken from older individuals would be expected to have less division potential because they have already accumulated a certain degree of dysdifferentiation and are therefore more sensitive or have less dysdifferentiation processes to accumulate before division stops. Greater division potential is predicted from cells derived from longer-lived species because, as predicted from the special hypothesis, cells from longer-lived species are inherently more stable in terms of maintaining their proper state of differentiation. Additional support for this is that cells taken from longer-lived species are less likely to transform spontaneously.[265] In addition, Hornsby and co-workers have shown the importance of antioxidants in stabilizing the differentiated state of cells placed in tissue culture.[222-225]

Thus, taking cells from an animal and placing them in culture is predicted to mimic changes that normally occur in vivo as a function of age and to consequently produce similar effects. The cessation of division would accordingly not be a result of an accumulation of damage nor a result of a genetic program of death but would be predicted to occur by the activation of normal mechanisms for shutting down division, such as the production of an inhibitor of division.[531,532] In this sense, the stopping of division is considered to be a highly probable event in cell dysdifferentiation, perhaps for the same reason that division is frequently the most sensitive parameter of a cell to radiation and chemical mutagens.

### D. All Cells are Mortal

The use of the term "normal cells" (cells undergoing a finite division potential) and "immortal cells" (cells that are transformed and have unlimited proliferation potential) are frequently confusing in terms of their relevance to gerontological research. The use of these terms to describe a property of these two cell types implies that, once an understanding of why the cancer cells are immortal is gained, we can use this knowledge to extend life span. Clearly, longer-lived species do not have cells more similar to the properties of transformed cells. Most importantly, however, is the question of how immortal are transformed cells. Could we also call *E. coli* and single-cell eukaryotic organisms immortal if, on culture, division potential appears to be indefinite? To answer such questions, *E. coli* was grown under fixed-culture conditions.[1] This is where cells were attached to the bottom side of a nitrocellulose membrane with growth media flowing through the membrane. The cells were fixed and hanging from the membrane, being bathed by the media. Cell-to-cell contact was prevented and division was not inhibited. On cell division, only one of the daughter cells was washed away from the membrane and the other daughter cell remained attached. Samples of cells were taken periodically to determine viability and growth rate. Under these conditions, a finite division potential and life span was found for the culture, which was about 6 to 7 days. The apparent immortality of the freely dividing culture of *E. coli* as it is normally grown was attributed to a small population of stem-like cells which carried no mutations and consequently were the most rapidly dividing. Random accumulation of mutation throughout the population of cells was postulated to result in the increasingly long division time. As division time increased, these cells were gradually diluted out by the more rapidly dividing cells. The relative rate of division to the rate of mutation was postulated to be such that a finite number of rapidly dividing cells with nomutations were always maintained. A mean mutational load in the population would exist which could account for the observed skewed distribution of division times. Death of the culture would be predicted by this model if selection for the most rapidly dividing cells was inhibited, as was the case when the cells were fixed to the membrane or, if by dilution, the mutation-free cells were eliminated from the population. A similar experiment to test for the possible finite proliferation potential of normal and transformed eukaryotic mammalian cell lines was postulated. Little difference is seen in the basic concept described here and the committed-cell hypothesis later postulated by Holliday and co-workers.[533,534] The fixed *E. coli* experiments described here should be considered to be very preliminary in nature and it is possible that other factors may have resulted in their cessation of division. The experiments are reviewed here to stimulate a more critical inquiry of what constitutes immortality of cultures and in the hope that these preliminary experiments might stimulate the continuation of such studies.

Other studies have indicated that if cells are not dividing they are dying.[1] *E. coli*, for example, is always in a state of dividing or dying. No means have ever been developed to my knowledge to maintain the vitality of a cell indefinitely in the nondividing state. Thus, there appears to be no immortal cells, only immortal populations.

The idea that conjugation may play a role in cell survival and might be involved in immortality of cell cultures is an interesting one, but it should be remembered that in *Paramecium*, although there are strains that do require conjugation for continuous proliferation, other strains exist that have unlimited proliferation potential without conjugation.[535] In fact, a useful model system of longevity would be to compare such strains that do and do not have finite division potential in terms of learning what the differences might be at the LDP level. Such studies may be of value, in addition to studying age-dependent changes in *Paramecium*.

## IX. EVALUATION OF TOXIC HAZARDS TO HUMAN

### A. Deriving a Theoretical Basis

The special hypothesis of aging and longevity predicts that longer-lived species are more resistant to natural endogenous agents which act to destabilize their cells from a proper state of differentiation. Mechanisms acting to stabilize the differentiated state are predicted to be DNA repair, free radical scavengers, detoxification processes, heavy metal-chelating agents, and so forth. In addition to natural endogenous agents,[536,537] many recently introduced environmental toxins are also carcinogenic[538] and may therefore act to accelerate dysdifferentiation and thus the aging processes. Because longer-lived species have a lower probability of cancer occurring as a function of time, it was proposed that the mechanism(s) causing most types of cancer are the same as those causing aging. Consequently, the mechanisms governing aging rate are the same as those that reduce the incidence rate of cancer in longer-lived species.[11] Thus, agents enhancing cancer incidence would be predicted to enhance aging rate and work by destabilizing the proper differentiated state of cells.

LDPs are predicted to work in part by providing cells with protection against endogenous as well as exogenous toxic agents. If this is true, then human cells should be found to be inherently more resistant to a number of agents known to alter states of differentiation, such as mutagens and carcinogens. In addition to the SOD correlation with MLP, a few other studies are consistent with this prediction. Also, cells from longer-lived species have a lower probability of spontaneous transformation in in vitro cell culture conditions.[265,539] In fact, human cells have never been observed in culture to undergo spontaneous transformation, whereas this is very common for mouse cells. The studies of Schwartz and co-workers have indicated cells taken from longer-lived species and grown in culture activate the precarcinogens DMBA and BP at a lower level.[284,285] Also, there is data indicating that cells from longer-lived species have higher levels of UV DNA repair levels.[261,273,274,277]

A clear implication of such studies is that shorter-lived species such as mice and rats would be expected to be more sensitive to environmental toxic agents than longer-lived species such as man. Thus, in evaluating such toxic agents to assess their long-term as well as short-term effects to human, these considerations may prove important.[540] Frequently, because humans are exposed to a toxic agent for a longer period of time than shorter-lived species, safe toxicity levels are reduced below that found to be safe for shorter-lived species. No consideration has ever been taken of the experimental animals' inherent life span potential in the calculation of safe levels of toxins to humans.[538,541,542] Such considerations could result in humans being found substantially more resistant to a number of toxic agents than is now believed to be the case. In this regard, it should be noted that a common assumption is that if cellular aging processes are involved with the age-dependent increase of cancer, then an age-dependent increase in a cell's sensitivity to transformation should occur.[543] This is of course not necessary. What should be tested is a correlation of a cell's sensitivity to transformation by carcinogens as a function of the species' MLP.

### B. Methods of Evaluation

One means of testing the validity of this suggestion is to determine the toxicity of a given agent using cells from primates having different MLPs. Cell viability, transformation frequency, and sister chromatid exchange frequency in response to a given toxin or mutagen would be typical parameters to measure. A number of shorter-lived primates could be used for these studies, and from these values, an extrapolation made to humans. It would be expected that sensitivity to the toxins would decrease with increased MLP. Another test would be the ability of primate species as a function of life span potential to metabolize and/or detoxify known carcinogenic agents. This could be conducted on whole animals, measuring the metabolic by-products of carcinogens in the urine[544] or hydrocarbon by-products in the breath.[501] The relative ability of the mixed function oxidase system to detoxify given carcinogens could also be evaluated using small liver samples obtained from the primate species or by using early-passage normal diploid tissue cultures of primate species.

In these studies, it would be important to remember that resistance to high acute doses of toxic agents are less likely to be a function of MLP than are low levels given over a long time period. Another consideration is not only to seek a correlation of toxicity values to MLP but also to maximum calorie consumption (MCC). For example, since it was found for primates that SOD = K(MCC) resistance to low levels of $O_2^-$ would be expected to correlate with MCC and not MLP. The MCC correlation indirectly takes into account the size differences in species, which represents another interesting but related problem of toxicity evaluation. A smaller animal usually has a shorter life span, a higher specific metabolic rate and fewer cells at risk. With two animals of the same size and consequently the same SMR, but one having a longer life span, the longer-lived animal would be predicted to have the higher resistance to toxins. On the other hand, with two animals of different sizes but having the same life span potentials, the sensitivity per cell to toxins might also be predicted to be equal. But perhaps the larger animal needs a higher level of protection because more cells are at risk. For example, if cancer originates from a single cell and longer-lived species have a lower incidence of cancer on a per cell basis, then the cells from the larger animal, even though it has the same life span, may be much more resistant to transformation.

Experiments to answer such questions would appear to be fundamental, not only in determining a better rationale for the evaluation of toxic agents to humans using shorter-lived species, but also in learning of the *natural* processes which have evolved to control the onset frequency of cancer.

## X. INTELLECTUAL DETERMINANT GENES

The two major developments that occurred during the evolution of hominids leading to human are considered to be the increase of longevity and the increase of intellectual capacity. Both of these processes have been proposed to have increased at very rapid rates, reaching a peak rate about 100,000 years ago.[34] In terms of the evolution of longevity, a special hypothesis was proposed, suggesting: (1) specific longevity determinant genes exist which govern aging rate, (2) these genes exist in all mammalian species, and (3) evolution of increased MLP occurred by genetic changes in regulatory genes altering their timing and degree of expression.

Similarly, the evolution of human intellectual capacity is proposed to have occurred by identical mechanisms, that is (1) specific intellectual genes exist which govern intellectual capacity, (2) these genes exist in all mammalian species, and (3) the evolution of greater intellectual capacity occurred by genetic changes in regulatory genes altering their timing and degree of expression.

From the high rate of evolution of longevity and the high degree of similarity of the primate species at all levels of biological function, it was predicted that relatively few regulatory genes exist controlling the timing and degree of expression of the postulated LDPs. For these same reasons, few regulatory genes are also proposed to exist which control the timing and degree of expression of the intellectual determinant genes.

It is, of course, recognized that many of the genetic changes involved in the coevolution of longevity and intellectual capacity may be overlapping in nature; that is, one type of change resulted in both an enhancement of longevity and of intellectual capacity. For example, high uric acid values appear to correlate well with both longevity in different primate species and with intellectual capacity.[309,318-320] Also, simply a larger brain size in relation to body size is likely to have played a role in the evolution of higher intellectual capacity, and this occurred by alterations in genes linked with control of developmental rate and neoteny parameters.[4] However, levels of biochemical determinants of intellectual capacity are also likely to be involved. In parallel to longevity, two types of intellectual determinant genes are proposed: those associated with developmentally linked processes and those associated with continuously acting processes.

Little is known about the genetics and biochemistry which determine the magnitude of intellectual functions or how such processes might be studied.[544] However, a method similar to that proposed for the screening of potential LDGs might also be of value in screening of potential intellectual determinant genes. In most cases, animals of greater longevity (particularly the primates) have greater intellectual capacity,[545] so screening for intellectual determinant genes could be made as a function of MLP. Potential intellectual determinant processes that could be tested by this method are specific metabolic rate of brain tissues[546] and the plasma and brain tissue levels of the many different neuropeptides, neurotransmitters, and enzymes known to be important in neuronal and neuroendocrine processes.[547-549]

Advantage could also be taken of the remarkable individual differences existing within a species' population in intellectual capacity. In human, for example, a comparison of levels of potential intellectual determinant processes could be made between individuals having unusually high I.Q. levels, mathematical abilities, musical abilities, or photographic memories with individuals having average abilities in these categories. Similar studies could be extended to those of abnormally low intellectual levels and of individuals suffering from disorders resembling accelerated aging, such as senile dementia and Alzheimer's disease.[550] By generating a broad data base, comparative studies of this type could result in identifying some of the processes essential for maintaining normal intellectual functions and of means to help correct abnormal situations.

## ACKNOWLEDGMENTS

The interest and sharing of unpublished papers with Kenneth Munkres, Roy Walford, Philip Hartman, Peter Hornsby, David Harrison, Rolf Martin, and Donald Ingram is deeply appreciated. The unusual patience shown by George Roth in waiting for the manuscript is also appreciated. Much of the recent laboratory data presented here, in addition to drawing the figures and typing the manuscript, is the result of the dedicated efforts of Edith Cutler. Her assistance was made possible by support received from the Paul Glenn Foundation for Medical Research.

## REFERENCES

1. **Cutler, R. G.,** Transcription of reiterated DNA sequence classes throughout the life span of the mouse, in *Advances in Gerontology Research,* Vol. 4, Strehler, B. L., Ed., Academic Press, New York, 1972, 219.
2. **Cutler, R. G.,** Redundancy of information content in the genome of mammalian species as a protective mechanism determining aging rate, *Mech. Ageing Dev.,* 2, 381, 1973.
3. **Cutler, R. G.,** Evolution of human longevity and the genetic complexity governing aging rate, *Proc. Natl. Acad. Sci. USA,* 72, 4664, 1975.
4. **Cutler, R. G.,** Evolution of longevity in primates, *J. Human Evol.,* 5, 169, 1976.
5. **Cutler, R. G.,** Cross-linkage hypothesis of aging: DNA adducts in chromatin as a primary aging process, in *Aging, Carcinogenesis, and Radiation Biology,* Smith, K. C., Ed., Plenum Press, New York, 1976, 443.
6. **Cutler, R. G.,** Nature of aging and life maintenance processes, in *Interdisciplinary Topics in Gerontology,* Cutler, R. G., Ed., S. Karger, Basel, 1976, 83.
7. **Ono, T. and Cutler, R. G.,** Age-dependent relaxation of gene repression: Increase of endogenous murine leukemia virus-related and globin-related RNA in brain and liver of mice, *Proc. Natl. Acad. Sci. USA,* 75, 4431, 1978.

8. **Cutler, R. G.,** Evolutionary biology of senescence, in *The Biology of Aging,* Behnke, J. A., Finch, C. E., Moment, G. B., Eds., Plenum Press, New York, 1978, 311.
9. **Cutler R. G.,** Evolution of longevity in ungulates and carnivores, *Gerontology,* 25, 69, 1979.
10. **Cutler, R. G.,** Evolution of human longevity: A critical overview, *Mech. Ageing Dev.,* 9, 337, 1979.
11. **Tolmasoff, J. M., Ono, T., and Cutler, R. G.,** Superoxide dismutase: Correlation with life span and specific metabolic rate in primate species, *Proc. Natl. Acad. Sci. USA,* 77, 2777, 1980.
12. **Cutler, R. G.,** Evolution of human longevity, in *Advances in Pathobiology 7. Aging, Cancer and Cell Membranes,* Borek, C., Fenoglio, C. M., and King, D. W., Eds., Thieme-Stratton, Inc., New York, 1980, 43.
13. **Cutler, R. G.,** Life span extension, in *Aging: Biology and Behavior,* McGaugh, J. L. and Kiesler, S. B., Eds., Academic Press, New York, 1981, in press.
14. **Cutler, R. G.,** *The Dysdifferentiative Hypothesis of Mammalian Aging and Longevity,* Raven Press, New York, 1982, in press.
15. **Haldane, J. B. S.,** Evolution: past and future, *Atl. Month.,* 179, 45, 1947.
16. **Medawar, P. B.,** The definition and measurement of senescence, in *Ciba Foundation Colloq. on Ageing, Vol. I. General Aspects,* Wolstenholme, G. E. W. and Cameron, M. P., Eds., Little, Brown, Boston, 1955, 4.
17. **Medawar, P. B.,** *The Uniqueness of the Individual,* Methuen and Co., Ltd., London, 1957.
18. **Williams, G. C.,** Pleiotropy, natural selection, and the evolution of senescence, *Evolution,* 11, 398, 1957.
19. **Hamilton, W. D.,** The moulding of senescence by natural selection, *J. Theo. Biol.,* 12, 12, 1966.
20. **Maynard Smith, J.,** A theory of aging, *Nature (London),* 184, 956, 1959.
21. **Maynard Smith, J.,** Review lectures on senescence I. The causes of ageing, *Proc. R. Soc. London, Ser. B,* 157, 115, 1962.
22. **Maynard Smith, J.,** Theories of aging, in *Topics in the Biology of Aging,* Krohn, P. L., Ed., Interscience, New York, 1966, 1.
23. **Beer, G. de,** *Embryos and Ancestors,* Oxford University Press, London, 1958.
24. **Schultz, A. H.,** Characters common to higher primates and characters specific for man, *Q. Rev. Biol.,* 2, 259, 1936.
25. **Schultz, A. H.,** Ontogenetic specializations of man, *Arch. Julius Klaus Stiflung,* 24, 197, 1949.
26. **Schultz, A. H.,** The physical distinctions of man, *Proc. Am. Philos. Soc.,* 94, 428, 1950.
27. **Schultz, A. H.,** Age changes in primates and their modifications in man, in *Human Growth,* Tanner, J., Ed., Pergamon Press, London, 1960, 1.
28. **Schultz, A. H.,** Changing views on the nature and interrelations of the higher primates, *Emory Univ. Primate Res. Center Newslett.,* 3, 15, 1966.
29. **Schultz, A. H.,** The recent hominoid primates, in *Perspectives on Human Evolution,* Vol. 1, Washburn, S. L. and Jay, P. C., Eds., Holt, Rinehart and Winston, New York, 1968, 122.
30. **Wilson, A. C., Sarich, V. M., and Maxson, L. R.,** The importance of gene rearrangement in evolution: Evidence from studies on rates of chromosomal, protein, and anatomical evolution, *Proc. Natl. Acad. Sci. USA,* 71, 3028, 1974.
31. **King, M. C. and Wilson, A. C.,** Evolution at two levels in humans and chimpanzees, *Science,* 188, 107, 1976.
32. **Wilson, A. C.,** Gene regulation in evolution, in *Molecular Evolution,* Ayala, F. J., Ed., Sinauer Associates, Inc., Sunderland, Mass., 1976, 225.
33. **Bush, G. L., Case, S. M., Wilson, A. C., and Patton, J. L.,** Rapid speciation and chromosomal evolution in mammals, *Proc. Natl. Acad. Sci. USA,* 74, 3942, 1977.
34. **Wilson, A. C., Carlson, S. S., and White, T. J.,** Biochemical evolution, *Ann. Rev. Biochem.,* 46, 573, 1977.
35. **Cherry, L. M., Case, S. M., Kunkel, J. G., and Wilson, A. C.,** Comparisons of frogs, humans, and chimpanzees, *Science,* 204, 434, 1979.
36. **Gould, S. J.,** Allometry in primates, with emphasis on scaling and the evolution of the brain, *Contrib. Primatol.,* 5, 244-292, 1975.
37. **Gould, S. J.,** Geometric similarity in allometric growth; A contribution to the problem of scaling in the evolution of size, *Am. Naturalist,* 105, 113, 1971.
38. **Gould, S. J.,** Human babies as embryos, *Natural History,* 85, 22, 1976.
39. **Gould, S.J.,** The child as man's real father, *Natural History,* 84, 18, 1976.
40. **Gould, S. J.,** *Ontogeny and Phylogeny,* The Belknap Press, Cambridge, Mass., 1977.
41. **Sacher, G. A.,** Relation of lifespan to brain and body weight in mammals, in *Ciba Foundation Colloq. on Ageing,* Vol. 5, Wolstenholme, G. E. W. and O'Connor, C. M., Eds., Churchill Press, London, 1959, 115.
42. **Sacher, G. A.,** The dimensionality of the life span, in *The Biology of Aging,* Strehler, B. L., Ed., A.I.B.S., Washington, D.C., 1960, 251.
43. **Sacher, G. A.,** The effect of physiologic fluctuations on mortality and aging, in *The Biology of Aging,* Strehler, B. L., Ed., A.I.B.S., Washington, D.C., 1960, 246.

44. **Sacher, G. A.,** The role of physiological fluctuations in the aging process and the relation of longevity to the size of the central nervous system, in *Aging and Levels of Biological Organization,* Brues, A. M. and Sacher, G. A., Eds., University of Chicago Press, Chicago, 1962, 266.
45. **Sacher, G. A.,** On longevity regarded as an organized behavior: the role of brain structure, in *Contribution to the Psychobiology of Aging,* Kastenbaum, R., Ed., Springer, New York, 1965, 99.
46. **Sacher, G. A.,** Abnutzungstheorie, in *Perspectives in Experimental Gerontology,* Shock, N. W., Ed., Charles C Thomas, Springfield, Ill., 1966, 326.
47. **Sacher, G. A.,** Molecular versus systemic theories on the genesis of ageing, *Exp. Gerontol.,* 3, 265, 1968.
48. **Sacher, G. A.,** Allometric and factorial analysis of brain structure in insectivores and primates, in *The Primate Brain,* Noback, C. R. and Montagna, W., Eds., Appleton-Century-Crofts, New York, 1970, 245.
49. **Monod, J.,** *Chance and Necessity,* A. A. Knopf, New York, 1971.
50. **Wilson, E. O.,** *Sociobiology,* Belknap Press, Cambridge, Mass., 1975.
51. **Strehler, B. L.,** *Time, Cells, and Aging,* Academic Press, New York, 1977.
52. **Lamb, M. J.,** *Biology of Aging,* J. Wiley & Sons, New York, 1977.
53. **Kohn, R. R.,** *Principles of Mammalian Aging,* Prentice-Hall, Inc., Englewood Cliff, N.J., 1978.
54. **Comfort, A.,** *The Biology of Senescence,* Elsevier, New York, 1978.
55. **Medvedev, Zh. A.,** Error theories of aging, in *Perspectives in Experimental Gerontology,* Shock, N. W., Ed., Charles C Thomas, Springfield, Ill., 1966, 336.
56. **Orgel, L. E.,** The maintenance of the accuracy of protein synthesis and its relevance to ageing: a correction, *Proc. Natl. Acad. Sci. USA,* 67, 1476, 1970.
57. **Orgel, L. E.,** Ageing of clones of mammalian cells, *Nature (London),* 243, 441, 1973.
58. **Medvedev, Zh. A.,** Error theories of ageing, in *Sonderdruck aus: Alternstheorien,* Platt, D., Ed., Schatauer, Verlag, 1975.
59. **Harman, D.,** Aging: a theory based on free radical and radiation chemistry, *J. Geront.,* 11, 298, 1956.
60. **Harman, D.,** Role of free radicals in mutation, cancer, aging, and the maintenance of life, *Rad. Res.,* 16, 753, 1962.
61. **Harman, D.,** Prolongation of life: role of free radical reactions in aging, *J. Am. Geriatr. Soc.,* 17, 721, 1969.
62. **Leibovitz, B. E., Siegel, B. V.,** Aspects of free radical reactions in biological systems: aging, *J. Geront.,* 35, 45, 1980.
63. **Curtis, H. J.,** *Biological Mechanisms of Aging,* Charles C Thomas, Springfield, Ill., 1966.
64. **Curtis, H. J.,** Genetic factors in aging, *Adv. Genetics,* 16, 305, 1971.
65. **Walford, R. L.,** Immunological theory of aging: current status, *Fed. Proc. Fed. Am. Soc. Exp. Biol.,* 33, 2020, 1974.
66. **Doolittle, W. F. and Sapienza, C.,** Selfish genes, the phenotype paradigm and genome evolution, *Nature (London),* 284, 601, 1980.
67. **Orgel, L. E. and Crick, F. H. C.,** Selfish DNA: the ultimate parasite, *Nature (London),* 284, 604, 1980.
68. **Orgel, L. E., Crick, F. H. C., and Sapienza, C.,** Selfish DNA, *Nature (London),* 288, 645, 1980.
69. **Hirsch, G. P.,** Spontaneous mutations balance reproductive selective advantage and genetically determine longevity, *Mech. Ageing Dev.,* 9, 355, 1979.
70. **Denckla, W. D.,** A time to die, *Life Sci.,* 16, 31, 1975.
71. **Washburn, S. L.,** Longevity in primates, in *Aging: Biology and Behavior,* McGaugh, J. L. and Kiesler, S. B., Eds., Academic Press, New York, 1981, in press.
72. **Lovejoy, C. W.,** The origin of man, *Science,* 211, 341, 1981.
73. **Lindstedt, S. L. and Calder, W. A.,** Body size, physiological time, and longevity of homeothermic animals, *Q. Rev. Biol.,* 56, 1, 1981.
74. **Dilman, V. M.,** Age-associated elevation of hypothalamic threshold to feedback control, and its role in development, ageing and disease, *Lancet,* 1, 1211, 1971.
75. **Dilman, V. M. and Anisimov, V. N.,** Hypothalamic mechanisms of ageing and of specific age pathology. I. Sensitivity threshold of hypothalamo-pituitary complex to homeostatic stimuli in the reproductive system, *Exp. Gerontol.,* 14, 161, 1979.
76. **Dilman, V. M., Ostroumova, M. N., and Tsyrlina, E. V.,** Hypothalamic mechanism of ageing and of specific age pathology. II. On the sensitivity threshold of hypothalamo-pituitary complex to homeostatic stimuli in adaptive homeostasis, *Exp. Gerontol.,* 14, 175, 1979.
77. **Dilman, V. M., Bobrov, J. F., Ostroumova, M. N., Lvovich, E. G., Vishnevsky, A. S., Anisimov, V. N., and Vasiljeva, I. A.,** Hypothalamic mechanisms of ageing and of specific age pathology. III. Sensitivity threshold of hypothalamo-pituitary complex to homeostatic stimuli in energy systems, *Exp. Gerontol.,* 14, 217, 1979.

78. **Dilman, V. M. and Berstein, L. M.**, Hypothalamic mechanisms of ageing and of specific age pathology. IV. Sensitivity threshold of the hypothalamo-pituitary complex to homeostatic inhibition by thyroid, *Exp. Gerontol.*, 14, 225, 1979.
79. **Dilman, V. M.**, Hypothalamic mechanisms of ageing and of specific age pathology. V. A model for the mechanism of human specific age pathology and natural death, *Exp. Gerontol.*, 14, 287, 1979.
80. **Cutler, R. G.**, Stabilization of the differentiated state of cells: Possible role of the major histocompatibility complex loci, *The Gerontologist*, 20, 88, 1980.
81. **Cutler, R. G.**, Life span determinant mechanisms: identification and genetic regulation of cellular integrity maintenance processes, *Abstr. Xii Intern. Congr. Geront.*, Hamburg, Germany, 272, 1981.
82. **Sugimura, T., Matsushima, T., Kawachi, T., Kogure, K., Tanaka, T., Miyake, S., Hozumi, M., Sato, S., and Sato, H.**, Disdifferentiation and decarcinogenesis, *Gann Monogr. Can. Res.*, 3, 31, 1972.
83. **Uriel, J.**, Cancer, retrodifferentiation, and the myth of Faust, *Cancer Res.*, 36, 4269, 1976.
84. **Taketa, K., Watanabe, A., and Kosaka, K.**, Undifferentiated gene expression in liver injuries, in *Onco-Developmental Gene Expression*, Fishman, W. H. and Sell, S., Eds., Academic Press, New York, 1976, 219.
85. **Ursprung, H., Ed.**, *The Stability of the Differentiated State*, Springer-Verlag, New York, 1968.
86. **Kidson, C.**, DNA repair in differentiation, in *DNA Repair Mechanisms*, Hanawalt, P. C., Friedberg, E. S., and Fox, C. F., Eds., Academic Press, New York, 1978, 761.
87. **Kirkwood, T. B. L.**, Evolution of ageing, *Nature (London)*, 270, 301, 1977.
88. **Gershon, D.**, Current status of age altered enzymes: Alternative mechanisms, *Mech. Ageing Dev.*, 9, 189, 1979.
89. **Sinex, F. M.**, The molecular genetics of aging, in *Handbook of the Biology of Aging*, Finch, C. E. and Hayflick, L., Eds., van Nostrand Reinhold, Co., New York, 1977, 37.
90. **Miquel, J., Economos, A. C., Fleming, J., and Johnson, J. E.**, Mitochondrial role in cell aging, *Exp. Gerontol.*, 15, 575, 1980.
91. **Dover, G. and Doolittle, W. F.**, Modes of genome evolution, *Nature (London)*, 288, 646, 1980.
92. **Straus, D. S.**, Somatic mutation, cellular differentiation, and cancer causation, *J. Natl. Cancer Inst.*, 67, 233, 1981.
93. **Harris, H.**, Some thoughts about genetics, differentiation, and malignancy, *Somatic Cell Genet.*, 5, 923, 1979.
94. **Fahmy, M. J. and Fahmy, O. G.**, Intervening DNA insertions and the alteration of gene expression by carcinogens, *Cancer Res.*, 40, 3374, 1980.
95. **Fahmy, M. J. and Fahmy, O. G.**, Altered control of gene activity in the soma by carcinogens, *Mutation Res.*, 72, 165, 1980.
96. **Braun, A. C.**, An epigenetic model for the origin of cancer, *Q. Rev. Biol.*, 56, 33, 1981.
97. **Pall, M. L.**, Gene-amplification model of carcinogenesis, *Proc. Natl. Acad. Sci. USA*, 78, 2465, 1981.
98. **Ohno, S.**, Gene duplication, junk DNA, intervening sequences and the universal signal for their removal, *Rev. Brasiliera Genet.*, 3, 99, 1980.
99. **Trosko, J. E. and Chang, C.-C.**, The role of radiation and chemicals in the induction of mutations and epigenetic changes during carcinogenesis, *Adv. Rad. Biol.*, 9, 1, 1981.
100. **Rubner, M.**, Probleme des wachstums und der lebensdauer, in *Gesellschaft fur Innere Medizine und Kinderheilkunde*, Vol. 7, Mitteilungen, Beiblatt, Wien, 1908, 58.
101. **Pearl, R.**, *The Rate of Living*, Knopf, New York, 1928.
102. **Pryor, W. A.**, The role of free radical reactions in biological systems, in *Free Radicals in Biology*, Vol. 1, Pryor, W. A., Ed., Academic Press, New York, 1976, 1.
103. **Michelson, A. M., McCord, J. M., and Fridovich, I., Eds.**, *Superoxide and Superoxide Dismutases*, Academic Press, New York, 1977.
104. **Hayaishi, O. and Asada, K., Eds.**, *Biochemical and Medical Aspects of Active Oxygen*, University Park Press, Baltimore, 1977.
105. **de Duve, C. and Hayaishi, O., Eds.**, *Tocopherol, Oxygen and Biomembranes*, Elsevier/North Holland Biomedical Press, Amsterdam, 1978.
106. **Chance, B., Sies, H., and Boveris, A.**, Hydroperoxide metabolism in mammalian organs, *Physiol. Rev.*, 59, 527, 1979.
107. **Del Maestro, R.**, The Influence of Oxygen Derived Free Radicals on In Vitro and In Vivo Model Systems, Ph.D. thesis, Uppsala University, 1979.
108. *Oxygen Free Radicals and Tissue Damage*, Ciba Foundation Symp. 65, Elsevier, Excerpta Medical North Holland, Amsterdam, 1979.
109. **Sohal, R. S., Ed.**, *Age Pigments*, Elsevier, Amsterdam, 1981.
110. **Yagi, S., Ed.**, *Lipid Peroxide in Biology and Medicine*, Academic Press, New York, 1981.
111. **Holley, R. W.**, Control of animal cell proliferation, in *J. Supramol. Str.*, 13, 191, 1980.
112. **Cameron, I. L. and Thrasher, J. D., Eds.**, *Cellular and Molecular Renewal in the Mammalian Body*, Academic Press, New York, 1971.

113. **Kent, S.**, Cell division and aging, *Geriatrics,* 33, 81, 1978.
114. **Rook, A.**, Endocrine influences on hair growth, *Br. Med. J.,* 1, 609, 1965.
115. **Adachi, K.**, The metabolism and control mechanism of human hair follicles, *Curr. Probl. Derm.,* 5, 37, 1973.
116. **Hamilton, J. B. and Mestler, G. E.**, Mortality and survival: comparison of eunuchs with intact men and women in a mentally retarded population, *J. Gerontol.,* 24, 395, 1969.
117. **Roth, G. S.**, Hormone action during aging: Alterations and mechanisms, *Mech. Ageing Dev.,* 9, 497, 1979.
118. **Roth, G. S.**, Hormone receptor changes during adulthood and senescence. Significance for aging research, *Fed. Proc. Fed. Am. Soc. Exp. Biol.,* 38, 1910, 1979.
119. **Roth, G. S.**, Changes in hormone binding and responsiveness in target cells and tissues during aging, in *Explorations in Aging,* Cristofalo, V. J., Roberts, J., and Adelman, R. C., Eds., Plenum Press, New York, 1975, 195.
120. **Roth, G. S.**, Altered biochemical responsiveness and hormone receptor changes during aging, preprint.
121. **Roth, G. S., Schocken, D. D., and Chang, W.-C.**, Changes in hormone action during aging: the role of target tissue hormone receptors and neuroendocrine regulatory mechanisms, preprint.
122. **Cutler, R. G.**, Thyroid hormone receptors in the brain of rat as a function of age and hypophysectomy, in *Brain Neurotransmitters and Receptors in Aging and Age-Related Disorders,* Enna, S. J., Samorajski, T., and Beer, B., Eds., Raven Press, New York, 1981.
123. **Huberman, E., Heckman, C., and Langenbach, R.**, Stimulation of differentiated functions in human melanoma cells by tumor-promoting agents and dimethyl sulfoxide, *Cancer Res.,* 39, 2618, 1979.
124. **Dix, D. and Cohen, P.**, On the role of aging in cancer incidence, *J. Theo. Biol.,* 83, 163, 1980.
125. **Cairns, J.**, Differentiation and cancer, *Differentiation,* 13, 67, 1979.
126. **Samaan, N. A.**, Ectopid hormone producing tumors, in *Influences of Hormones in Tumor Development,* Vol. 1, Kellen, J. A. and Holf, R., Eds., CRC Press, Boca Raton, Fla., 1979, 95.
127. **Criss, W. E.**, A review of isozymes in cancer, *Cancer Res.,* 31, 1523, 1971.
128. **Schapira, F.**, Isozymes and cancer, *Adv. Cancer Res.,* 18, 77, 1973.
129. **Knox, W. E.**, *Enzyme Patterns in Fetal, Adult and Neoplastic Rat Tissues,* S. Karger, Basel, 1976.
130. **Cone, C. D.**, Unified theory on the basic mechanism of normal mitotic control and oncogenesis, *J. Theo. Biol.,* 30, 151, 1971.
131. **Cone, C. D.**, The role of the surface electrical transmembrane potential in normal and malignant mitogenesis, *Ann. N.Y. Acad. Sci.,* 238, 420, 1974.
132. **Cone, C. D. and Cone, C. M.**, Evidence of normal mitosis with complete cytokinesis in central nervous system neurons during sustained depolarization with ouabain, *Exp. Neurol.,* 60, 41, 1978.
133. **Cone, C. D.**, Ionically mediated induction of mitogenesis in CNS neurons, *Ann. N.Y. Acad. Sci.,* 339, 115, 1980.
134. **Zs.-Nagy, I.**, The role of membrane structure and function in cellular aging: a review, *Mech. Ageing Dev.,* 9, 237, 1979.
135. **McClure, H. M.**, Neoplasia in Rhesus monkeys, in *The Rhesus Monkey II. Management, Reproduction and Pathology,* Bourne, G. H., Ed., Academic Press, New York, 1975, 369.
136. **McClure, H. M.**, Tumors in nonhuman primates: observations during a six-year period in the Yerkes Primate Center colony, *Am. J. Phys. Anthrop.,* 38, 425, 1973.
137. **Totter, J. R.**, Spontaneous cancer and its possible relationship to oxygen metabolism, *Proc. Natl. Acad. Sci. USA,* 77, 1763, 1980.
138. **Hartman, P. E.**, Metaplasias, *Genetics,* 91, s45, 1979.
139. **Hartman, P. E.**, Nitrates and nitrites: ingestion, pharmacodynamics and toxicology, in *Chemical Mutagens. Principles and Methods for Their Detection,* Vol. 7, de Serres, F. J. and Hollaender, Eds., Plenum Press, New York, 1981, in press.
140. **Farber, E. and Cameron, R.**, The sequential analysis of cancer development, *Adv. Cancer Res.,* 31, 125, 1980.
141. **Ponder, B. A. J.**, Genetics and cancer, *Biochim. Biophys. Acta,* 605, 369, 1980.
142. **Hay, E. D.**, Dedifferentiation and metaplasia in vertebrate and invertebrate regeneration, in *The Stability of the Differentiated State,* Ursprung, H., Ed., Springer-Verlag, New York, 1968, 85.
143. **Nandy, K.**, Brain-reactive antibodies in serum of germ-free mice, *Mech. Ageing Dev.,* 1, 133, 1972.
144. **Nandy, K., Fritz, F. B., and Threatt, J.**, Specificity of brain-reactive antibodies in serum of old mice, *J. Gerontol.,* 30, 269, 1975.
145. **Nandy, K.**, Significance of brain-reactive antibodies in serum of aged mice, *J. Gerontol.,* 30, 412, 1975.
146. **Nandy, K.**, Immune reactions in aging brain and senile dementia, in *The Aging Brain and Senile Dementia,* Nandy, K. and Sherwin, I., Eds., Plenum Press, New York, 1976, 181.
147. **Huebner, R. and Todaro, G.**, Oncogenes of RNA tumor viruses as determinants of cancer, *Proc. Natl. Acad. Sci. USA,* 64, 1087, 1969.

148. **Gajdusek, D.**, Slow virus infection and activation of latent infections in aging, in *Advances in Gerontology Research,* Vol. 4, Strehler, B. L., Ed., Academic Press, New York, 1972, 201.
149. **Tovey, M. G.**, Viral latency and its importance in human disease, *Pathol. Biol.,* 28, 631, 1980.
150. **Nathanson, N.**, Slow viruses and chronic disease: the contribution of epidemiology, *Public Health Rep.,* 95, 436, 1980.
151. **Weinberg, R. A.**, Origins and roles of endogenous retroviruses, *Cell,* 22, 643, 1980.
152. **Moore, D. H., Long, C. A., Vaidya, A. B., Sheffield, J. B., Dion, A. S., and Lasfargues, E. Y.**, Mammary tumor viruses, *Adv. Cancer Res.,* 29, 347, 1979.
153. **Pincus, T.**, The endogenous murine type C viruses, in *Molecular Biology of RNA Tumor Viruses,* Stephenson, J. R., Ed., Academic Press, New York, 1980, 77.
154. **Todaro, G. J.**, Interspecies transmission of mammalian retroviruses, in *Molecular Biology of RNA Tumor Viruses,* Stephenson, J. R., Ed., Academic Press, New York, 1980, 47.
155. **Field, E. J.**, Slow virus infections of the nervous system, *Intern. Rev. Exp. Pathol.,* 8, 130, 1969.
156. **Field, E. J. and Peat, A.**, Intranuclear inclusions in neurones and glia: a study in the ageing mouse, *Gerontologia,* 17, 129, 1971.
157. **Field, E. J. and Shenton, B. K.**, Emergence of new antigens in ageing tissues, *Gerontologia,* 19, 211, 1973.
158. **Field, E. J.**, Immunological assessment of ageing: emergence of scrapie-like antigens, *Age and Ageing,* 7, 28, 1978.
159. **Koproski, H.**, Possible role of herpes virus in the chronic CNS diseases, in *Persistent Viruses,* Stevens, J. G., Todaro, G. J., and Fox, C. F., Eds., Academic Press, New York, 1978, 691.
160. **Florine, D. L., Ono, T., Cutler, R. G., and Getz, M. J.**, Regulation of endogenous murine leukemia virus-related nuclear and cytoplasmic RNA complexity in C57BL/6J mice of increasing age, *Cancer Res.,* 40, 519, 1980.
161. **Getz, M. J., Elder, P. K., and Moses, H. L.**, Complexity and abundance of murine leukemia virus-related nuclear and messenger RNA sequences in mouse embryo cell lines which are differentially sensitive to carcinogen-induced virus activation, *Cancer Res.,* 39, 321, 1979.
162. **Getz, M. J. and Florine, D. L.**, Age-related changes in the expression of endogenous mouse C-type RNA tumor virus genes, in *Biological Mechanisms in Aging,* Schimke, R. T., Ed., National Institute on Aging, NIH Pub. No. 81-2194, 1981, 226.
163. **Kenyon, C. J. and Walker, G. C.**, DNA-damaging stimulate gene expression at specific loci in *Escherichia coli, Proc. Natl. Acad. Sci. USA,* 77, 2819, 1980.
164. **Kollar, E. J. and Fisher, C.**, Tooth induction in chick epithelium: expression of quiescent genes for enamel synthesis, *Science,* 207, 993, 1980.
165. **Barrett, J. C., Wong, A., and McLachlan, J. A.**, Diethylstilbestrol induces neoplastic transformation without measurable gene mutation at two loci, *Science,* 212, 1402, 1981.
166. **Hancock, R. L., Forrester, P. I., Lorscheider, F. L., Lai, P. C. W., and Hay, D. M.**, Ethionine-induced activation of embryonic genes, in *Onco-Developmental Activation of Embryonic Genes,* Fishman, W. H. and Sell, S., Eds., Academic Press, New York, 1976, 247.
167. **Enomoto, K., Dempo, K., Mori, M., and Onoe, T.**, Demonstration of embryonic-type hemoglobin in extramedullary hematopoietic cells in the liver during experimental liver carcinogenesis by 3′-methyl-4-dimethylaminoazobenzene, *Cancer Res.,* 40, 1769, 1980.
168. **Groudine, M. and Weintraub, H.**, Activation of cellular genes by avian RNA tumor viruses, *Proc. Natl. Acad. Sci. USA,* 77, 5351, 1980.
169. **Cho, H. Y. and Rhim, J. S.**, Cycloheximide-dependent reversion of human cells transformed by MSV and chemical carcinogen, *Science,* 205, 691, 1979.
170. **Sperling, L. and Weiss, M. C.**, Chromatin repeat length correlates with phenotypic expression in hepatoma cells, their dedifferentiated variants, and somatic hybrids, *Proc. Natl. Acad. Sci. USA,* 77, 3412, 1980.
171. **Wisniewski, H. M., Narang, H. K., and Terry, R. D.**, Neurofibrillary tangles of paired helical filaments, *J. Neurol. Sci.,* 27, 173, 1976.
172. **Terry, R. D.**, The fine structure of neurofibrillary tangles in Alzheimer's disease, *J. Neuropath. Exp. Neurol.,* 8, 629, 1963.
173. **Terry, R. D.**, Some biological aspects of the aging brain, *Mech. Ageing Dev.,* 14, 191, 1980.
174. **Wisniewski, H. M. and Soifer, D.**, Neurofibrillary pathology: current status and research perspectives, *Mech. Ageing Dev.,* 9, 119, 1979.
175. **Tomlinson, B. E.**, Morphological changes and dementia in old age, in *Aging and Dementia,* Smith, W. L. and Kinsbourne, M., Eds., Spectrum Pub., Inc., Jamaica, N.Y., 1977, 25.
176. **Scheirel, M. E., Lindsay, R. D., Tomiyasu, U., and Scheibel, A. B.**, Progressive dendritic changes in aging human cortex, *Exp. Neurol.,* 47, 392, 1975.
177. **Feldman, M. L.**, Dendritic changes in aging rat brain: pyrimidal cell dendrite length and ultrastructure, in *The Aging Brain and Senile Dementia,* Nandy, K. and Sherwin, I., Eds., Plenum Press, New York, 1976, 23.

178. **Richardson, A.,** A comprehensive review of the scientific literature on the effect of aging on protein synthesis, in *Biological Mechanisms in Aging,* Schimke, R. T., Ed., National Institute on Aging, NIH Pub. No. 81-2194, 1981, 339.
179. **Finch, C. E.,** Enzyme activities, gene function and ageing in mammals (review), *Exp. Gerontol.,* 7, 53, 1972.
180. **Brown, D. D.,** Gene expression in eukaryotics, *Science,* 211, 667, 1981.
181. **Davidson, E. H. and Britten, R. J.,** Regulation of gene expression: possible role of repetitive sequences, *Science,* 204, 1052, 1979.
182. **Wold, B. J., Klein, W. H., Hough-Evans, B. R., Britten, R. J., and Davidson, E. H.,** Sea urchin embryo mRNA sequences expressed in the nuclear RNA of adult tissues, *Cell,* 14, 941, 1978.
183. **Tsai, S. Y., Tsai, M.-J., Lin, C.-T., and O'Malley, B. W.,** Effect of estrogen on ovalbumin gene expression in differentiated nontarget tissues, *Biochemistry,* 18, 5726, 1979.
184. **Caplan, A. I. and Ordahl, C. P.,** Irreversible gene repression model for control of development, *Science,* 201, 120, 1978.
185. **Rutter, W. J.,** Control of cellular differentiation: overview, *Ann. N. Y. Acad. Sci.,* 339, 263, 1980.
186. **Holliday, R. and Pugh, J. E.,** DNA modification mechanisms and gene activity during development, *Science,* 187, 226, 1975.
187. **Razin, A. and Riggs, A. D.,** DNA methylation and gene function, *Science,* 210, 604, 1980.
188. **Cutler, R. G.,** Transcription of unique and reiterated DNA sequences in mouse liver and brain tissues as a function of age, *Exp. Gerontol.,* 10, 37, 1975.
189. **Hill, B. T.,** Influence of age on chromatin transcription in murine tissue using an heterologous and an homologous RNA polymerase, *Gerontology,* 22, 111, 1976.
190. **Cutler, R. G.,** Alterations with age in the informational storage and flow systems of the mammalian cell, in *Genetic Effects on Aging,* Bergsma, D. and Harrison, D. E., Eds., A. R. Liss, Inc., New York, 1978, 463.
191. **Mays, L. L.,** Post-transcriptional modification of RNA in aging organisms, in *Biological Mechanisms in Aging,* Schimke, R. T., Ed., National Institute on Aging, NIH Pub. No. 81-2194, 1981, 366.
192. **Romavon, G. A. and Banyushin, B. F.,** Intragenome specificity of DNA methylation in animals. Tissue specificity and variation in the methylation of repeated sequences due to aging, carcinogenesis, and hormonal induction, *Molec. Biol.,* 14, 279, 1980.
193. **Farquhar, M. N., Kosky, K. J., and Omenn, G. S.,** Gene expression in brain, in *Aging in Nonhuman Primates,* Bowden, D. M., Ed., Van Nostrand Reinhold, New York, 1979, 71.
194. **Grady, L. J., Campbell, W. P., and North, A. B.,** Nonrepetitive DNA transcription in normal and regenerating rat liver, *Nucleic Acids Res.,* 7, 259, 1979.
195. **Grouse, L. D., Schrier, B. K., Letendre, C. H., and Nelson, P. G.,** RNA sequence complexity in central nervous system development and plasticity, *Curr. Top. Dev. Biol.,* 16, 381, 1980.
196. **Colman, P. D., Kaplan, B. B., Osterburg, H. H., and Finch, C. E.,** Brain poly(A) during aging: stability of yield and sequence complexity in two rat strains, *J. Neurochem.,* 34, 335, 1980.
197. **Grady, L. J. and Campbell, W. P.,** Ageing studies in rat liver I. Complexity of RNA from two to ten months of age, *Mech. Ageing Dev.,* 15, 415, 1981.
198. **Dean, R., Ono, T., Socher, S., and Cutler, R. G.,** Age-dependent changes in endogenous viral and host gene expression in AKR and C57BL/6J mice, *The Gerontologist,* 19, 62, 1979.
199. **Finch, C. E.,** The regulation of physiological changes during mammalian aging, *Q. Rev. Biol.,* 51, 49, 1976.
200. **Hegner, D.,** Age-dependence of molecular and functional changes in biological membrane properties, *Mech. Ageing Dev.,* 14, 101, 1980.
201. **Pacifici, M., Fellini, S. A., Holtzer, H., and DeLuca, S.,** Changes in the sulfated proteoglycans synthesized by "ageing" chondrocytes. I. Dispersed cultured chondrocytes and *in vivo* cartilages, *J. Biol. Chem.,* 256, 1029, 1981.
202. **Heron, D. S., Shinitzky, M., Hershkowitz, M., and Samuel, D.,** Lipid fluidity markedly modulates the binding of serotonin to mouse brain membranes, *Proc. Natl. Acad. Sci. USA,* 77, 7463, 1980.
203. **Hughes, B. A., Roth, G. S., and Pitha, J.,** Age-related decrease in repair of oxidative damage to surface sulfhydryl groups on rat adipocytes, *J. Cell Physiol.,* 103, 349, 1980.
204. **Rosen, R.,** Structural stability, alternate descriptions and information, *J. Theo. Biol.,* 63, 19, 1976.
205. **Rosen, R.,** Feedforwards and global system failure: a general mechanism for senescence, *J. Theo. Biol.,* 74, 579, 1978.
206. **Rosen, R.,** Cells and senescence, *Intern. Rev. Cytol.,* 54, 161, 1978.
207. **Rosen, R.,** Dynamical aspects of senescence, in *Biological Mechanisms in Aging,* Schimke, R. T., Ed., National Institute on Aging, NIH Pub. No. 81-2194, 1981, 108.
208. **Goldstein, S. and Singal, D. P.,** Loss of reactivity of HL-A antigens in clonal populations of cultured human fibroblasts during aging *in vitro, Exp. Cell Res.,* 75, 278, 1972.
209. **Goldstein, S. and Singal, D. P.,** Absence of detectable HL-A antigens on cultured fibroblasts in progeria, *J. Clin. Invest.,* 52, 2259, 1973.

210. **Goldstein, S., Lin, C. C., and Singal, D. P.**, Immunological selection of HL-A variants of cultured progeric fibroblasts and their identification by quinacrine fluorescence, *Exp. Cell Res.*, 89, 451, 1974.

211. **Robertson, O. H. and Wexler, B. C.**, Hyperplasia of the adrenal cortical tissue in Pacific salmon (*Genus Oncorhynchus*) and rainbow trout (*Salmo gairdnerii*) accompanying sexual maturation and spawning, *Endocrinology*, 65, 225, 1959.

212. **Robertson, O. H. and Wexler, B. C.**, Histological changes in the organs and tissues of migrating and spawning Pacific salmon (Genus *Oncorhynchus*), *Endocrinology*, 66, 222, 1960.

213. **Robertson, O. H.**, Prolongation of the life span of kokanee salmon (*Oncorhynchusnerka kennerlyi*) by castration before beginning of gonad development, *Proc. Natl. Acad. Sci. USA*, 47, 609, 1961.

214. **Robertson, O. H., Krupp, M. A., Thomas, S. F., Favour, C. B., Hane, S., and Wexler, B. C.**, Hyperadrenocorticism in spawning migratory and nonmigratory rainbow trout *(Salmo gairnerii)*; comparison with Pacific salmon *(Genus Oncorhynchus)*, *Gen. Comp. Endocrin.*, 1, 473, 1961.

215. **Robertson, O. H., Wexler, B. C., and Miller, B. F.**, Degenerative changes in the cardiovascular system of the spawning Pacific salmon *(Oncorhynchus tshawytscha)* *Circ. Res.*, 9, 826, 1961.

216. **Robertson, O. H. and Wexler, B. C.**, Histological changes in the pituitary gland of the Pacific salmon (Genus *Oncorhynchus)* accompanying sexual maturation and spawning, *J. Morphol.*, 110, 171, 1962.

217. **Hane, S., Robertson, O. H., Wexler, B. C., and Krupp, M. A.**, Adrenocortical response to stress and ACTH in Pacific salmon *(Oncorhynchus tsawytscha)* and steelhead trout *(Salmo gairnerii)* at successive stages in the sexual cycle, *Endocrinology*, 78, 791, 1966.

218. **Van Citters, R. L. and Watson, N. W.**, Coronary disease in spawning steelhead trout, *Salmo gairnerii*, *Science*, 159, 105, 1968.

219. **Wexler, B. C.**, Comparative aspects of hyperadrenocorticism and aging, in *Hypothalamus, Pituitary and Aging*, Everitt, A. V. and Burgess, J. A., Eds., Charles C Thomas, Springfield, Ill., 1976, 333.

220. **Wodinsky, J.**, Hormonal inhibition of feeding and death in octopus: control by optic gland secretion, *Science*, 198, 948, 1977.

221. **Berdyshev, G. D. and Protsenko, N. A.**, Current theories of the mechanism of the postspawning death of Pacific salmon, *Hydrobiological J.*, 8, 85, 19.

222. **Hornsby, P. J., Simonian, M. H., and Gill, G. N.**, Aging of adrenocortical cells in culture, *Intern. Rev. Cytol.*, 10, 131, 1979.

223. **Hornsby, P. J.**, Regulation of cytochrome P-450-supported 11$\beta$-hydroxylation of deoxycortisol by steroids, oxygen, and antioxidants in adrenocortical cell cultures, *J. Biol. Chem.*, 255, 4020, 1980.

224. **Hornsby, P. J. and Gill, G. N.**, Regulation of responsiveness of cultured adrenal cells to adrenocorticotropin and prostaglandin $E_1$: cell density, cell division, and inhibitors of protein synthesis, *Endocrinology*, 108, 183, 1981.

225. **Hornsby, P. J. and Gill, G. N.**, Regulation of glutamine and pyrivate oxidation in cultured adrenocortical cells by cortisol, antioxidants, and oxygen: effects of cell proliferation, *J. Cell. Physiol.*, in press, 1981.

226. **Everitt, A. V. and Burgess, J. A.**, *Hypothalamus, Pituitary and Aging*, Charles C Thomas, Springfield, Ill., 1976.

227. **Everitt, A. V., Syedsman, N. J., and Jones, F.**, The effects of hypophysectomy and continuous food restriction, begun at ages 70 and 400 days, on collagen aging, proteinuria, incidence of pathology and longevity in the male rat, *Mech. Ageing Dev.*, 12, 161, 1980.

228. **Everitt, A. V.**, The neuroendocrine system and aging, *Gerontology*, 26, 108, 1980.

229. **Bilder, G. E. and Denckla, W. D.**, Restoration of ability to reject xenografts and clear carbon after hypophysectomy of adult rats, *Mech. Ageing Dev.*, 6, 153, 1977.

230. **Denckla, W. D.**, Interactions between age and the neuroendocrine and immune systems, *Fed. Proc. Fed. Am. Soc. Exp. Biol.*, 37, 1263, 1978.

231. **Parker, R. J., Berkowitz, B. A., Lee, C.-H., and Denckla, W. D.**, Vascular relaxation, aging and thyroid hormones, *Mech. Ageing Dev.*, 8, 397, 1978.

232. **Scott, M., Bolla, R., and Denckla, W. D.**, Age-related changes in immune function of rats and the effect of long-term hypophysectomy, *Mech. Ageing Dev.*, 11, 127, 1979.

233. **Miller, J. K., Bolla, R., and Denckla, W. D.**, Age-associated changes in initiation of ribonucleic acid synthesis in isolated rat liver nuclei, *Biochem. J.*, 188, 55, 1980.

234. **Landfield, P. W., Rose, G., Sandles, L., Wohlstadter, T. C., and Lynch, G.**, Patterns of astroglial hypertrophy and neuronal degeneration in the hippocampus of aged, memory-deficient rats, *J. Gerontology*, 32, 3, 1977.

235. **Landfield, P. W.**, An endocrine hypothesis of brain aging and studies on brain-endocrine correlations and monosynaptic neurophysiology during aging, in *Advances in Experimental Medicine and Biology, Vol. 113, Parkinson's Disease II. Aging and Neuroendocrine Relationships*, Finch, C. E., Potter, D. E., and Kenney, A. D., Eds., Plenum Press, New York, 1978, 179.

236. **Landfield, P. W., Waymire, J. C., and Lynch, G.**, Hippocampal aging and adrenocorticoids: quantitative correlations, *Science*, 202, 1098, 1978.

237. **Landfield, P. W.**, Correlative studies of brain neurophysiology and behavior during aging, in *The Psychobiology of Aging: Problems and Perspectives,* Stein, D. G., Ed., Elsevier North Holland, Amsterdam, 1980, 227.
238. **Landfield, P. W., Sundberg, D. K., Smith, M. S., Eldridge, J. C., and Morris, M.**, Mammalian aging: theoretical implications of changes in brain and endocrine systems during mid- and late-life in rats, *Peptides,* 1, 185, 1980.
239. **Landfield, P. W., Baskin, R. K., and Pitler, T. A.**, Brain aging correlates: retardation by hormonal-pharmacological treatments, *Science,* 214, 581, 1981.
240. **Goodrick, C. L.**, Effects of long-term voluntary wheel exercise on male and female Wistar rats. I. Longevity, body weight, and metabolic rate, *Gerontology,* 26, 22, 1980.
241. **Schwartz, A. G. and Perantoni, A.**, Protective effect of dehydroepiandrosterone against aflatoxin $B_1$- and 7,12-dimethylbenz(a)anthracene-induced cytotoxicity and transformation in cultured cells, *Cancer Res.,* 35, 2482, 1975.
242. **Schwartz, A. G.**, Inhibition of spontaneous breast cancer formation in female C3H($A^{vy}$/a) mice by long-term treatment with dehydroepiandrosterone, *Cancer Res.,* 39, 1129, 1979.
243. **Cutler, G. B., Glenn, M., Bush, M., Hodgen, G. D., Graham, C. E., and Loriaux, D. L.**, Adrenarche: a survey of rodents, domestic animals, and primates, *Endocrinology,* 103, 2112, 1978.
244. **De Peretti, E. and Forest, M. G.**, Unconjugated dehydroepiandrosterone plasma levels in normal subjects from birth to adolescence in human; the use of a sensitive radioimmunoassay, *J. Clin. Endocrinol. Metab.,* 43, 982, 1976.
245. **Oertel, G. W., Menzel, P., and Bauke, D.**, Effects of dehydroepiandrosterone and its conjugates upon the activity of glucose-6-phosphate dehydrogenase, *Clin. Chim. Acta,* 27, 197, 1970.
246. **Demopoulos, H. B.**, Personal communication.
247. **Demopoulos, H. B., Flamm, E. S., Pietronigro, D. D., and Seligman, M. L.**, The free radical pathology and the microcirculation in the major central nervous system disorders, *Acta Physiol. Scand.,* Suppl. 492, 91, 1980.
248. **Walton, J. R. and Packer, L.**, Free radical damage and protection: relationship to cellular aging and cancer, in *Vitamin E: A Comprehensive Treatise,* Machlin, L. J., Ed., M. Dekker, New York, 1980, 495.
249. **Jakoby, W. B., Ed.**, *Enzymatic Basis of Detoxification,* Academic Press, New York, 1980.
250. **Kimball, R. F.**, DNA repair and its relationship to mutagenesis, carcinogenesis and cell death, in *Cell Biology, Vol. 2, A Comprehensive Treatise,* Prescott, D. M. and Goldstein, L., Eds., Academic Press, New York, 1969, 440.
251. **Hanawalt, P. C., Cooper, P. K., Ganesan, A. K., and Smith, C. A.**, DNA repair in bacteria and mammalian cells, *Ann. Rev. Biochem.,* 48, 783, 1979.
252. **Hartman, P. E.**, Bacterial mutagenesis: review of new insights, *Env. Mutagenesis,* 2, 3, 1980.
253. **Apffel, C. A.**, Nonimmunological host defenses: a review, *Cancer Res.,* 36, 1527, 1976.
254. **Del Maestro, R. F.**, An approach to free radicals in medicine and biology, *Acta Physiol. Scand. Suppl.,* 492, 153, 1980.
255. **Del Maestro, R. F., Thaw, H. H., Bjork, J., Planker, M., and Arfors, K.-E.**, Free radicals as mediators of tissue injury, *Acta Physiol. Scand. Suppl.,* 492, 43, 1980.
256. **Oshino, N. and Chance, B.**, A survey of factors involved in cellular oxygen toxicity, in *Biochemical and Medical Aspects of Active Oxygen,* Hayaishi, O. and Asada, K., Eds., University Park Press, Baltimore, 1977, 191.
257. **Goldberg, A. L. and Dice, J. F.**, Intracellular protein degradation in mammalian and bacterial cells. I., *Ann. Rev. Biochem.,* 43, 835, 1974.
258. **Goldberg, A. L. and St. John, A. C.**, Intracellular protein degradation in mammalian and bacterial cells. II, *Ann. Rev. Biochem.,* 45, 747, 1976.
259. **Goldberg, A. L., Tischler, M., DeMartino, G., and Griffin, G.**, Hormonal regulation of protein degradation and synthesis in skeletal muscle, *Fed. Proc. Fed. Am. Soc. Exp. Biol.,* 39, 31, 1980.
260. **Cutler, R. G.**, Redundancy of critical genes in mammalian species of different maximum life spans, *The Gerontologist,* 12, 40, 1972.
261. **Hart, R. W. and Setlow, R. B.**, Correlation between deoxyribonucleic acid excision-repair and life-span in a number of mammalian species, *Proc. Natl. Acad. Sci. USA,* 71, 2169, 1974.
262. **Tice, R. R.**, Aging and DNA-repair capability, in *The Genetics of Aging,* Schneider, E. L., Ed., Plenum Press, New York, 1978, 53.
263. **Painter, R. B.**, The action of ultraviolet light on mammalian cells, in *Photophysiology,* Vol. 5, Giese, A. C., Ed., Academic Press, New York, 1970, 169.
264. **Rauth, A. M.**, Effects of ultraviolet light on mammalian cells in culture, *Curr. Top. Rad. Res.,* 6, 197, 1970.
265. **Diatloff-Zito, C., Deschavanne, P. J., Loria, E., Malaise, E. P., and Macieira-Coelho, A.**, Comparison between the radiosensitivity of human, mouse and chicken fibroblast-like cells using short-term endpoints, *Intern. J. Rad. Biol.,* 39, 419, 1981.

266. **Szumiel, I.**, Intrinsic radiosensitivity of proliferating mammalian cells, *Adv. Rad. Biol.*, 9, 281, 1981.

267. **Arlett, C. F. and Harcourt, S. A.**, Survey of radiosensitivity in a variety of human cell strains, *Cancer Res.*, 40, 926, 1980.

268. **Nilsson, S. and Johansson, I.**, Induction and repair of DNA strand breaks in human cell-lines with different radiosensitivity, *Intern. J. Rad. Biol.*, 39, 107, 1981.

269. **Thacker, J. and Cox, R.**, Mutation induction and inactivation in mammalian cells exposed to ionising radiation, *Nature (London)*, 258, 429, 1975.

270. **Shaeffer, J., El-Mahdi, A. M., and Karr, B. M.**, DNA-repair in mammary tumor cell lines with different x-ray sensitivities, *Experientia*, 35, 190, 1979.

271. **Kakunaga, T. and Crow, J. D.**, Cell variants showing differential susceptibility to ultraviolet light-inducing transformation, *Science*, 209, 505, 1980.

272. **Lipetz, P. D.**, DNA superstructure, differentiation, and aging, in *Biological Mechanisms in Aging*, Schimke, R. T., Ed., National Institute on Aging, N.I.H. Pub. No. 81-2194, 1981, 290.

273. **Francis, A. A., Lee, W. H., and Regan, J. D.**, The relationships of DNA excision repair of ultraviolet-induced lesions to the maximum life span of mammals, *Mech. Ageing Dev.*, 16, 181, 1981.

274. **Bergmann, K., Walford, R. L., Esra, G. N., and Hall, K. Y.**, A correlation of repair of UV-induced DNA damage and maximum lifespan in primate lymphocytes, in *Thematic Sessions. XII Intern. Congr. Gerontol.*, Vol. 2, 1981, 125.

275. **Peleg, L., Raz, E., and Ben-Ishaf, R.**, Changing capacity for DNA excision repair in mouse embryonic cells *in vitro*, *Exp. Cell Res.*, 104, 301, 1976.

276. **Bertazzoni, U., Stefanini, M., Noy, G. P., Giulotto, E., Nuzzo, F., Falaschi, A., and Spadari, S.**, Variations of DNA polymerases-$\alpha$ and -$\beta$ during prolonged stimulation of human lymphocytes, *Proc. Natl. Acad. Sci. USA*, 73, 785, 1976.

277. **Hart, R. W., Sacher, G. A., and Hoskins, T. L.**, DNA repair in short- and a long-lived rodent species, *J. Gerontol.*, 34, 808, 1979.

278. **Kato, H., Harada, M., Tsuchiya, K., and Moriwaki, K.**, Absence of correlation between DNA repair in ultraviolet irradiated mammalian cells and life span of the donor species, *Jpn. J. Genet.*, 55, 99, 1980.

279. **Woodhead, A. D. and Setlow, R. B.**, DNA repair and longevity in three species of cold-blooded vertebrates, *Exp. Gerontol.*, 15, 301, 1980.

280. **Chetsanga, C. J. and Lindahl, T.**, Release of 7-methylguanine residues whose Imidazole rings have been opened from damaged DNA by a DNA glycosylase from *Escherichia coli*, *Nucleic Acids Res.*, 6, 3673, 1979.

281. **Margison, G. P. and Pegg, A. E.**, Enzymatic release of 7-methylguanine from methylated DNA by rodent liver extracts, *Proc. Natl. Acad. Sci. USA*, 78, 861, 1981.

282. **Singer, B. and Brent, T. P.**, Human lymphoblasts contain DNA glycosylase activity excising N-3 and N-7 methyl and ethyl purines but not $O^6$-alkylguanines and 1-alkyladenines, *Proc. Natl. Acad. Sci. USA*, 78, 856, 1981.

283. **Roderick, T. H.**, The response of twenty-seven inbred strains of mice to daily doses of whole-body x-irradiation, *Rad. Res.*, 20, 631, 1963.

284. **Schwartz, A. G.**, Correlation between species life span and capacity to activate 7,12-dimethylbenz(a)anthracene to a form mutagenic to a mammalian cell, *Exp. Cell Res.*, 94, 445, 1975.

285. **Schwartz, A. G. and Moore, C. J.**, Inverse correlation between species life span and capacity of culture fibroblasts to bind 7,12-dimethylbenz(a)anthracene to DNA, *Exp. Cell Res.*, 109, 448, 1977.

286. **Schwartz, A. G. and Moore, C. J.**, Inverse correlation between species life span and capacity of cultured fibroblasts to metabolize polycyclic hydrocarbon carcinogens, *Fed. Proc. Fed. Am. Soc. Exp. Biol.*, 38, 1989, 1979.

287. **Murad, F., Mittal, C. K., Arnold, W. P., Katsuki, S., and Kimura, H.**, Guanylate cyclase: activation by azide, nitro compounds, nitric oxide, and hydroxyl radical and inhibition by hemoglobin and myoglobin, in *Advances in Cyclic Nucleotide Research*, Vol. 9, George, W. J. and Ignarro, L. J., Eds., Raven Press, New York, 1978, 145.

288. **Murad, F., Arnold, W. P., Mittal, C. K., and Braughler, J. M.**, Properties and regulation of guanylate cyclase and some proposed functions for cyclic GMP, in *Advances in Cyclic Nucleotide Research*, Vol. 11, George, W. J. and Ignarro, L. J., Eds., Raven Press, New York, 1979, 175.

289. **Arnold, W. P., Aldred, R., and Murad, F.**, Cigarette smoke activates guanylate cyclase and increases guanosine 3′,5′-monophosphate in tissues, *Science*, 198, 934, 1977.

290. **Vesely, D. L. and Hill, D. E.**, Estrogens and progesterone increase fetal and maternal guanylate cyclase activity, *Endocrinology*, 107, 2104, 1980.

291. **DeRubertis, F. R. and Craven, P. A.**, Cyclic nucleotides in carcinogenesis: Activation of the guanylate cyclase-cyclic GMP system by chemical carcinogens, in *Advances in Cyclic Nucleotide Research*, Vol. 12, George, W. J. and Ignarro, L. J., Eds., Raven Press, New York, 1980, 97.

292. **Baba, A., Lee, E., Ohta, A., Tatsuno, T., and Iwata, H.**, Activation of adenylated cyclase of rat brain by lipid peroxidation, *J. Biol. Chem.*, 256, 3679, 1981.

293. **Earp, H. S.**, The role of insulin, glucagon, and cAMP in the regulation of hepatocyte guanylate cyclase activity, *J. Biol. Chem.*, 255, 8979, 1980.
294. **Crouch, R. K., Gandy, S. E., Kimsey, G., Galbraith, R. A., Galbraith, G. M. P., and Buse, M. G.**, The inhibition of islet superoxide dismutase by diabetologenic drugs, *Diabetes*, 30, 235, 1981.
295. **Brandwein, H. J., Lewicki, J. A., and Murad, F.**, Reversible inactivation of guanylate cyclase by mixed disulfide formation, *J. Biol. Chem.*, 256, 2958, 1981.
296. **Willett, J. D., Rahim, I., Geist, M., and Zuckerman, B. M.**, Cyclic nucleotide exudation by nematodes and the effects on nematode growth, development and longevity, *Age*, 3, 82, 1980.
297. **Lehnert, S.**, Modification of postirradiation survival of mammalian cells by intracellular cyclic AMP, *Rad. Res.*, 62, 107, 1975.
298. **Lehnert, S.**, Relation of intracellular cyclic AMP to the shape of mammalian cell survival curves, in *Cell Survival After Low Doses of Radiation: Theoretical and Clinical Implications*, Alper, T., Ed., J. Wiley & Sons, New York, 1975, 266.
299. **Lehnert, S.**, Radioprotection of mouse intestine by inhibitors of cyclic AMP phosphodiesterase, *Int. J. Rad. Oncol. Biol. Phys.*, 5, 825, 1979.
300. **Lehnert, S.**, Modification of radiation response of CHO cells by methol-isobutyl xanthine 1. Reduction of $D_o$, *Rad. Res.*, 78, 1, 1979.
301. **Dubravsky, N. B., Hunter, N., Mason, K., and Withers, H. R.**, Dibutryl cyclic adenosine monophosphate: effect on radiosensitivity of tumors and normal tissues in mice, *Radiology*, 126, 799-802, 1978.
302. **Beatty, C. H., Herrinton, P. T., Hoskins, M. K., and Bocek, R. M.**, Guanylate cyclase activity in the skeletal muscle of adult (6-11 yr) and aged (over 20 yr) male rhesus monkeys, *Age*, in press, 1981.
303. **Walford, R. L. and Tam, C. F.**, Lymphocyte biochemistry in relation to immune function in aging: Cyclic nucleotides and purine salvage pathways, in *Biological Mechanisms in Aging*, Schimke, R. T., Ed., National Institute on Aging, NIH Pub. No. 81-2194, 1981, 517.
304. **Sohal, R. S.**, personal communication.
305. **Talbott, J. H. and Yu, T. F.**, *Gout and Uric Acid Metabolism*, G. Thieme, Stuttgart, 1976.
306. **Wyngaarden, J. B. and Kelley, W. N.**, *Gout and Hyperuricemia*, Grune & Stratton, New York, 1976.
307. **Seegmiller, J. E.**, Disorders of purine and pyrimidine metabolism, in *Contemporary Metabolism*, Vol. 1, Freinkel, N., Ed., Plenum Press, New York, 1979, 1.
308. **Keilin, J.**, The biological significance of uric acid and guanine excretion, *Biol. Rev.*, 34, 265, 1959.
309. **Ames, B. N., Cathcart, R., Schwiers, E., and Cochstein, P.**, Uric acid: an antioxidant defense in humans against oxidant- and radical-caused aging and cancer. A hypothesis, *Proc. Natl. Acad. Sci. USA*, 78, 6858, 1981.
310. **Fanelli, G. M. and Beyer, K. H.**, Uric acid in nonhuman primates with special reference to its renal transport, *Ann. Rev. Pharmacol.*, 14, 355, 1974.
311. **Bernirschke, K., Garner, F. M., and Jones, T. C., Eds.**, *Pathology of Laboratory Animals*, Springer-Verlag, Basel, 1978.
312. **Jukes, T. H. and King, J. L.**, Evolutionary loss of ascorbic acid synthesizing ability, *J. Human Evol.*, 4, 85, 1975.
313. *Homo sapiens ascorbicus*, a biochemical corrected robust human mutant, *Med. Hypoth.*, 5, 711, 1979.
314. **Lewin, S.**, *Vitamin C: Its Molecular Biology and Medical Potential*, Academic Press, New York, 1976.
315. **Bielski, B. H. J., Richter, H. W., and Chan, P. C.**, Some properties of the ascorbate free radical, *Ann. N.Y. Acad. Sci.*, 258, 231, 1975.
316. **Robinson, A. B. and Richheimer, S. L.**, Instability and function: ascorbic acid and glutaminyl and asparaginyl residues, *Ann. N.Y. Acad. Sci.*, 258, 314, 1975.
317. **Chatterjee, I. B., Majumder, A. K., Nandi, B. K., and Subramanian, N.**, Synthesis and some major functions of vitamin C in animals, *Ann. N.Y. Acad. Sci.*, 258, 24, 1975.
318. **Solyom, L., Enesco, H. E., and Beaulieu, C.**, The effect of RNA, uric acid and caffein on conditioning and activity in rats, *J. Psychiatr. Res.*, 6, 175, 1968.
319. **Mueller, E. F., Kasl, S. V., Brooks, G. W., and Cobb, S.**, Psychological correlates of serum urate levels, *Psychological Bull.*, 73, 238, 1970.
320. **Park, K.-S. and Asaka, A.**, Plasma and urine uric acid levels: heritability estimates and correlation with IQ, *Jpn. J. Human Genet.*, 25, 193, 1980.
321. **Rounds, D. E.**, RNA as a protective agent against irradiation of cell cultures, *Ann. N.Y. Acad. Sci.*, 95, 994, 1961.
322. **Odens, M.**, Prolongation of the life span in rats, *J. Am. Geriatr. Soc.*, 21, 450, 1973.
323. **Gardner, T. S.**, The possible roles of oral yeast ribonucleic acid (Y-RNA) in geriatrics and gerontology, *Gerontologia*, 7, 109, 1963.

324. **Herman, J. B., Medalie, J. H., and Goldbourt, U.,** Diabetes and uric acid — a relationship investigated by the epidemiological method, in *Advances in Experimental Medicine and Biology, 41 B Purine Metabolism in Man,* Sperling O., de Vries, A., and Wyngaarden, J. B., Eds., Plenum Press, New York, 1973, 483.

325. **Sonka, J., Gregorova, I., and Krizek, V.,** Dehydroepiandrosterone in gout, *Steroids,* 4, 843, 1964.

326. **Sparagana, M. and Phillips, G.,** Dehydroepiandrosterone (3β-hydroxy-5-androsten-17-one) metabolism in gout, *Steroids,* 19, 477, 1972.

327. **Seegmiller, J. E., Watanabe, T., Shreier, M. H., and Waldmann, T. A.,** Immunological aspects of purine metabolism, in *Advances in Experimental Medicine and Biology, 76 A, Purine Metabolism in Man II. Regulation of Pathways and Enzyme Defects,* Muller, M. M., Kaiser, E., and Seegmiller, J. E., Eds., Plenum Press, New York, 1976, 412.

328. **Townsley, J. D. and Pepe, G. J.,** Serum dehydroepiandrosterone and dehydroepiandrosterone sulphate in baboon *(Papio papio)* pregnancy, *Acta Endocrinol.,* 85, 415, 1981.

329. **Snipes, C. A., Forest, M. G., and Migeon, C. J.,** Plasma androgen concentrations in several species of old and new world monkeys, *Endocrinology,* 85, 941, 1969.

330. **Peto, R., Doll, R., Buckley, J. D., and Sporn, M. B.,** Can dietary β-carotene materially reduce human cancer rates? *Nature (London),* 290, 201, 1981.

331. **Altman, P. C. and Dittmer, D. S., Eds.,** *Blood and Other Body Fluids,* FASEB, Washington, D.C., 1961.

332. **Spector, I.,** Animal longevity and protein turnover rate, *Nature (London),* 249, 66, 1974.

333. **Cutler, R. G. and Wulf, J. H.,** Protein synthesis fidelity and altered protein as a function of age and aging rate indifferent wild-type rodent species, in *10th Intern. Congr. Geront. Vol. II. Congr. Abstr. Sectional Sessions,* Jerusalem, Israel, 1975, 11.

334. **Allison, A. C.,** Turnovers of erythrocytes and plasma proteins in mammals, *Nature (London),* 188, 37, 1960.

335. **Berlin, N. I.,** Life span of the red cell, in *The Red Blood Cell,* Bishop, C. and Surgenor, Eds., Academic Press, New York, 1964, 423.

336. **Landaw, S. A.,** Biological aspects of senescence in red cells, in *Experiments in Aging Research Special Review Program in Biology,* Elias, M. F., Eleftheriou, B. E., and Elias, P. K., Eds., Bar Harbor, Maine, 1976, 304.

337. **Altman, P. L. and Dittmer, D. S., Eds.,** *Biological Data Book,* Vol. 1, FASEB, Bethesda, Md., 1972.

338. **Huser, H.-J.,** *Atlas of Comparative Primate Hematology,* Academic Press, New York, 1970.

339. **Harman, D.,** Prolongation of the normal lifespan and inhibition of spontaneous cancer by antioxidants, *J. Gerontol.,* 16, 247, 1961.

340. **Harman, D.,** Free radical theory of aging: effect of free radical reaction inhibitors on the mortality rate of male $LAF_1$ mice, *J. Gerontol.,* 23, 476, 1968.

341. **Harman, D., Eddy, D. E., Noffsinger, J.,** Free radical theory of aging: inhibition of amyloidosis in mice by antioxidants; possible mechanism, *J. Am. Geriat. Soc.,* 24, 203, 1976.

342. **Harman, D., Heidrick, M. L., and Eddy, D. E.,** Free radical theory of aging: effect of free-radical-reaction inhibitors on the immune system, *J. Am. Geriatr. Soc.,* 25, 400, 1977.

343. **Harman, D.,** Free radical theory of aging: nutritional implication, *Age,* 1, 143, 1978.

344. **Harman, D. and Eddy, D. E.,** Free radical theory of aging: beneficial effect of adding antioxidants to the maternal mouse diet on life span of offspring: possible explanation of the sex difference in longevity, *Age,* 2, 109, 1979.

345. **Harman, D.,** Free radical theory of aging: beneficial effect of antioxidants on the life span of male NZB mice; role of free radical reactions in the deterioration of the immune system with age and in the pathogenesis of systemic lupus erythematosus, *Age,* 3, 64, 1980.

346. **Kohn, R.,** Effect of antioxidants on life-span of C57BL mice, *J. Gerontol.,* 26, 378, 1971.

347. **Wattenburg, L. W.,** Inhibitors of chemical carcinogens, *J. Env. Pathol. Toxicol.,* 3, 35, 1980.

348. **Benson, A. M., Hunkeler, M. J., and Talalay, P.,** Increase of NAD(P)H:quinone reductase by dietary antioxidants: possible role in protection against carcinogenesis and toxicity, *Proc. Natl. Acad. Sci. USA,* 77, 5216, 1980.

349. **Cumming, R. B. and Walton, M. F.,** Modification of the acute toxicity of mutagenic and carcinogenic chemicals in the mouse by prefeeding with antioxidants, *Food Cosmet. Toxicol.,* 11, 547, 1973.

350. **Robinson, J. R., Felton, J. S., Levitt, R. C., Thorgeirsson, S. S., and Nebert, D. W.,** Relationship between "aromatic hydrocarbon responsiveness" and the survival times in mice treated with various drugs and environmental compounds, *Molec. Pharmacol.,* 11, 850, 1975.

351. **Reddy, V. N., Giblin, F. J., and Matsuda, H.,** Defense system of the lens against oxidative damage, in *Red Blood Cell and Lens Metabolism,* Srivastava, S. K., Ed., Elsevier/North Holland, Amsterdam, 1980, 139.

352. **Zigler, J. S. and Goosey, J.,** Aging of protein molecules: Lens crystallins as a model system, *Trends Biochem. Sci.,* 6, 133, 1981.

353. **Baroques, J., Gregori, C., and Schapira, F.**, Aging of aldolase and pyruvate kinase in eye lens, in *Ageing of the Lens*, Regnault, F., Hockwin, O., and Courtois, Y., Eds., Elsevier/North Holland, Amsterdam, 1980, 63.
354. **Reiss, U. and Gershon, D.**, Methionine sulfoxide reductase: a novel protective enzyme in liver and its potentially significant role in aging, in *Liver and Aging*, Kitani, K., Ed., Elsevier/North Holland, Amsterdam, 1979, 35.
355. **Brot, N., Weissbach, L., Werth, J., and Weissbach, H.**, Enzymatic reduction of protein-bound methionine sulfoxide, *Proc. Natl. Acad. Sci. USA*, 78, 2155, 1981.
356. **Martin, R., Likton, A., and Salthe, S. N.**, Coordination of separate, inducible repair mechanisms into a single, comprehensive, cellular repair program may have been necessary for the evolution of life cycles which include aging and rejuvenation, *Age*, in press, 1981.
357. **Lima-de-Faria, A.**, Classification of genes, rearrangements and chromosomes according to the chromosome field, *Hereditas*, 93, 1, 1980.
358. **Hassan, H. M. and Fridovich, I.**, Superoxide, hydrogen peroxide, and oxygen tolerance of oxygen-sensitive mutants of *Escherichia coli*, *Rev. Infect. Dis.*, 1, 357, 1979.
359. **Munkres, K. D.**, Biochemical genetics of ageing of *Neurospora crassa* and *Podospora anserina*. A review, in *Age Pigments*, Sohal, R. S., Ed., Elsevier/North Holland, Amsterdam, 1981, in press.
360. **Munkres, K. D., Furtek, C. A., and Rana, R. S.**, Genetics of cellular longevity in Neurospora. II. A superogene cluster, *Age*, in press, 1981.
361. **Munkres, K. D., Rana, R. S., Goldstein, E., and Furtek, C. A.**, Cellular longevity determinant genes control superoxide dismutase, catalase, glutathione peroxidase, cytochrome peroxidase, and ascorbate free-radical reductase in Neurospora, *Age*, in press, 1981.
362. **O'Brien, S. J.**, *Genetic Maps*, Vol. 1, Lab. of Viral Carcinogenesis, NCI, Bethesda, Md., 1980.
363. **Lin, P.-F. and Ruddle, F. H.**, Murine DNA repair gene located on chromosome 4, *Nature (London)*, 289, 191, 1981.
364. **Hoffman, H. A. and Grieshaber, C. K.**, Genetic studies of murine catalase: regulation of multiple forms of kidney catalase, *Biochem. Genet.*, 14, 59, 1976.
365. **Gasser, D. L., Mele, L., Lees, D. D., and Goldman, A. S.**, Genes in mice that affect susceptibility to cortisone-induced cleft palate are closely linked to Ir genes on chromosomes 2 and 17, *Proc. Natl. Acad. Sci. USA*, 78, 3147, 1981.
366. **Nebert, D. W. and Jensen, N. M.**, The Ah locus: genetic regulation of the metabolism of carcinogens, drugs, and other environmental chemicals by cytochrome P-450-mediated monoxigenases, *Crit. Rev. Biochem.*, 6, 401, 1979.
367. **Bulfield, G.**, Molecular genetics of the mouse, *Nature (London)*, 288, 114, 1980.
368. **Womack, J. E., Yan, D. L. S., and Potier, M.**, Gene for neuroaminidase activity of mouse chromosome 17 near H-2: pleiotropic effects of multiple hydrolases, *Science*, 212, 63, 1981.
369. **Gill, T. J. and Kunz, H. W.**, Gene complex controlling growth and fertility linked to the major histocompatibility complex in the rat, *Am. J. Pathol.*, 96, 185, 1979.
370. **Barnett, E. V., Chia, D., Fahey, J. L., Gatti, R. A., Gossett, T. C., Grossman, H., Hibrawi, H., Medici, M. A., Motola, M., Naeim, F., Sparkes, R. S., Spina, C., Tam, C., Van Lancker, J. L., and Walford, R. L.**, Immunological and biochemical studies of Down's syndrome as a model of accelerated aging, in *Immunological Aspects of Aging*, Segre, D. and Smith, L., Eds., Marcel Dekker, in press.
371. **Baret, A., Baeteman, M. A., Mattei, J. F., Michel, P., Broussolle, B., and Giraud, F.**, Immunoreactive Cu SOD and Mn SOD in the circulating blood cells from normal and trisomy 21 subjects, *Biochem. Biophys. Res. Comm.*, 98, 1035, 1981.
372. **Erickson, R. P., Lewis, S. E., and Slusser, K. S.**, Conservation of autosomal gene synteny groups in mouse and man, *Nature (London)*, 274, 160, 1978.
373. **Sinet, P.-M., Lejeune, J., and Jerome, H.**, Trisomy 21 (Down's syndrome) and glutathione peroxidase, hexose monophosphate shunt and I.Q., *Life Sci.*, 24, 29, 1979.
374. **Smith, G. S. and Walford, R. L.**, Influence of the main histocompatibility complex on ageing in mice, *Nature (London)*, 270, 727, 1977.
375. **Smith, G. S. and Walford, R. L.**, Influence of the H-2 and H-1 histocompatibility systems upon life span and spontaneous cancer incidences in congenic mice, in *Genetic Effects on Aging*, Bergsma, D. and Harrison, D. E., Eds., A. R. Liss, Inc., New York, 1978, 281.
376. **Walford, R. L.**, Multigene families, histocompatibility systems, transformation, meiosis, stem cells, and DNA repair, *Mech. Ageing Dev.*, 9, 19, 1979.
377. **Walford, R. L. and Bergmann, K.**, Influence of genes associated with the main histocompatibility complex on deoxyribonucleic acid excision repair capacity and bleomycin sensitivity in mouse lymphocytes, *Tissue Antigens*, 14, 336, 1979.
378. **Novak, R., Bosze, Z., Matkovics, B., and Fachet, J.**, Genes affecting superoxide dismutase activity linked to the histocompatibility complex in H-2 congenic mice, *Science*, 207, 86, 1980.
379. **Meruelo, D. and Edidin, M.**, Association of mouse liver adenosine 3′:5′-cyclic monophosphate (cyclic AMP) levels with histocompatibility-2 genotype, *Proc. Natl. Acad. Sci. USA*, 72, 2644, 1975.

380. **Lafuse, W., Meruelo, D., and Edidin, M.,** The genetic control of liver cAMP levels in mice, *Immunogenetics,* 9, 57, 1979.

381. **Meruelo, D. and Edidin, M.,** The biological function of the major histocompatibility complex: Hypotheses, in *Contemporary Topics in Immunobiology,* Vol. 9, Marchalonis, J. J. and Cohen, N., Eds., Plenum Press, New York, 1980, 231.

382. **Lafuse, W. and Edidin, M.,** Influence of the mouse major histocompatibility complex, H-2, on liver adenylate cyclase activity and on glucogon binding to liver cell membranes, *Biochemistry,* 19, 49, 1980.

383. **Chirkov, Yu., Chesnokova, L. P., Sobolev, A. L., and Lomonosov, M. V.,** Effect of radioprotectors on cAMP-dependent protein phosphorylation, *Biull. Eksper. Biol. Medit.,* 87, 230, 1979.

384. **Copeland, F. S.,** Mechanisms of radioprotection-a review, *Photochem. Photobiol.,* 28, 839, 1978.

385. **Baker, G. T.,** Age-dependent arginine phosphokinase activity changes in male vestigial and wild-type *Drosphila melanogaster, Gerontologia,* 21, 203, 1975.

386. **Bartosz, G., Leyko, W., and Fried, R.,** Superoxide dismutase and life span of *Drosophila melanogaster, Experientia,* 35, 1193, 1979.

387. **Gatt, M., Pimpinelli, S., and Baker, B. S.,** Relationships among chromatid interchanges, sister chromatid exchanges, and meiotic recombination in *Drosophila melanogaster, Proc. Natl. Acad. Sci. USA,* 77, 1575, 1980.

388. **Nebert, D. W.,** Multiple forms of inducible drug-metabolizing enzymes: A reasonable mechanism by which any organism can cope with adversity, *Molec. Cellular Biochem.,* 27, 27, 1979.

389. **Braun, W. E.,** *HLA and Disease: A Comprehensive Review,* CRC Press, Boca Raton, Fla., 1979.

390. **DeWolf, W. C., Dupont, B., and Yunis, E. J.,** HLA and disease: current concepts, *Human Pathol.,* 11, 332, 1980.

391. **Snell, G. D.,** Recent advances in histocompatibility immunogenetics, *Adv. Genet.,* 20, 291, 1979.

392. **Snell, G. D.,** Studies in histocompatibility, *Science,* 213, 172, 1981.

393. **Beighlie, D. J. and Teplitz, R. L.,** Repair of UV damaged DNA in systemic lupus erythematosus, *J. Rheumatol.,* 2, 149, 1975.

394. **Rister, M., Bauermeister, K., Gravert, U., and Gladtke, E.,** Superoxide-dismutase deficiency in rheumatoid arthritis, *Lancet,* 1, 1904, 1978.

395. **Walford, R. L., Weidruch, R. H., Gottesman, S. R. C., and Tam, C. F.,** The immunopathology of aging, *Ann. Rev. Geront. Geriatr.,* in press.

396. **Szeihberg, A., Golan, R., Ben-Ezzer, J., Sarova-Pinhas, I., and Kindler, D.,** Glutathione peroxidase activity in various types of blood cells in multiple sclerosis, *Acta Neurol. Scand.,* 63, 67, 1981.

397. **Jensen, G. E., Gissel-Nielsen, G., and Clausen, J.,** Leucocyte glutathione peroxidase activity and selenium level in multiple sclerosis, *J. Neurol. Sci.,* 48, 61, 1980.

398. **Wu, J.-Y., Welch, K. M. A., and Duncan, C. C.,** Abnormal protein patterns in multiple sclerosis, *Neurochem. Res.,* 4, 811, 1979.

399. **Arlett, C. F. and Lehmann, A. R.,** Human disorders showing increased sensitivity to the induction of genetic damage, *Ann. Rev. Genet.,* 12, 95, 1978.

400. **Martin, G. M.,** Genetic heterogeneity: implications for the pathobiology of aging in man, in *Biological Mechanisms in Aging,* Schimke, R. T., Ed., National Institute on Aging, NIH Pub. No. 81-2194, 1981, 4.

401. **Sinet, P. M., Lavelle, F., Michelson, A. M., and Jerome, H.,** Superoxide dismutase activities of blood platelets in trisomy 21, *Biochem. Biophys. Res. Comm.,* 67, 904, 1975.

402. **Ambani, L. M., Van Woert, M. H., and Murphy, S.,** Brain peroxidase and catalase in Parkinson's disease, *Arch. Neurol.,* 32, 114, 1975.

403. **Serfass, R. E. and Ganther, H. E.,** Defective microbicidal activity in glutathione peroxidase-deficient neutrophils of selenium-deficient rats, *Nature (London),* 255, 640, 1975.

404. **Gerli, G. C., Beretta, L., Bianchi, M., Pellegatta, A., and Agostoni, A.,** Erythrocyte superoxide dismutase, catalase and glutathione peroxidase activities in $\beta$-thalassaemia (major and minor), *Scand. J. Haematol.,* 25, 87, 1980.

405. **Gandy, S. E., Galbraith, R. A., Crouch, R. K., Buse, M. G., and Galbraith, G. M. P.,** Superoxide dismutase in human islets of langerhans, *N. Eng. J. Med.,* 304, 1547, 1981.

406. **Gerli, G. C., Beretta, L., Bianchi, M., and Agostoni, A.,** Erythrocyte superoxidase dismutase, catalase and glutathione peroxidase in conditions of augmented oxidant stress, *Bull. Europ. Physiopathol. Respir.,* 17, 201, 1981.

407. **Stone, W. L. and Dratz, E. A.,** Increased glutathione S-transferase activity in antioxidant-deficient rats, *Biochim. Biophys. Acta,* 631, 1980.

408. **Garver, J. J., Estop, A. M., Khan, P. M., Balner, H., and Pearson, P.L.,** Evidence of similar organization of the chromosomes carrying the major histocompatibility complex in man and other primates, *Cytogenet. Cell Genet.,* 27, 238, 1980.

409. **McClay, D. R. and Gooding, L. R.,** Involvement of histocompatibility antigens in embryonic cell recognition events, *Nature (London),* 274, 367, 1978.

410. **Alton, A. K., Silver, L. M., Artzt, K., and Bennett, D.**, Molecular analysis of the genetion relationship of trans interacting factors at the T/t complex, *Nature (London)*, 288, 368-370, 1980.
411. **Portugal, F. H.**, Histocompatibility antigens and cytoskeletal elements, *Nature (London)*, 279, 102-103, 1979.
412. **Monroy, A. and Rosati, F.**, The evolution of the cell-cell recognition system, *Nature (London)*, 278, 165, 1979.
413. **Hirai, T., Yamamoto, Y., and Hamaoka, T.**, Relationship between carcinoembryonic antigen and major histocompatibility antigens on cultured human carcinoma cells, *J. Immunol.*, 124, 2765, 1980.
414. **Gresser, I.**, On the varied biologic effects of interferon, *Cell. Immunol.*, 34, 406, 1977.
415. **Bocci, V.**, Is interferon produced in physiologic conditions? *Med. Hypoth.*, 6, 735, 1980.
416. **Vesely, D. L. and Cantell, K.**, Human interferon enhances guanylate cyclase activity, *Biochem. Biophys. Res. Comm.*, 96, 574, 1980.
417. **Ortaldo, J. R. and McCoy, J. L.**, Protective effects of interferon in mice previously exposed to lethal irradiation, *Rad. Res.*, 81, 262, 1980.
418. **Renton, K. W. and Mannering, G. J.**, Depression of hepatic cytochrome P-450-dependent monoxygenase systems with administered interferon inducing agents, *Microsomes and Drug Oxidation, Biochem. Pharm. Suppl.* 2, 484, 1977.
419. **Tan, Y. H.**, Chromosome 21 and the cell growth inhibitory effect of human interferon preparations, *Nature (London)*, 260, 141, 1976.
420. **Maroun, L. E.**, Interferon action and chromosome 21 trisomy, *J. Theo. Biol.*, 86, 603, 1980.
421. **Pottathil, R., Chandrabose, K. A., Cuatrecasas, P., and Lang, D. J.**, Establishment of the intermediated antiviral state: possible role of superoxide dismutase, *Proc. Natl. Acad. Sci. USA*, 78, 3343, 1981.
422. **Dausset, J. and Contu, L.**, Is the MHC a general self-recognition system playing a major unifying role in an organism? *Human Immunol.*, 1, 5, 1980.
423. **Gill, T. J.**, Structure and function of major histocompatibility complex, *Arch. Pathol. Lab. Med.*, 104, 559, 1980.
424. **Richardson, J. S., Richardson, D. C., Thomas, K. A., Silverton, E. W., and Davies, D. R.**, Similarity of three-dimensional structure between the immunoglobulin domain and the copper, zinc superoxide dismutase subunit, *J. Molec. Biol.*, 102, 221, 1976.
425. **Bernacerraf, B.**, Role of MCH gene products in immune regulation, *Science*, 212, 1229, 1981.
426. **Dryer, S. E., Dryer, R. L., and Autor, A. P.**, Enhancement of mitochondrial, cyanide-resistant superoxide dismutase in the livers of rats treated with 2,4-dinitrophenol, *J. Biol. Chem.*, 255, 1054, 1980.
427. **Johnson, H. D., Kintner, L. D., Kibler, H. H.**, Effects of 48°F and 83°F on longevity and pathology of male rats, *J. Gerontol.*, 18, 29, 1963.
428. **Johnson, H. A. and Pavelec, M.**, Thermal injury due to normal body temperature, *Am. J. Pathol.*, 66, 557, 1972.
429. **Johnson, H. A. and Pavelec, M.**, Thermal noise in cells. A cause of spontaneous loss of cell function, *Am. J. Pathol.*, 69, 119, 1972.
430. **Martin, G. M.**, Genetic syndromes in man with potential relevance to the pathology of aging, in *Genetic Effects on Aging*, Bergsma, D. and Harrison, D. E., Eds., Alan R. Liss, Inc., New York, 1978, 5.
431. **Brown, W. T.**, Human mutations affecting aging — a review, *Mech. Ageing Dev.*, 9, 325, 1979.
432. **Martin, G. M.**, Genetic and evolutionary aspects of aging, *Fed. Proc. Fed. Am. Soc. Exp. Biol.*, 38, 1962, 1979.
433. **Tappel, A., Fletcher, B., and Deamer, D.**, Effect of antioxidants and nutrients on lipid peroxidation fluorescent products and aging parameters in the mouse, *J. Gerontol.*, 28, 415, 1973.
434. **Davies, J. E. W., Ellery, P. M., and Hughes, R. E.**, Dietary ascorbic acid and life span of guinea-pigs, *Exp. Gerontol.*, 12, 215, 1977.
435. **Blackett, A. D. and Hall, D. A.**, The effects of vitamin E on mouse fitness and survival, *Gerontology*, 27, 133, 1981.
436. **Lippman, R. D.**, The prolongation of life: a comparison of antioxidants and geroprotectors versus superoxide in human mitochondria, *J. Gerontol.*, 36, 550, 1981.
437. **Hassan, H. M. and Fridovich, I.**, Induction of the manganese-containing superoxide dismutase (MnSOD) in *Escherichia coli* by compounds capable of intracellular generation of $O_2$, *Fed. Proc. Fed. Am. Soc. Exp. Biol.*, 37, 1425, 1978.
438. **Dalrymple, G. V., Sanders, J. L., Baker, M. L., and Wilkinson, K. P.**, The effect of 2,4-dinitrophenol on the repair of radiation injury by L cells, *Rad. Res.*, 37, 90, 1969.
439. **Little, J. B. and Williams, J. R.**, Enhancement of survival of irradiated plateau phase cells by dinitrophenol: effect of dose-rate and cell strain, *Rad. Res.*, 66, 90, 1976.
440. **Laval, F.**, Effect of uncouplers on radiosensitivity and mutagenicity in x-irradiated mammalian cells, *Proc. Natl. Acad. Sci. USA*, 77, 2702, 1980.

441. **Kenyon, C. J. and Walker, G. C.**, Expression of the *E. coli* uvrA gene is inducible, *Nature (London)*, 289, 808, 1981.
442. **Jeggo, P., Defais, M., Samson, L., and Schendel, P.**, An adaptive response of *E. coli* to low levels of alkylating agent: comparison with previously characterized DNA repair pathways, *Molec. Gen. Genet.*, 157, 1, 1977.
443. **Samson, L. and Cairns, J.**, A new pathway for DNA repair in *Escherichia coli, Nature (London)*, 267, 281, 1977.
444. **Schendel, P. F., Defais, M., Jeggo, P., Samson, L., and Cairns, J.**, Pathways of mutagenesis and repair in *Escherichia coli* exposed to low levels of simple alkylating agents, *J. Bacteriol.*, 135, 466, 1978.
445. **Robins, P. and Cairns, J.**, Quantitation of the adaptive response to alkylating agents, *Nature (London)*, 280, 74, 1979.
446. **Sarasin, A. R. and Hanawalt, P. C.**, Carcinogens enhance survival of UV-irradiated simian virus 40 in treated monkey kidney cells: induction of a recovery pathway? *Proc. Natl. Acad. Sci. USA*, 75, 346, 1978.
447. **Durrant, L. G., Margison, G. P., and Boyle, J.**, Pretreatment of Chinese hamster V79 cells with MNU increases survival without affecting DNA repair or mutagenicity, *Carcinogenesis*, 2, 55, 1981.
448. **Samson, I. and Schwartz, J. I.**, Evidence for an adaptive DNA repair pathway in CHO and human skin fibroblast cell lines, *Nature (London)*, 287, 861, 1980.
449. **Petrovic, V. M., Gudz, T., and Saicic, Z.**, Selective effect of noradrenalin on superoxide dismutase activity in the brown adipose tissue and liver of the rat, *Experientia*, 37, 14, 1981.
450. **Del Villano, B. C., Miller, S. I., Schachter, L. P., and Tischfield, J. A.**, Elevated superoxide dismutase in black alcoholics, *Science*, 207, 991, 1980.
451. **Fuentes, O. R.**, Enhancement of rat liver catalase activity dietary cholesterol, *Life Sci.*, 23, 2039, 1978.
452. **Reddy, J., Chiga, M., and Svobada, D.**, Stimulation of liver catalase synthesis in rats by ethyl-$\alpha$-$\varrho$-chlorophenoxisobutyrate, *Biochem. Biophys. Res. Comm.*, 43, 318, 1971.
453. **Bartosz, G., Leyko, W., and Fried, R.**, Is superoxide dismutase a physiological radioprotector? *Experientia*, 35, 1194, 1979.
454. **Stevens, J. B. and Autor, A. P.**, Oxygen-induced synthesis of superoxide dismutase and catalase in pulmonary macrophages of neonatal rats, *Lab. Invest.*, 37, 470, 1977.
455. **Smith-Sonneborn, J.**, DNA repair and longevity assurance in *Paramecium tetraurelia, Science*, 203, 1115, 1979.
456. **Klass, M. R. and Smith-Sonneborn, J.**, Studies on DNA content, RNA synthesis, and DNA template activity in aging cells of *Paramecium aurelia, Exp. Cell Res.*, 98, 63, 1976.
457. **Sonneborn, T. M. and Dippell, R. V.**, Cellular changes with age in Paramecium, in *The Biology of Aging*, Strehler, B. L., Ed., AIBS, Washington, D. C., 1960, 285.
458. **Ducoff, H. S.**, Causes of death in irradiated adult insects, *Biol. Rev.*, 47, 211, 1972.
459. **Sacher, G. A.**, Life table modification and life prolongation, in *Handbook of the Biology of Aging*, Finch, C. E. and Hayflick, L., Eds., Van Nostrand Reinhold, New York, 1977, 582.
460. **Allen, R. G. and Sohal, R. S.**, The effects of irradiation on the mortality, metabolic rate, lipid peroxidation potential and fluorescent age pigment concentration in the housefly, *Musca domestica, Age*, in press.
461. **Fleming, J. E., Yengoyan, L. S., and Miquel, J.**, Rate of living in Drosphila: effects of various antioxidants on life span and oxygen consumption, *Age*, in press.
462. **Lippman, R., Agren, A., and Uhlen, M.**, Vitamin E derivatives which may increase antioxidant protection on the inner mitochondrial membrane, *Age*, in press.
463. **Brawn, K. and Fridovich, I.**, Superoxide radical and superoxide dismutases: threat and defense, *Acta Physiol. Scand.*, 492, 9, 1980.
464. **Bacq, Z. M. and Alexander, P.**, *Fundamentals of Radiobiology*, Pergamon Press, New York, 1971.
465. **Terzi, M.**, Comparative analysis of inactivating efficiency of radiation of different organisms, *Nature (London)*, 191, 461, 1961.
466. **Sparrow, A. H., Underbrink, A. G., and Sparrow, R. C.**, Chromosomes and cellular radiosensitivity. I. The relationship of $D_o$ to chromosome volume and complexity in seventy-nine different organisms, *Rad. Res.*, 32, 915, 1967.
467. **Koval, T. M.**, Relative responses of mammalian and insect cells, in *Radiation Biology in Cancer Research*, Meyn, R. E. and Withers, H. R., Eds., Raven Press, New York, 1980, 169.
468. **Fernandes, G., Yunis, E. J., and Good, R. A.**, Influence of diet on survival of mice, *Proc. Natl. Acad. Sci. USA*, 73, 1279, 1976.
469. **Young, V. R.**, Diet as a modulator of aging and longevity, *Fed. Proc. Fed. Am. Soc. Exp. Biol.*, 38, 1994, 1979.
470. **Weindruch, R. H., Kristie, J. A., Cheney, K. E., and Walford, R. L.**, Influence of controlled dietary restriction on immunologic function and aging, *Fed. Proc. Fed. Am. Soc. Exp. Biol.*, 38, 2007, 1979.

471. **McCay, C. M., Maynard, L. A., Sperling, G., and Barnes, L. L.,** Retarded growth, life span, ultimate body size, and age changes in the albino rat after feeding diets restricted in calories, *J. Nutr.*, 18, 1, 1939.
472. **McCay, C. M., Crowell, M. F., and Maynard, L. A.,** The effect of retarded growth upon the length of lifespan and upon the ultimate body size, *J. Nutr.*, 10, 63, 1935.
473. **Carlson, A. and Hoelzel, F.,** Apparent prolongation of the life span of rats by intermittent fasting, *J. Nutr.*, 31, 363, 1946.
474. **Carlson, A. and Hoelzel, F.,** Prolongation of the lifespan of rats by bulk-formers in the diet, *J. Nutr.*, 36, 27, 1948.
475. **Berg, B. N.,** Nutrition and longevity in the rat. I. Food intake in relation to size, health and fertility, *J. Nutr.*, 71, 242, 1960.
476. **Berg, B. N. and Simms, H. S.,** Nutrition and longevity in the rat. II. Longevity and onset of disease with different levels of food intake, *J. Nutr.*, 71, 255, 1960.
477. **Barrows, C.,** Nutrition, aging and genetic program, *Am. J. Clin. Nutr.*, 25, 829, 1972.
478. **Ross, M. H.,** Nutrition and longevity in experimental animals, in *Nutrition and Aging,* Winick, M., Ed., John Wiley & Sons, New York, 1976, 43.
479. **Jose, D. G., Stutman, O., and Good, R. A.,** Long term effects on immune function of early nutritional deprivation, *Nature (London)*, 241, 57, 1973.
480. **Good, R. A., West, A., and Fernandes, G.,** Nutritional modulation of immune responses, in *Fed. Proc. Fed. Am. Soc. Exp. Biol.*, 39, 3098, 1980.
481. **Levin, P., Janda, J. K., Joseph, J. A., Ingram, D. K., and Roth, G. S.,** Dietary restriction retards the age-associated loss of rat striatal dopaminergic receptors, *Science*, 214, 561, 1981.
482. **Wulf, J. H. and Cutler, R. G.,** Altered protein hypothesis of mammalian aging processes. I. Thermal stability of glucose-6-phosphate dehydrogenase in C57BL/6J mouse tissue, *Exp. Gerontol.*, 10, 101, 1975.
483. **Ross, M. and Braes, G.,** Lasting influence of early caloric restrictions on prevalence of neoplasms in the rat, *J. Natl. Cancer Inst.*, 47, 1095, 1971.
484. **Murray, J. and Murray, A.,** Toward a nutritional concept of host resistance to malignancy and intracellular infection, *Persp. Biol. Med.*, 24, 290, 1981.
485. **Young, V. R., Perera, W. D., Winterer, J. C., and Scrimshaw, N. S.,** Protein and amino acid requirements of the elderly, in *Nutrition and Aging,* Winick, M., Ed., John Wiley & Sons, New York, 1976, 77.
486. **Coleman, D. L.,** Obesity genes: beneficial effects in heterozygous mice, *Science*, 203, 663, 1979.
487. **Harrison, D.,** personal communication.
488. **Adelman, R. C.,** Loss of adaptive mechanisms during aging, *Fed. Proc. Fed. Am. Soc. Exp. Biol.*, 38, 1968, 1979.
489. **Meredith, P. J. and Walford, R. L.,** Autoimmunity, histocompatibility, and aging, *Mech. Ageing Dev.*, 9, 61, 1979.
490. **Finch, C. E., Felicio, L. S., Flurkey, K., Gee, D. M., Mobbs, C., Nelson, J. F., and Osterburg, H. H.,** Studies on ovarian-hypothalamic-pituitary interactions during reproductive aging in C57BL/6J mice, *Peptides*, 1, 163, 1980.
491. **Sinex, F. M.,** Cross-linkage and aging, in *Advances in Gerontology Research,* Vol. 1, Strehler, B. L., Ed., Academic Press, New York, 1964, 165.
492. **Hruza, Z. and Hlavackova, V.,** Effect of environmental temperature and under-nutrition on collagen ageing, *Exp. Gerontol.*, 4, 169, 1969.
493. **Everitt, A. V. and Delbridge, L.,** Two phases of collagen ageing in the tail tendon of hypophysectomized rats, *Exp. Gerontol.*, 7, 45, 1972.
494. **Hamlin, C. R., Kohn, R. R., and Luschin, J. H.,** Apparent accelerated aging of human collagen in diabetes mellitus, *Diabetes*, 24, 902, 1975.
495. **Deyl, Z., Juricova, M., Rosmus, J., and Adam, M.,** Aging of the connective tissue: Collagen cross linking in animals of different species and equal age, *Exp. Gerontol.*, 6, 227, 1971.
496. **Kao, K. Y. T., Hitt, W. E., and Leslie, J. G.,** The intermolecular cross-links in uterine collagens of guinea pig, pig, cow, and human beings, *Proc. Soc. Exp. Biol. Med.*, 151, 385, 1976.
497. **Hamlin, C. R., Lischin, J. H., and Kohn, R. R.,** Aging of collagen: comparative rates in four mammalian species, *Exp. Gerontol.*, 15, 393, 1980.
498. **Harrison, D. E., Archer, J. R., Sacher, G. A., and Boyce, F. M.,** Tail collagen aging in mice of thirteen different genotypes and two species: relationship to biological age, *Exp. Gerontol.*, 13, 63, 1978.
499. **Bada, J. L. and Brown, S. E.,** Amino acid racemization in living mammals; biochronological applications, *Trends Biochem. Sci.*, 5, 111, 1980.
500. **Oberley, L. W. and Buettner, G. R.,** Role of superoxide dismutase in cancer: a review, *Cancer Res.*, 39, 1141, 1979.

501. **Tappel, A. L. and Dillard, C. J.,** *In vivo* lipid peroxidation: measurement via exhaled pentane and protection by vitamin E, *Fed. Proc. Fed. Am. Soc. Exp. Biol.,* 40, 174, 1981.

502. **Sacher, G. A. and Trucco, E.,** The stochastic theory of mortality, *Ann. N.Y. Acad. Sci.,* 96, 985, 1962.

503. **Havighurst, R. J. and Sacher, G. A.,** Prospects of lengthening life and vigor, in *Extending the Human Life Span: Social Policy and Social Ethics,* Neugarten, B. L. and Havighurst, R. J., Eds., National Science Foundation, NSF/RA 770123, 1977, 13.

504. **Shock, N. W.,** Physiologic aspects of aging, *J. Am. Diatetic Assoc.,* 56, 491, 1970.

505. **Hayflick, L.,** Aging under glass, *Exp. Gerontol.,* 5, 291, 1970.

506. **Hayflick, L.,** The cellular basis for biological aging, in *Handbook of the Biology of Aging,* Finch, C. E. and Hayflick, L., Eds., Van Nostrand Reinhold Co., New York, 1977, 159.

507. **Hayflick, L.,** Recent advances in the cell biology of aging, *Mech. Ageing Dev.,* 14, 59, 1980.

508. **Nichols, W. W. and Murphy, D. G., Eds.,** *Differentiated Cells in Aging Research,* Academic Press, New York, 1979.

509. **Gershon, D., Gershon, H., Jacobus, S., Reiss, U., and Reznick, A.,** The accumulation of faulty enzyme molecules in aging cells, in *Metabolic Interconversion of Enzymes,* Shaltiel, S., Ed., Springer-Verlag, Berlin, 1976, 227.

510. **Bell, E., Marek, L. F., Levinstone, D. S., Merrill, C., Sher, S., Young, I. T., and Eden, M.,** Loss of division potential *in vitro:* aging or differentiation? *Science,* 202, 1158, 1978.

511. **Bell, E., Marek, L., Sher, S., Merrill, C., Levinstone, D., and Young, I.,** Do diploid fibroblasts in culture age? in *Differentiated Cells in Aging Research,* Nichols, W. W. and Murphy, D. G., Eds., Academic Press, New York, 1979, 1.

512. **Norwood, T.,** personal communication.

513. **Stein, G.,** personal communication.

514. **Goldstein, S.,** personal communication.

515. **Hornsby, P.,** personal communication.

516. **Holland, J. J., Kohne, D., and Doyle, M. V.,** Analysis of virus replication in ageing human fibroblast cultures, *Nature (London),* 245, 316, 1973.

517. **Pitha, J., Adams, R., and Pitha, P. M.,** Viral probe into the events of cellular *(in vitro)* aging, *J. Cell. Physiol.,* 83, 211, 1974.

518. **Tomkins, G. A., Stanbridge, E. J., and Hayflick, L.,** Viral probes of aging in the human diploid cell strain WI-38, *Proc. Soc. Exp. Biol. Med.,* 146, 385, 1974.

519. **Harley, C. B., Pollard, J. W., Chamberlain, J. W., Stanners, C. P., and Goldstein, S.,** Protein synthetic errors do not increase during aging of cultured human fibroblasts, *Proc. Natl. Acad. Sci. USA,* 77, 1885, 1980.

520. **Wojtyk, R. I. and Goldstein, S.,** Fidelity of protein synthesis does not decline during aging of cultured human fibroblasts, *J. Cell. Physiol.,* 103, 299, 1980.

521. **Stanley, J. F., Pye, D., and MacGregor, A.,** Comparison of doubling numbers attained by cultured animal cells with life span of species, *Nature (London),* 255, 158, 1975.

522. **Rohme, D.,** Evidence for a relationship between longevity of mammalian species and life spans of normal fibroblasts *in vitro* and erythrocytes *in vivo, Proc. Natl. Acad. Sci. USA,* 78, 5009, 1981.

523. **Saksela, E. and Moorhead, P. S.,** Aneuploidy in the degenerative phase of serial cultivation of human cell strains, *Proc. Natl. Acad. Sci. USA,* 50, 390, 1963.

524. **Shmookler Reis, R. J. and Goldstein, S.,** Loss of reiterated DNA sequences during serial passage of human diploid fibroblasts, *Cell,* 21, 739, 1980.

525. **Paul, J.,** *Cell and Tissue Culture,* Churchill Livingston, London, 1975.

526. **Bissell, M. J.,** The differentiated state of normal and malignant cells or how to define a normal cell in culture, *Int. Rev. Cytology,* Bourne, G. H. and Danielli, J. F., Eds., Academic Press, New York, 1980.

527. **Barnes, D. and Sato, G.,** Serum-free cell culture: a unifying approach, *Cell,* 22, 649, 1980.

528. **Kontermann, K. and Bayreuther, K.,** The cellular aging or rat fibroblasts *in vitro* is a differentiation process, *Gerontology,* 25, 261, 1979.

529. **Leblond, C. P.,** The life history of cells in renewing systems, *Am. J. Anatomy,* 160, 113, 1981.

530. **Deschatrette, J.,** Dedifferentiated variants of a rat hepatoma: partial reversion induced by cell aggregation, *Cell,* 22, 501, 1980.

531. **Yanishevsky, R. M. and Stein, G. H.,** Ongoing DNA synthesis continues in young human diploid cells (HDC) fused to senescent HDC, but entry into S phase is inhibited, *Exp. Cell Res.,* 126, 469, 1980.

532. **Smith, J. R. and Whitney, R. G.,** Intraclonal variation in proliferative potential of human diploid fibroblasts: stochastic mechanism for cellular aging, *Science,* 207, 82, 1980.

533. **Kirkwood, T. B. L. and Holliday, R.,** Commitment to senescence: a model for the finite and infinite growth of diploid and transformed human fibroblasts in culture, *J. Theo. Biol.,* 53, 481, 1975.

534. **Kirkwood, T. B. L. and Holliday, R.,** A stochastic model for the commitment of human cells to senescence, in *Biomathematics and Cell Kinetics,* Valleron, A.-J. and Macdonald, P. D. M., Eds., Elsevier-North/Holland Biomedical Press, Amsterdam, 1978, 161.
535. **Sonneborn, T. M.,** Enormouse differences in length of life of closely related ciliates and their significance, in *The Biology of Aging,* Strehler, B. L., Ed., AIBS, Washington, D.C., 1960, 289.
536. **Fishbein, L.,** Environmental sources of chemical mutagens. II. Synthetic mutagens, in *Advances in Modern Toxicology, Vol. 5, Mutagenesis,* Flamm, W. G. and Mehlman, M. A., Eds., John Wiley & Sons, New York, 1978, 257.
537. **Miller, E. C. and Miller, J. A.,** Naturally occurring chemical carcinogens that may be present in foods, in *Intern. Rev. Biochem. Vol. 27, Biochem. of Nutrition 1,* Neuberger, A. and Jukes, T. H., Eds., University Park Press, Baltimore, 1979, 123.
538. **Weisberger, J. H. and Williams, G. M.,** Carcinogen testing: current problems and new approaches, *Science,* 214, 401, 1981.
539. **Macieira-Coelho, A., Diatloff, C., and Malaise, E.,** Concept of fibroblast aging *in vitro:* implication for cell biology, *Gerontology,* 23, 290, 1977.
540. **Peto, R.,** Epidemiology, multistage models, and short-term mutagenicity tests, in *Origins of Human Cancer, Book C.,* Hiatt, H. H., Watson, J. D., and Winsten, J. A., Eds., Cold Spring Harbor, New York, 1977, 1403.
541. **Hiatt, H. H., Watson, J. D., and Winsten, J. A., Eds.,** *Origins of Human Cancer, Book C, Human Risk Assessment,* Cold Spring Harbor, New York, 1977.
542. **Campbell, T. C.,** Chemical carcinogens and human risk assessment, *Fed. Proc. Fed. Am. Soc. Exp. Biol.,* 39, 2467, 1980.
543. **Peto, R., Roe, F. J. C., Lee, P. N., Levy, L., and Clack, J.,** Cancer and ageing in mice and men, *Br. J. Cancer,* 32, 411, 1975.
544. **DeFries, J. C., Vanderberg, S. G., and McClearn, G. E.,** Genetics of specific cognitive abilities, *Ann. Rev. Genet.,* 10, 179, 1976.
545. **Hahn, M. E., Jensen, C., and Dukek, B. C.,** *Development and Evolution of Brain Size,* Academic Press, New York, 1979.
546. **Sokoloff, L., Fitzgerald, G. G., and Kaufman, E. E.,** Cerebral nutrition and energy metabolism, *Nutrition and the Brain,* 1, 87, 1977.
547. **Guillemin, R.,** Peptides in the brain: the new endocrinology of the neuron, *Science,* 202, 390, 1978.
548. **Snyder, S. H.,** Brain peptides as neurotransmitters, *Science,* 209, 976, 1980.
549. **Anderson, G. H.,** Diet, neurotransmitters and brain function, *Br. Med. Bull.,* 37, 95, 1981.
550. **Enna, S. J., Samorajski, T., and Beer, B., Eds.,** *Brain Neurotransmitters and Receptors in Aging and Age-Related Disorders,* Raven Press, New York, 1981.

Chapter 3

# GENETIC ALTERATION AND THE PATHOLOGY OF AGING

Evan C. Hadley

## TABLE OF CONTENTS

## I. INTRODUCTION

The idea that acquired genetic alteration may be related to aging has a certain intuitive appeal and has been proposed by several authors.[17,24,32,55,110-113,165,166] The essential role of the genome in cellular replicative and synthetic processes suggests that its alteration might contribute to many age-related diseases and impairments in function. The appeal of this idea wanes considerably, however, when one turns from the global and hard-to-define concept of "aging" in general to various specific phenomena that occur in organisms as they grow older. This chapter examines the evidence regarding the etiologic role of genetic alteration in various age-related changes, and some experiments that might be done to clarify or rule out such a role. The focus is on age-related diseases or impairment of function in man in particular.

## II. WHICH AGING PROCESSES MIGHT BE CAUSED BY GENETIC ALTERATION?

Table 1 lists a collection of disorders of aging in man. The list is not intended to be comprehensive, but rather to convey the diversity of pathologic conditions associated with age. It might be argued that this list merely comprises "diseases of aging" and not "normal" changes with age. However, though the separation of disease-related from age-related effects is indeed critical, the focus in this review is on age-associated pathology, which is clearly an important aspect of aging research. After all, the development of these age-associated pathologies is in a sense a part of "normal" aging: an individual who failed to develop any of these changes in old age would be quite abnormal indeed.

Even the most rabid enthusiast for a theory of genetic alteration would have to admit that at present the evidence for its contribution to any of these diseases, with the exception of cancer, is either very slim or nonexistent. Indeed it would seem too much to ask for any single process, genetic alteration included, to require it to explain all or even most of the listed disorders. It might be argued that, while these disorders may have diverse etiologies, genetic damage somehow causes some kind of overall "impairment of function" which increases susceptibility to them. The nature of this impairment, and how it might lead to increased susceptibility, has been generally left unclear. There are indeed types of impairment at the subcellular, cellular tissue, organ, and/or organism level that could indeed produce increased susceptibility to specific diseases. Some examples might include: cell loss from tissues, impaired mitochondrial function, impairment of the sodium pump, impairment of cell proliferative capacity, impaired ribosomal function, impaired microtubule function, impaired pulmonary, renal, or cardiac function, impaired body temperature regulation, etc., *ad infinitum*. There is evidence for some of these changes occurring with age and some evidence that they may predispose to disease. (For example, impaired cell proliferative capacity in the immune system has been suggested as a factor in decreased resistance to infections in old age.) As yet, there is very little evidence for or against the idea that these changes stem from genetic alteration of any sort.

How might one go about looking for connections between an age-associated disorder and genetic alteration? A classic technique of detecting a factor's etiologic role in disease consists of looking for: (1) the presence of the factor in cases of the disease (preferably demonstrated before symptomatic onset of the disease) and (2) the absence of the factor in nonvictims of the disease. This demonstration may be either absolute (all cases having the factor, no controls having it) or statistical (cases having a higher level of the factor than controls, or a higher percentage of cases having the factor than controls). Genetic alteration has not been shown in this way to contribute to any age-

**Table 1**
**DISEASES OR IMPAIRMENTS OF FUNCTION ASSOCIATED WITH AGING**

Amyloidosis (some types)
Atherosclerosis (cardiovascular and peripheral)
Benign prostatic hypertrophy
Cancer (most types)
Cataract ("senile" type)
Diverticulosis
Emphysema
Gingival recession
Glaucoma
Hypothermia (increased susceptibility)
Impaired wound and fracture healing
Infection (increased susceptibility to certain types e.g. pneumonia, urinary tract)
Maturity-onset diabetes melitus
Osteoarthritis
Osteoporosis
Parkinson's Disease
Polycythemia vera
Presbyopia
Chronic renal failure
Senile dementia, Alzheimer's type
Senile macular degeneration
Temporal arteritis
Urinary incontinence

associated disease. (Certain cancers come closest.) Indeed, many types of genetic alteration have not yet been demonstrated in vivo, except under experimental conditions designed to induce them.

(At this point it is perhaps important to point out one criterion that need *not* be required of a particular genetic alteration to be considered as a factor in a particular disease of aging: the alteration need not increase with age. Much effort has been directed at finding age-related changes in certain alterations, and an age-related increase of a particular alteration in cases of some disorder of aging would certainly suggest a causal role for this change. However, increased *steady-state* levels of an alteration (e.g., strand breaks, base adducts) throughout the life span could produce the same effect through an increased predisposition to mutation, cell death, or other harmful consequence.)

Section III deals with studies on genetic alteration under normal conditions in vivo and the direct evidence relating these alterations to age and disease. As mentioned above, judged by the criterion of direct association with age-associated diseases, the data on genetic alterations as a causal factor are slim. Section IV deals with more indirect lines of evidence that have led to speculation on the role of genetic alteration in age-associated diseases.

## III. DIRECT EVIDENCE OF GENETIC DAMAGE IN AGING AND DISEASE

When considering genetic damage as a possible cause of a disease, it is clearly useful to know what specific genetic damage one has in mind. As is shown in Table 2, there is no shortage of possibilities. Most of these lesions have been produced and observed under experimental conditions (irradiation, administration of carcinogens, etc.) However, with a few exceptions, there is little direct data on their prevalence or functional significance in intact organisms under normal circumstances or specific disease conditions. Those lesions which have been observed under "normal" circumstances, and

## Table 2
## GENETIC LESIONS AT VARIOUS LEVELS OF ORGANIZATION[a]

I. Base Lesions (2,5,130)
- A. Missing bases (apurinic-apyrimidinic site)
- B. Incorrect bases
  1. Mispaired bases (including U substitution for T)
  2. Products of malfunction of normal enzymatic base methylation systems (inappropriate methylation or nonmethylation)
  3. Nonenzymatic base adducts (3,45,55) (e.g., polycyclic hydrocarbons, alkyl groups)
  4. Deamination products (uracil, hypoxanthine, xanthine) (4)
  5. Products of transmigration of *N*-glycosidic bond (4) (e.g., neoguanosine)
  6. Products of free radical attack (12) (e.g., 5,6-dihydroxy-5,6-dihydrothymidine)
- C. Pyrimidine dimers

II. Phosphate lesions (triesters, etc.) (31)

III. Deoxyribose lesions (11)
- A. Products of free radical attack (e.g., 2-deoxy-O-glyceropentos-4-ulose)
- B. Protein (and other?) adducts to deoxyribose at AP sites (8)
- C. Cleavage of deoxyribose C-C bonds

IV. Strand breaks (single and double) (11,13,14)
- A. Cleavage of 5′ phosphate
- B. Cleavage of 3′ phosphate
- C. Cleavage of ribose C-C skeleton
- D. Simultaneous release of sugar(s) and base(s)

V. Strand gaps

VI. Areas of denaturation (including strand separation)

VII. Interstrand cross-links (130)

VIII. Gene loss (18-20)

IX. Gene excess (e.g., via amplification)

X. Insertion of foreign DNA (e.g., viral)

XI. Loss of appropriate tertiary structure (e.g., changes in superhelicity)

XII. Loss of appropriate organization at nucleosome or higher level (28)

XIII. Inappropriate modification of nucleoprotein (32,43)

XIV. Chromosome aberrations and aneuploidy (15,16,108)

[a] References indicate reviews on specific lesions, or papers on lesions not thoroughly covered by reviews.

which show some change with age have been the subject of a recent comprehensive review.[17] Unfortunately, the number of types of damage studied is quite small in relation to the range of potential damage (see Table 2).

### A. Base Lesions

There are essentially no data directly demonstrating the presence in higher eukaryotes under normal conditions of any base, phosphate, or deoxyribose lesion, with two possible exceptions: one study has reported an increase with age in oligopeptides covalently bound to DNA (40) in rat liver. However, this report left many methodologic questions unanswered regarding identification of the adducts and the possibility of artificial adduct formation during purification. Another study reported the presence of histones covalently bound to sugars at apurinic-apyrimidinic sites via ε-amino groups on lysine residues.[39] In this case as well, as the investigators have noted, questions remain about the possibility of these products forming during the purification procedure, and other possible artifacts.

Two severe problems facing searchers for the appearance of base, sugar, and/or phosphate lesions under normal conditions in vivo are the questions of (1) what lesions to look for and (2) how to detect them at the very low frequencies in which they are likely to be found. At this point there is not much information on which to make an educated guess as to what base lesions, if any, are most likely to be present. Apurinic-apyrimidinic (AP) sites, uracil substitution for cytosine, and pyrimidine dimers (in light-exposed areas) have received attention stemming from data strongly suggesting their apparent rapid formation in vivo and the presence of specific endonucleases or *N*-glycosylases directed at these alterations.[2,5,130] However, available data do not rule out any of the other types of base, sugar, or phosphate lesions outlined in Table 2 as an important source of genetic alteration. Of particular interest, perhaps, are the damage products of free radical attack (e.g., dihydrodihydroxythymidine and altered sugars). At present the evidence for free radical involvement in this kind of damage comes from the radiation biology literature. Though there is accumulating evidence for the importance of species such as superoxide and hydroxyl radical in vivo under normal circumstances, little is known about the DNA damage (if any) they produce. In view of the successful search for other damage-specific endonucleases and/or *N*-glycosylases, it might be worthwhile to undertake a similar search for analogous enzymatic activity directed against specific products of free radical attack. Such enzymes, if found, obviously would be of considerable use in assaying for the presence of this type of damage in vivo under normal circumstances.

Another type of lesion that may be of importance consists of base adducts formed by endogenous body compounds, dietary constituents, and/or pharmacologic and other chemical agents, or metabolites of any of these three groups. There is a considerable literature on adduct formation in vivo by certain dietary constituents (e.g., aflatoxins) administered to animals experimentally. Ethical questions obviously limit this approach in humans. However, such a demonstration could be made in human subjects exposed in the course of daily life to adduct-forming agents. To date such a demonstration has only been made in cases of unusual exposure to high concentrations of such agents.[161] However, with techniques of sufficient sensitivity, adducts formed under more typical conditions might be demonstrated. There are data indicating that such normal body constituents as estrone[162] and dopamine[163] can be metabolized to adduct-forming species. The search for adducts of this type might be fruitful, particularly in tissues in which the potential adduct-forming compounds are most highly concentrated.

To detect lesions at the very low frequency at which they are likely to occur may require techniques of very high sensitivity and specificity. This chapter does not address the many technical problems hampering the performance and interpretation of studies on lesions of this type. However, it may be worthwhile to broadly review the recurrent problem of adequate sensitivity in looking for damage of this type in normal in vivo circumstances: in the broadest sense, potential techniques for measurement of DNA lesions fall into one of the three classes or combinations thereof:

- Direct "visualization" of the lesion (e.g., by electron microscopy)
- Selective tagging of the lesion (e.g., by radioisotopes, fluorescent ligands, etc.)
- Using some property of the lesion that alters (or can be made to alter) its physical behavior or that of the DNA or nucleoprotein surrounding it.

Viewed from this perspective the more common techniques of base lesion detection, such as chromatographic separation of labeled base adducts, and density gradient centrifugation or alkaline elution after specific "repair" endonuclease exposure, are but a few of the potential strategies which could be employed. Further, these techniques have particularly severe limitations in the investigation of DNA lesions occurring under normal circumstances in man. Ethical considerations obviously limit the extent to which radiolabeled DNA-damaging agents can be administered, and density gradient or alkaline elution techniques have not yet demonstrated sufficient sensitivity to detect endonuclease-sensitive lesions at the low frequency at which they would be expected to occur spontaneously in vivo. However, only a few endonucleases and tissues have been tested, and this approach could be sufficiently sensitive in certain instances to measure spontaneous damage reliably.

On the other hand, other approaches offer more potential sensitivity. One that is already gaining increasing favor is the use of "repair" endonuclease-treated nucleoids in the measurement of base damage.[164] This approach greatly amplifies the signal from a base lesion by causing the sedimentation behavior of a very large amount of DNA to be altered by endonuclease nicking at the lesion site. This approach has not yet significant application in the measurement of "spontaneous" damage, but its apparent high sensitivity makes it a strong candidate for this kind of work. It is even conceivable that the principle underlying the nucleoid technique could be pushed even further if even larger DNA structures could be isolated intact and their changes in sedimentation after endonuclease treatment were measurable. Other measures of strand breakage in nucleoids besides sedimentation changes (e.g., superhelicity) are also potentially applicable to this problem.

Another approach for detection of base damage which does not require use of radiolabeled ligands is radioimmunoassay.[1,150] The measurement of base damage by this approach, which offers the potential for very high sensitivity, is still in its very early stages. Mass-analyzed ion kinetic energy spectrometry[44] also offers the potential for detecting altered bases with great sensitivity. A third approach which does not require the use of radiolabeled ligands in vivo is the use of specific chemical properties of the damage to allow the formation of radiolabeled covalent ligands after the tissue sample has been isolated. The rare examples of this type of approach include the attachment of labeled thymidine at free ends at putative strand breaks in fixed tissue sections,[33] and the use of tritrated borohydride to introduce label into histone-deoxyribose adducts formed at previously apurinic sites.[8] It might be possible to measure other lesions (e.g., AP sites) by using radiolabeled covalent ligands of high affinity and specificity to tag them after tissue isolation.

### B. Strand Lesions

Among several studies on strand breaks[6,7,9,33,35-37,41,42] most, but not all, show some increase with age. These studies have been conducted in various tissues of rodents and dogs; to date there are no human studies. The presence of single stranded regions of DNA has also been examined. Such regions could reflect either local areas of denaturation or gap lesions on one nucleotide strand. Increases with age in single-strandedness in several tissues have been reported in several mouse tissues[35-37] together with an increase in strand breaks. Contradictory findings have been reported,[167] and a study in human ovary also failed to show any changes in single-strandedness with age.[46] Increases with age in single-strandedness have also been reported in mouse brain and liver using a histochemical technique.[34]

One must bear in mind that not all strand breaks or single-stranded regions are damage; they are an integral part of DNA replication and repair. Furthermore, it has never been conclusively shown what, if any, impairment in DNA function they cause, since available DNA strand-breaking agents (e.g., gamma radiation) produce other lesions which may result in many of their cytotoxic, mutagenic, and carcinogenic effects. This issue may be approached by comparisons of the cellular effects of agents differing in the ratio of strand breaks to other lesions produced. The problem is even more difficult in regard to single-stranded regions, since no agent to induce their formation has been developed.

There is little literature on the presence of interstrand cross-links. The presence of "hairpin" structures in DNA from mouse brain and liver[29] was seen to increase with age. The susceptibility of these structures to proteolysis led to the conjecture that they might represent protein interstrand cross-links. The functional significance of this type of structure is undetermined. Similarly, in hybridization studies, partial reversal of age-associated "loss" of ribosomal DNA from various tissues of old mice by denaturation and stringent proteolytic treatment of the DNA[22] has been interpreted as reflecting the presence of protein cross-links rendering DNA inaccessible to the RNA probe. Demonstration of interstrand cross-links in human skin by an interesting electron microscopic technique has been reported[30] though there may be difficulties in interpretation and quantification of results. The technique has not yet been used in any age-related studies.

As noted above, some hybridization studies have reported a decrease in ribosomal genes with age in various tissues from several species, including man.[18-20,22] Whether this "loss" is primarily due to increasing inaccessibility with age of rDNA under routine hybridization conditions[22] or to actual disappearance of rDNA sequences is not clear. In either case the functional significance of such changes is unknown.

### C. Chromatin Lesions

The primitive state of knowledge regarding higher-level organization of chromatin renders attempts to measure and interpret "damage" at this level very hazardous. To date, such studies have been confined to nucleosome organization. A study in human brain[47] found an increase in nucleosome repeat length and a decrease in susceptibility to micrococeal nuclease. A study in rat brain which separated neurons from glial elements found an increase in nucleosome repeat length with age in the former but not the latter, and a decreased susceptibility to staphylococcal nuclease digestion in both.[109] Studies in various tissues of the mouse[48] revealed no change in repeat length or micrococcal nuclease susceptibility. To repeat a by-now familiar refrain, the functional significance of these changes in chromatin organization are still completely unclear. Similar considerations apply to the results of studies on quantitative changes in composition and turnover of components of chromatin.[146-149]

There is also a body of indirect evidence pointing to some as-yet-undetermined structural change(s) in chromatin with age. This evidence comes mainly from three types of studies: chromatin melting curves,[24-27,32,49,85] studies on extractability of chromatin proteins in various salt concentrations,[24,49-51] and studies on chromatin template activity.[49,51-53] Age-related changes in the amino acid composition of peptides remaining after exhaustive deproteinization of DNA[54] and in chromatin sulfhydryl and -s-s- groups[10,83] have also been described.

Studies on beef thymus[27] and rodent liver[24,26,49-51] showing an increase with age in chromatin (but not DNA) melting temperature, a decrease in template activity, and a decreasing extractability of nucleoprotein by high salt suggested the possibility of some age-related change in nucleoprotein-DNA interaction which could interfere with transcription and/or replication. However, dissimilar results have been abstained in other tissues.[52,53] All these studies raise technical and interpretative questions. For example, it is difficult to draw conclusions about the functional state of chromatin in intact cells from the template activity observed with the particular RNA polymerases used in these studies. However, it is interesting to note that in some aspects the pattern of the aging studies in cell-free systems corresponds roughly to the pattern of aging studies of RNA synthesis in intact cells. For example, rat liver, which generally has been found to show the aforementioned physiochemical changes,[49,50] also appears to show a decline in cellular RNA synthesis.[56] In salivary gland, where little or no age-related physiochemical change was observed, little or no change in RNA synthesis in the intact tissue was seen.[53]

Even in those tissues which show a decline in translation, together with physiochemical changes in chromatin, it remains to be seen whether this association is only circumstantial or whether indeed some alteration in nucleoprotein-DNA interactions is responsible for inhibition of transcription and/or replication. More detailed understanding of the structural basis of the physiochemical changes may help in clarifying this question.

A methodologic caveat which applies to virtually all the studies in the preceding sections is the problem of the appearance of "lesions" as an artifactual result of events during tissue isolation and purification. This is particularly difficult in studies in tissues from intact organisms. Though attempts were made in some studies to address this problem, no study has conclusively ruled out the possibility that age-related "changes" in fact reflected events during tissue processing and not in vivo conditions. Though, of course, this is very hard to rule out completely, more controls (examining the effect of various homogenization and incubation conditions, for example) could be employed.

The analysis of age changes in these studies is also complicated by the heterogeneity of cell types found in most tissues. Changes observed in homogenized tissues could merely reflect shifts in the proportions of various cell types. Though techniques of obtaining pure cell populations are improving, they have not been used extensively in this field. Histochemical, immunocytochemical, or ultrastructural techniques of demonstrating genetic lesions are an ideal approach to the problem,[5] and have been employed in studies of strand breaks,[33] single-stranded regions,[34] interstrand cross links,[30] and pyrimidine dimers.[38] Important methodologic questions and problems in quantitation with these approaches remain unsolved.[5,30,34]

### D. Chromosomal Lesions

There is extensive literature on the relationship of chromosomal lesions to various diseases. This field is obviously far too enormous to encompass in this review, which is confined to the narrower issue of the acquisition of chromosomal abnormalities with age, and their role, if any, in diseases of aging. This has been the subject of a recent review.[15] Only a limited number of tissues have been studied, predominantly regenerating liver,[57-61] bone marrow,[62,63,74-76,89,143,150] and peripheral blood lymphocytes stimulated to divide in vitro.[23,64-74,78-84,86,87] One study has examined short-term cultures from human ovary.[77]

Studies on regenerating liver have primarily focused on the production of chromosome breaks and dicentric chromosomes and have shown a linear increase with age at a rate inversely related to the life span of several species investigated (mouse, hamster, dog). In this system there exists the concern that age- and species-associated differences may reflect differences in response to the stimuli for regeneration (e.g., partial hepatectomy) rather than pre-existing genetic damage. One reassuring consideration is that the same pattern is seen in several studies, despite the fact that a variety of stimuli for regeneration were used.

Human chromosomal aging data is almost exclusively confined to studies of bone marrow and peripheral blood lymphocytes. Though contradictory studies exist[64,80,81] the overall picture emerging from the peripheral lymphocyte studies suggests an age-associated increase in aneuploidy (especially 45,X; more rarely 47,XXX) in women, and to a lesser extent (45,X) in men.[23,66,68-73,78,79,82] Among autosomal chromosomes there is a suggestion of preferential loss or gain of chromosome 21.[60] Since the above studies were cross-sectional, some of the age changes could be attributed to selection effects. In a six-year longitudinal study, however, an increase in hypodiploidy was seen in women but not in men.[93]

Several investigators have also examined structural chromosome and chromatid abnormalities in peripheral lymphocytes.[23,64,65,69,87,88] Though the age trend in specific abnormalities varies from study to study, the overall picture suggests increases in both chromatid and isochromatid breaks in both sexes. One study[66] found a statistically significant increase in stable abnormalities (e.g., translocations).

It has been noted many times that the degree of aneuploidy and/or structural abnormalities seen in tissue culture may reflect the response of the cells to the in vitro conditions of mitogenic stimulation rather than any in vivo lesion. A common approach to this problem has been the comparison of abnormalities in cells from the same donor at various intervals after establishing the culture.[66,69,71] Different studies using this approach have yielded differing results with respect to aneuploidy, showing either an increase, no change, or a decrease with increased time in culture. Thus this question is still quite unclear. Other strategies (e.g., varying the degree of exposure to light or the concentration of various media components) may be useful in this regard.

Studies in human bone marrow[74-76] suggest an age-associated increase in men with 45,X. The results in women, are as yet, inconclusive. The bone marrow series included many patients being evaluated for suspected hematologic disorders. Though the investigators addressed this problem, the possibility of artifactitious relationships (e.g., due to X-ray exposure, medication use, etc.) remains.

With regard to chromosomal structural abnormalities in bone marrow, there are virtually no data on changes with age in man. The data from experimental animals is conflicting.[62,63,84,89,143] However, the predominant picture is of an increase with age in the same abnormalities seen to increase with age in peripheral blood. A comparative study of several species has shown an inverse correlation between species life span and the rate of increase with age in spontaneous bone marrow aberrations.[143]

The number of sister chromatid exchanges have been used as an indicator of genetic damage. Studies on rodent bone marrow, cultured skin fibroblast lines from human donors, and mitogen-stimulated human peripheral blood lymphocytes all indicate no change in spontaneous sister chromatid exchanges as a function of donor age.[88]

Chromosomal structural abnormalities and aneuploidy are the only acquired genetic lesions that have been systematically studied in relation to disease. The vast majority of this work pertains to cancer, and is too extensive to cover here, but has been the subject of numerous reviews.[90-92,139] The following general conclusions have emerged:

1. Most, but not all malignancies have chromosomal abnormalities.
2. In a large number of malignancies, the same abnormalities are found in a high proportion of malignant cells from an affected individual, though the specific abnormality may vary among individuals with the same malignancy.
3. In certain malignancies (e.g., chronic myelogenous leukemia) the same abnormality is found both in the vast majority of malignant cells within an individual and among a high proportion of individuals with the same disorder.
4. Alterations associated with particular malignancies are type-specific. That is, for example, the abnormality found in chronic myelogenous leukemia differs from that in Burkitts's lymphoma.

These findings obviously suggest an etiologic role for chromosomal damage in carcinogenesis. However, as has been noted repeatedly, what has been missing is the demonstration that the chromosomal lesion preceded rather than followed the appearance of malignancy. There is a fairly large body of evidence strongly suggesting that this is so, but it comes largely from in vitro models, from rare human syndromes, or from unusual exposure to radiation or carcinogens. Karyotypic abnormalities have been noted in "premalignant" condition such as carcinoma *in situ* of the cervix, polycythemia vera, and colonic polyps. The development of karyotypically abnormal clones has been reported in patients treated with thorium dioxide sol[94] and $^{32}P$,[95] but obviously these subjects and their exposure are very atypical of the mass population at risk for cancer. Further, though abnormal clones were observed, a progression to malignancy was not. The demonstration of such a progression has yet to be made within a normal subject population and is fraught with difficulties. Nonetheless, it might be possible to follow a population of subjects heterogenous in their degree of karyotypic abnormality in a specific cell type, to examine longitudinal changes in abnormalities, and to relate the incidence of malignancy of that cell type to the degree of antecedent karyotypic abnormality. Presently, the technical problems of obtaining the most suitable tissues, screening a sufficient number of cells from a sufficient number of subjects, and interassay variation seriously limit the applicability of such an approach. One might solve some of the interassay problems by screening a much larger number of cells per individual; but this may have to wait for advances in cytophotometry or other techniques. The application of new banding techniques may also aid in revealing previously unobserved abnormalities in chromosomes from "normal" individuals. These approaches may help to evaluate the role of karyotypic abnormalities in carcinogenesis at an earlier stage than has previously been observed, and may serve as a guide in looking for specific gene products associated with malignant transformation.

Cell cloning techniques could be used to detect changes with age in the number of karyotypically abnormal cells having abnormal proliferative characteristics. Until recently, technical problems have confined this approach to a few cell types, but the development of new culture techniques, particularly for epithelial cells, may allow examination of this question in those cell populations most susceptible to cancer in man.

The other major disease of aging which has been related to karyotypic abnormality is senile dementia. Reports from two laboratories have indicated an unusually high degree of hypodiploidy in mitogen-stimulated peripheral blood lymphocytes from female (but not male) dementia patients relative to age-matched controls.[96-98] Patients with a probable diagnosis of arteriosclerotic dementia appeared to have the same degree of hypodiploidy as controls.[97] The most dramatic excess of hypodiploidy occurred in the demented subjects without a diagnosis of arteriosclerotic etiology. Since the majority of nonarteriosclerotic dementias in the elderly are of the Alzheimer type, this would appear to be the condition associated with excess hypodiploidy in these subjects. As has been noted,[99] however, these studies contain some uncertainty as to the accuracy of diagnosis, and the adequacy of matching cases and controls with respect to health, medication, nutrition, and other factors. Other workers have been unable to confirm the original findings.[66]

If the relationship between hypodiploidy and senile dementia of the Alzheimer type (SDAT) should hold up under controlled studies, it would raise some intriguing questions. The observed lesion is in lymphocytes. What this has to do, if anything, with the specific pathology of SDAT is obviously very unclear. One possibility is that as-yet-undefined chromatin damage (chemical, viral, etc.) is involved in both the development of the abnormal karyotype in lymphocytes and the loss of functional integrity of the neurons affected in Alzheimer's disease. Clearly a prime target to look for such damage would be the neurons involved, but as noted above, histopathologic techniques to study most of the recognized genetic lesions are not yet well developed, and studies of homogenized tissue even from well-defined target areas (e.g., hippocampal cortex) would face major problems because of the great number of cell types in brain tissue. One lesion that might be detected histologically may be the loss of the full neuronal complement of DNA. This possibility is suggested by the possible tendency toward hypodiploidy observed in the lymphocytes of many female SDAT victims. However, the possibility of an analogous change in brain cells is speculative at best.

Heston[107] has offered an hypothesis that may integrate the possible karyotypic abnormalities in SDAT with the neuronal pathology of the disease: incidence of Down's syndrome is high in relatives of non-Down's patients who have Alzheimer's disease and is particularly high in offspring of female relatives of Alzheimer's disease patients. Heston has conjectured that a familial abnormality in tubular and/or fibrillary protein organization could explain this phenomenon, since these proteins are closely involved both in the organization of mitosis and the deranged elements in Alzheimer's disease. Hence it is conceivable that the same lesion could lead to a predisposition to chromosomal nondisjunction with consequent aneuploidy, and to appearance of neurofibrillary tangles. The idea that this lesion could lead to other age-associated pathology is consistent with data showing increased risk for certain hematologic malignancies in relatives of Alzheimer patients[107] and increased risk for acceleration of many age-associated changes in young mothers of Down's syndrome subjects.[142]

This idea illustrates how a defect in extragenetic structures (e.g., tubules) could produce genetic alteration in one cell type (lymphocytes) while quite possibly producing no genetic change in neuronal tissue in SDAT. In this case, karyotypic abnormalities in lymphocytes, even if truly correlated with SDAT, could be an etiologic "red herring" and may actually be only the symptom of a primary tubular/fibrillary lesion.

## IV. OTHER EVIDENCE RELATING GENETIC ALTERATION TO AGE-ASSOCIATED DISEASES

In addition to the direct evidence discussed in the previous section, there is considerable evidence of other types which may be pertinent to the relationship of genetic alteration to age-associated disease. This evidence can be grouped into a few categories.

### A. Syndromes with High Susceptibility to Genetic Damage

(A variation on this theme is the study of heterozygotes not expressing the syndrome, but with some or all of its increased genetic susceptibility, e.g., ataxia telangiectasia heterozygotes.[124]) In evaluating this kind of evidence, certain considerations should be kept in mind.

The association of many age-related conditions (e.g., certain malignancies, dementia) with some syndromes having a high susceptibility to genetic damage has great heuristic value. However, it is risky to extrapolate too freely from these conditions, in which components of the organism's defense system against disease are often grossly deficient. Though genetic damage, by reaching levels far above those appearing in normals, may well become the crucial vector in the diseases seen in these syndromes, the situation in normals may be quite different. Here, genetic damage may be contained to low or trivial levels, well within the ability of other systems to deal with it. (In the case of cancer, such systems include immunologic surveillance mechanisms to destroy small numbers of malignant cells. In the case of dementia, an example might be synaptogenic plasticity, allowing reformation of pathways impaired by normal loss.) In normal individuals, such diseases of aging might appear only when other defenses began to fail. Even if the original "causal" event in such diseases *were* genetic alteration, failures in other systems (leading to the expression of that alteration only in old age) might prove more amenable to study and therapeutic intervention. In such a situation the discussion about which factor was the real "cause" of the disease would be largely semantic. The question of how much the disease might be prevented by lowering the degree of genetic damage vs. raising the performance of other protective systems is of course *not* semantic. Unfortunately, the evidence from the syndromes of grossly high susceptibility to DNA damage, for the reasons discussed above, cannot provide a conclusive answer.

Despite these caveats, it is still tempting to speculate on the implications of the data emerging from these syndromes. The two best characterized are xeroderma pigmentosum (XP) and ataxia telangiectasia (AT). XP may be stereotyped as a syndrome of "long-patch" repair deficiency, with impaired removal of dimers and bulky adducts such as polycyclic hydrocarbons. Ataxia telangiectasia subjects are hypersensitive to ionizing radiation, in part at least through deficiencies in "short-patch" repair processes, which also repair certain chemically-induced lesions, including many alkylation products.[120,138] AT patients have an unusually high incidence of spontaneous chromosome aberrations.[140]

These two diseases are far from being ideal "progeroid" models: many of their characteristics are unique and unlike any normal aging changes. Even in their aspects which mimic diseases of aging (malignancy, dementia, etc.) their specific characteristics differ from these diseases in the elderly. For example, the increased and accelerated malignancy in XP is entirely cutaneous, whereas in AT, there is an increased and accelerated incidence of lymphoreticular malignancy and (to a lesser extent) solid tumors of various types, including some commonly associated with age in normals. Thus the damage handled by "short patch", rather than "long patch", mechanisms may be a more likely suspect in the more common noncutaneous malignancies of aging. This damage appears to include smaller base adducts. There is as yet no information as to what specific adducts of this type (if any) occur in normal individuals.

As mentioned earlier, the histopathologic picture of dementias in repair-deficiency syndromes differs markedly from the common dementias of aging. Nonetheless, it remains of interest that in XP the severity of the dementia appears related to the severity of the repair defect[116] and possibly to the specificity of the defect: XP complementation group D victims, which show exceptionally severe neurological deficits and impairment of unscheduled DNA synthesis following UV irradiation, also seem to have an increased impairment in AP endonuclease function,[141] suggesting a possible role of AP sites in the development of their dementia.

The evidence from the syndromes of high susceptibility to genetic alteration can also serve a useful "negative" role. That is, if a syndrome exhibits grossly impaired protection against a certain class of alteration, and the syndrome does *not* exhibit accelerated or increased incidence of a particular disease of aging, this is a fairly good reason to believe that either (1) the alteration is not the "rate-limiting step" in the pathogenesis of the disease *or* (2) the alteration does not occur under normal circumstances in aging individuals. An example may be the deficiency seen in cells from xeroderma pigmentosum patients in excision repair of DNA adducts formed by polycyclic hydrocarbons and related compounds.[114,135] Since these patients do not appear to have an increased or accelerated incidence of noncutaneous malignancies, this evidence would suggest either that there is no formation of adducts of this type in normal individuals or that it is not the rate-limiting step in the development of noncutaneous malignancies. However, this kind of reasoning must be applied with caution since, from the trends in the growth of knowledge of DNA repair pathways, it seems likely that many more lesion-specific pathways will be revealed. Hence, for example, guesses as to whether a particular adduct is normally or abnormally removed in xeroderma subjects must still be rather tentative in most cases.

### B. "Progeroid" Syndromes and Diseases of Aging

There is a fair amount of this kind of evidence relating to the progeroid diseases such as Werner's syndrome, Hutchinson-Guilford progeria, Down's syndrome, and Cockayne's syndrome.[122] The much sparser literature on diseases of aging includes studies on Huntington's disease,[100] hypertension,[123] lung cancer,[125] and actinic keratoses.[145,151,152] This approach appears to be growing in popularity, and could be used in prospective studies, particularly on populations having unusually high risk for particular diseases. An aspect of genetic alteration that has been widely examined in this regard is susceptibility to viral transformation of cultured cells from individuals at risk for various proliferative disorders.[144]

The fact that a disease shows a high sensitivity to agents causing genetic damage is obviously no guarantee that this sensitivity reflects a lesion responsible for any or all of the other manifestations of that disease. There are two issues that must be addressed in regard to this point: (1) Since all known DNA damaging agents have other molecular targets besides DNA, abnormal sensitivity to the cytoxic effects of these agents does not prove that the preferentially damaged target is DNA. This must be shown experimentally. (2) Assuming that cells from a particular condition do sustain exceptionally high genetic damage by these agents, one should still refrain from concluding that the primary lesion in all cases is closely related to genetic alteration. Clearly the maintenance of genetic functional integrity ultimately depends in part on other cellular systems, e.g., energy production, osmotic equilibrium, maintenance of intracellular compartmentation, etc. Thus it would not be too surprising if a lesion in one of these systems resulted in abnormally high genetic damage by cerain cytotoxic agents. One obvious way of testing whether or not a particular kind of damage is in fact responsible for certain aspects of a disease is to see if they fail to appear if the source of the damage is removed. This has been done in the case of xeroderma pigmentosum, in which patients kept in a low-UV environment show reduced incidence of cutaneous malignancy. In most other "damage-susceptible conditions", however, knowledge of what damaging agents might actually be responsible for the disease is so scant that testing hypotheses by this approach would be premature, even if the experiment were technically feasible.

Evidence from progeroid conditions can serve a useful "negative" role in a manner analogous to that described above for the repair deficiency syndromes. If such a disorder has *no* demonstrable abnormal sensitivity to agents causing genetic alteration, this fact would argue against genetic alteration being a principal cause of its associated pathology. This point has been made by Tice.[157] One must, however, bear in mind that lack of increased sensitivity in a progeroid syndrome to agents producing genetic alteration does not logically imply that this sensitivity has no role in producing the pathologic changes in normals which are accelerated in the progeroids. Some factor other than high sensitivity may cause the acceleration of the condition in the progeroids, while genetic alteration itself is the underlying basis of the disease in normals. In addition, it is possible that a disease may be caused by a type of genetic alteration which is not produced by the commonly used probes for sensitivity to genetic damage or which is not detectable by current techniques. Such a condition would remain a "false negative" in this kind of testing until a suitable damaging agent or detection technique were found. Finally, a progeroid condition or age-associated disease might be caused by genetic alteration, but not show abnormal sensitivity to exogenous agents producing genetic alteration, if the fundamental defect was increased endogenous production of agents producing genetic alteration. There is evidence for such factors in Bloom's syndrome[159] and ataxia telangiectasia.

Despite all the above *caveats,* it remains striking that in several progressive degenerative neurologic diseases, including Huntington's disease,[100] ataxia telangiectasia,[101] hereditary olivopontocerebellar atrophy, and several others,[102,103] non-neuronal cells show abnormally high sensitivity to ionizing radiation. (Sensitivity of neuronal tissue has not been examined.) In some cases hypersensitivity to *N*-methyl-*N'*-nitro-*N*-nitrosoguanidine has been shown as well. Interestingly, in ataxia telangectasia and Huntington's disease the sensitivity to UV seems normal.

Though these findings demonstrate that neuronal degenerative disease may indeed be associated with increased susceptibility to DNA-damaging agents, they obviously must be interpreted with caution, especially when speculating on the relationship of such findings to the more common neural degenerative diseases of aging, for example senile dementia of the Alzheimer type (SDAT). None of the degenerative diseases thus far studied (including those with progressive dementia as a component) has any of the cytopathologic changes characteristic of SDAT. (This applies as well, as far as can be determined, to the progressive dementia associated with xeroderma pigmentosum, though the number of neuropathologic studies[105,106] is too small to yield much certainty on this point). A second distinction between SDAT and the above-mentioned disorders is that the latter are all strongly hereditary, generally showing simple autosomal dominant or recessive transmission. Though a rare familial form of Alzheimer's disease exists, and though there is a considerable familial tendency in SDAT, it clearly is not of the same hereditary nature as the degenerative disorders thus far associated with increased susceptibility to DNA damage. This obviously does not rule a relationship between DNA damage and SDAT, but it suggests that such a relationship, if any, may be even more complex than that seen in the hereditary disorders.

Before leaving the subject of the association of specific diseases and predisposition to genetic alteration, one obvious point to be stressed is that the overwhelming bulk of the data on this subject is from "case-control" studies. In these studies, the possibility always exists that differences in predisposition to genetic alteration between cases and controls are secondary to the symptom(s) of the disease and not vice versa.

### C. Interspecies Comparisons

The few studies of this type have examined unscheduled DNA synthesis following UV irradiation[126-129] and susceptibility to DNA damage by certain metabolically activated carcinogens.[131-133] Generally, unscheduled DNA synthesis correlated positively and metabolic activation of polycyclic hydrocarbons correlated negatively, with species life span.

In these studies, one must remember that these correlations may reflect other species factors besides longevity. This is suggested by recent results comparing fibroblasts from a number of primates (including man) with other species in their capacity to perform unscheduled DNA synthesis after UV irradiation[128] indicating that primates of widely differing life spans have similar high degrees of repair in this system. Though these are some methodologic problems in this work, it suggests that other interspecies correlations of life span with repair capacity[126] may in part reflect genetic differences unrelated to life span *per se*. However, among mice, the correlation of repair synthesis with life span holds up even among different strains of the same species.[127,129]

### D. Experimental Models of Genetic Damage and Diseases of Aging

One could clarify the role of genetic alteration by attempting to induce various diseases of aging (or diseases sufficiently like them to be used as models) by agents causing genetic damage. The problem could also be addressed by the converse strategy of examining the prophylactic effect of agents protecting against specific types of genetic damage. In addition, known or suspected etiologic or protective factors in diseases of aging could be examined for their capacity to produce or prevent genetic alteration. The overwhelming preponderance of work using these approaches has been on cancer.[45,134,137] The strategy has been used in relation to senile dementia of the Alzheimer type in a study demonstrating induction of unscheduled DNA synthesis by aluminum,[136] which has been suggested to play a role in the development of this disease.

## V. GENETIC ALTERATION AND "PRE-MORBID" CONDITIONS OF AGING

The previous two sections have outlined approaches which could provide information on the relationship of genetic alteration to diseases of aging. This section returns to a consideration mentioned earlier in this chapter — the notion that genetic alteration may contribute to these diseases, not by directly producing their specific pathophysiologic changes, but by producing some "pre-morbid" condition — some loss of function which predisposes to the development of a disease. The most obvious general lesions of this sort are (1) cell death, (2) impaired cell proliferation, and (3) impaired transcription. (The latter two lesions could appear either as inappropriate decreases or increases. Transcription could also be impaired by an increase in error frequency.) Data consistent with one or more of these processes have been found in aging studies of several tissues. In certain instances an association exists between one of these impairments and specific pathology. For example, increased cerebral cortical cell loss relative to age-matched controls has been demonstrated in senile dementia of the Alzheimer type[153] and decreased cell proliferation coexists with the decline in cellular immunity seen in the elderly,[154] while increased cell proliferation is found in benign prostatic hypertrophy.

Clearly, a major question that has yet to be conclusively answered is the contribution of genetic alteration to cell death or impaired proliferation or transcription in specific pathologic conditions. The problem of the role of genetic alteration in cell death is difficult, but not impossible to address. A major problem is that in terms of direct evidence of genetic damage, "dead cells tell no tales", or the tales they tell are hard to interpret, since genetic damage may be secondary to cell death. Further, though cell death may be an important process in many diseases of aging, the actual percentage of intact dead or dying cells in the pertinent tissue at any one time may be very low. Hence techniques of selectively examining moribund cells would have considerable advantage (though in many cases the problem of interpreting genetic damage as cause vs. effect would remain). By adaptation of vital staining techniques or other indices of viability combined with histologic assays of DNA damage, damage in dead or dying cells could be specifically identified. Another approach might be the use of cell sorting technology to get enriched populations of dead or dying cells on which to perform measurements of genetic damage. In this case as well, some type of vital staining could be the basis of cell separation; other properties which may correlate with viability (density, surface charge, etc.) may be of use. Obviously, such approaches are very speculative at this time, and it remains to be seen whether the requisite techniques can be developed, not to mention whether they will yield any useful information.

A strategy which has well served investigators in carcinogenesis might be usefully applied to this problem: much of the evidence for the role of genetic damage in carcinogenesis is based on comparative studies relating the carcinogenicity of a compound with the degree of genetic damage it produces vs. the degree of other types of damage. The high correlations of carcinogenicity with genetic damage, and the lesser correlations with other types of damage, are considered to be evidence for the important role of genetic damage in carcinogenesis. By analogy, one could undertake studies using factors causally implicated in diseases associated with specific cell loss, and determine to what extent their potency in producing the disease-specific cell loss correlated with genetic damage in those cells. The production of a high degree of genetic damage in the cell types involved in the disease vs. uninvolved cell types, a good correlation of the degree of genetic damage produced by a variety of agents with the degree of cell loss produced, and a *poor* correlation of other types of damage with this cell loss, would all imply a role for genetic damage in the development of the disease.

In looking for relationships between genetic alteration and impaired cell proliferation and/or transcription, strategies analogous to those discussed above for cell death may be useful. For example, techniques for obtaining enriched populations of dividing or nondividing cells are already in use.

One problem in relating genetic alteration to altered transcription is that such alterations may be confined to a subset of the genome. Differing rates of repair in different regions of chromatin[155,156] suggest that there may be considerable heterogeneity in the damage accumulated in different regions of chromatin, depending on their various structural and functional properties. If damage preferentially occurred in a particular subset of the genome, it clearly would be advantageous to look selectively at that subset. For example, it seems possible that actively transcribing genes might show altered rates of damage and/or repair. In examining a condition with a demonstrated or suspected impairment in transcription of a particular gene or genes, it would seem desirable to get enriched or purified preparations of that gene. Many such approaches would of course involve extensive processing and hence fail to detect many alterations (e.g., in tertiary structure) that could have selective effects on particular genes. Nonetheless, the approach could greatly increase the sensitivity toward certain lesions (e.g., base defects) if indeed they were concentrated in particular genes.

A final consideration bears on the potential complexities of the pathways which may relate genetic alteration to disease. Instead of leading directly to a disease, a class of genetic alterations may result in a second class of genetic alterations which produce the disease or cause still further changes which produce the disease. Studies on malignant transformation indicate that this may be a common event in carcinogenesis, with initial genetic damage producing changes in gene expression and chromosomal organization which result in overt malignancy only after a series of stages. If similar progressions exist in other disease of aging it would seem that "prospective" studies of the tissues eventually involved would be essential in clarifying the relationship of genetic alteration to the disease.

## ACKNOWLEDGMENTS

I am grateful to Drs. Jerry Williams and Kerry Dearfield for allowing me to read their review (Reference 17) prior to its publication, and to Janet Galvagna, Lisa Burall, Cheryl King, and Joanna Badinelli for their assistance in preparing this manuscript.

## REFERENCES

1. **Poirier, M. C., Yuspa, S. H., Weinstein, I. B., and Blobstein, S.,** Detection of carcinogen-DNA adducts by radioimmunoassay, *Nature (London)*, 270, 186, 1977.
2. **Lindahl, T.,** DNA glycosylases and endonucleases for apurinic/apyrimidinic sites and base excision repair, *Progr. Nucl. Acid Res. Mol. Biol.*, 22, 135, 1979.
3. **Roberts, J. J.,** The repair of DNA modified by cytotoxic, mutagenic, and carcinogenic compounds, *Adv. Radiat. Biol.*, 7, 211, 1978.

4. **Drake, J. W. and Baltz, R. H.**, The biochemistry of mutagenesis, *Ann. Rev. Biochem.*, 45, 11, 1976.
5. **Brash, D. E. and Hart, R. W.**, DNA damage and repair *in vivo, J. Environ. Pathobiol. Toxicol.*, 2, 79, 1978.
6. **Lett, J. T., Keng, P. C., and Sun, C.**, Rejoining of DNA strand breaks in nondividing cells irradiated *in situ*, in *DNA Repair Mechanisms (ICN-UCLA Symposia on Molecular and Cellular Biology 9)*, Hanawalt, P. C., Friedburg, E. C., and Fox, C. F., Eds., Academic Press, New York, 1978, 481.
7. **Wheeler, K. T. and Lett, J. T.**, On the possibility that DNA repair is related to age in non-dividing cells, *Proc. Natl. Acad. Sci. USA*, 71, 1862, 1974.
8. **Mirzabekov, A. D., Shick, V. V., Belyavsfy, A. V., and Bavyfin, S. G.**, Primary organization of nucleosome core particle of chromatin: sequence of histone arrangement along DNA, *Proc. Natl. Acad. Sci. USA*, 75, 4184, 1978.
9. **Ono, T., Okada, S., and Sugahara, T.**, Comparative studies of DNA size in various tissues of mice during the aging process, *Exp. Gerontol.*, 11, 127, 1976.
10. **Tas, S.**, Involvement of disulfide bonds in the condensed structure of facultative heterochromatin and implications on cellular differentiation and aging, *Gerontology*, 24, 358, 1978.
11. **Von Sonntag, C. and Schultz-Frohlinde, D.**, Radiation-induced degradation of the sugar in model compounds and in DNA, *Mol. Biol. Biochem. Biophys.*, 27, 204, 1978.
12. **Von Sonntag, C. and Schultz-Frohlinde, D.**, Radiation-induced degradation of the base-component in DNA and related substances — final products, *Mol. Biol. Biochem. Biophys.*, 27, 171—203, 1978.
13. **Ormerod, M. G.**, Radiation-induced strand breaks in the DNA of mammalian cells, in *Biology of Radiation Carcinogenesis*, Yuhas, J. M., Temnant, R. W., and Regan, J. D., Eds., Raven Press, New York, 1976, 67.
14. **Williams, J. R.**, DNA strand breaks: patterns of induction and rejoining in mammalian cells, in *DNA Repair Processes*, Nichols, W. W. and Murphy, D. G., Eds., Symposia Specialists, Miami, 1977, 73.
15. **Schneider, E. L.**, Cytogenetics of aging, in *The Genetics of Aging*, Schneider, E. L., Ed., Plenum Press, New York, 1978, 27.
16. **Hamerton, J. L.**, *Human Cytogenetics*, Academic Press, New York, 1971.
17. **Williams, J. R. and Dearfield, K. L.**, DNA damage and repair in aging mammals, in *CRC Handbook Series on Aging*, Section D, Biological Sciences, Vol. 1 (Biochemistry), Florini, J. R., Ed., 1981.
18. **Strehler, B. and Johnson, R.**, Loss of genes coding for rRNA in aging brain cells, *Nature (London)*, 240, 412, 1972.
19. **Strehler, B. L., Chang, M. P., and Johnson, L. K.**, Loss of hybridizable ribosomal DNA from human post-mitotic tissues during aging. I. Age-dependent loss in human myocardium, *Mech. Ageing Dev.*, 11, 371, 1979.
20. **Strehler, B. L., Chang, M. P., and Johnson, L. K.**, Loss of hybridizable ribosomal DNA from human post-mitotic tissues during aging II. Age-dependent loss in human cerebral cortex — hippocompal and somatosensory cortex comparison, *Mech. Ageing Dev.*, 11, 379, 1979.
21. **Gaubatz, J., Prashad, N., and Cutler, R. G.**, Ribosomal RNA gene dosage as a function of tissue and age for mouse and human, *Biochem. Biophys. Acta*, 418, 358, 1976.
22. **Gaubatz, J. S. and Cutler, R. G.**, Age-related differences in the number of ribosomal RNA genes of mouse tissues, *Gerontology*, 24, 179, 1978.
23. **Deknudt, A. and Leonard, A.**, Ageing and radiosensitivity of human somatic chromosomes, *Exp. Gerontol.*, 12, 237, 1977.
24. **Von Hahn, H. P.**, Structural and functional changes in nucleoprotein during the ageing of the cell, *Gerontologia*, 16, 116, 1970.
25. **Russell, A. P., Dowling, L. F., and Herrman, R. L.**, Age-related differences in mouse liver DNA melting and hydroxylapatite fractionation, *Gerontologia*, 16, 159, 1970.
26. **Kurtz, D. I., Russell, A. P., and Sinex, F. M.**, Multiple peaks in the derivative melting curve of chromatin from animals of varying age, *Mech. Ageing Dev.*, 3, 37, 1974.
27. **Pyhtila, M. J. and Sherman, F. G.**, Age-associated studies on thermal stability and template effectiveness of DNA and nucleoproteins from beef thymus, *Biochem. Biophys. Res. Comm.*, 31, 340, 1968.
28. **Hart, R. W., D'Ambrosio, S. M., Ng, K. J., and Modak, S. P.**, Longevity, stability and DNA repair, *Mech. Ageing Dev.*, 9, 203, 1979.
29. **Herrman, R. L., Dowling, L., Russell, A. P., and Bick, M. D.**, Age-related changes in a spontaneously reassociating fraction of mouse DNA, *Mech. Ageing Dev.*, 4, 181, 1975.
30. **Sondergaard, J., Lerche, A., Bohn, V., Lerche, V., and Wadsbov, S.**, DNA in psoriatic epidermis, *Derm. Venereol.*, 87, 59, 1979.
31. **Lawley, P. D.**, Effect of some chemical mutagens and carcinogens on nucleic acids, *Progr. Nucl. Acad. Res. Mol. Biol.*, 5, 89, 1966.

32. **Cutler, R. G.,** Cross-linkage hypothesis of aging; DNA adducts in chromatin as a primary aging process, in *Aging, Carcinogenesis, and Radiation Biology,* Smith, K. C., Ed., Plenum Press, New York, 1976, 443.
33. **Price, G. P., Modak, S. P., and Makinodan, T.,** Age-associated changes in the DNA of mouse tissue, *Science,* 171, 917, 1971.
34. **Nakanishi, K., Shima, A., Fukuda, M., and Fujita, S.,** Age associated increase of single-stranded regions in the DNA of mouse brain and liver cells, *Mech. Ageing Dev.,* 10, 273, 1979.
35. **Chetsanga, C. J., Boyd, V., Peterson, L., and Rushlow, K.,** Single-stranded regions in DNA of old mice, *Nature (London),* 253, 130, 1975.
36. **Chetsanga, C. J., Tuttle, M., and Jacoboni, A.,** Changes in structural integrity of heart DNA from aging mice, *Life Sci.,* 18, 1405, 1976.
37. **Chetsanga, C. J., Tuttle, M., Jacoboni, A., and Johnson, C.,** Age-associated structural alterations in senescent mouse brain DNA, *Biochem. Biophys. Acta,* 474, 180, 1977.
38. **Natali, P. C. and Tan, E. M.,** Immunological detection of thymidine photoproduct formation *in vivo, Radiat. Res.,* 46, 506, 1977.
39. **Sinex, F. M. and Gerstenfeld, L.,** Proteins in the aging nucleus, *Age,* 2, 125, 1979.
40. **Acharya, P. V. N.,** The isolation and partial characterization of age-correlated oligo-deoxyribo-ribonucleotides with covalently linked aspartyl-glutamyl polypeptides, *Johns Hopkins Med. J. Suppl.,* 1, 254, 1972.
41. **Masore, H. R., Bard, M. B., Nicolosi, R. J., and Samis, H. V.,** Changes in the structure of rat liver DNA relation to age, *Arch. Biochem. Biophys.,* 153, 736, 1972.
42. **Karran, P. and Ormerod, M. G.,** Is the ability to repair damage to DNA related to the proliferative capacity of a cell? The rejoining of x-ray induced strand breaks, *Biochem. Biophys. Acta,* 299, 54, 1973.
43. **Kornhauser, A.,** UV-induced DNA protein crosslinks *in vitro* and *in vivo, Photochem. Photobiol.,* 23, 457, 1976.
44. **Schoen, A. E., Cooks, R. G., and Webers, J. L.,** Modified bases characterized in intact DNA by mass-analyzed ion kinetic energy spectrometry, *Science,* 203, 1249, 1979.
45. **Smith, K. C., Ed.,** *Aging, Carcinogenesis and Radiation Biology: The Role of Nucleic Acid Addition Reactions,* Plenum Press, New York, 1975.
46. **Sheid, B., Pedrinan, L., Lu, T., and Nelson, T. H.,** Single-stranded regions in DNA from pre- and post-menopausal human ovaries, *Biochem. Biophys. Res. Comm.,* 66, 1131, 1975.
47. **Ermini, M., Moret, M. L., Reichlmeier, K., and Danne, T.,** Age-dependent structural changes in human chromatin, *Akt. Gerontol.,* 8, 675, 1978.
48. **Gaubatz, J., Ellis, M., and Chalkley, R.,** Nuclease digestion studies of mouse chromatin as a function of age, *J. Gerontol.,* 34, 672, 1979.
49. **Zhelabovskaya, S. and Berdyshev, G.,** Composition, template activity and thermostability of the liver chromatin in rats of various ages, *Exp. Gerontol.,* 7, 313, 1972.
50. **Berdyshev, G. D.,** Age-dependent changes of *in vitro* transcription activities of animals, *Interdiscip. Top. Gerontol.,* 10, 70, 1976.
51. **O'Meara, A. R. and Herrman, R. L.,** A modified mouse liver chromatin preparation displaying age-related differences in salt dissociation and template ability, *Biochem. Biophys. Acta,* 269, 419, 1972.
52. **Shirey, T. L. and Sobel, H.,** Compositional and transcriptional properties of chromatins isolated from cardiac muscle of young-mature and old dogs, *Exp. Gerontol.,* 7, 15, 1972.
53. **Stein, A. S., Wang, P. L., and Adelman, R. C.,** Age-dependent changes in the structure and function of mammalian chromatin. I. Variations in chromatin template activity, *Exp. Gerontol.,* 8, 123, 1973.
54. **Salser, J. S. and Balis, M. E.,** Alterations in deoxyribonucleic acid-bound amino acids with age and sex, *J. Gerontol.,* 27, 1, 1972.
55. **Smith, K. C.,** Chemical adducts to deoxyribonucleic acid. Their importance to the genetic alteration theory of aging, *Interdiscip. Top. Gerontol.,* 9, 16, 1976.
56. **Kreamer, W., Zarich, N., Liu, D. S. H., and Richardson, A.,** Effect of age on RNA synthesis by rat hepatocytes, *Exp. Gerontol.,* 14, 27, 1979.
57. **Stevenson, K. and Curtis, H.,** Chromosome aberrations in irradiated and nitrogen mustard treated mice, *Radiat. Res.,* 15, 774, 1961.
58. **Crowley, C. and Curtis, H. J.,** The development of somatic mutations in mice with age, *Proc. Natl. Acad. Sci. USA,* 49, 626, 1963.
59. **Curtis, H. J., Leith, J., and Tilley, J.,** Chromosomal aberrations in liver cells of dogs of different ages, *J. Gerontol.,* 21, 268, 1966.
60. **Curtis, H. J. and Miller, K.,** Chromosome aberrations in liver cells of guinea pigs, *J. Gerontol.,* 26, 292, 1971.
61. **Brooks, A. L., Mead, D. K., and Peters, R. F.,** Effect of aging on the frequency of metaphase chromosome aberrations in the liver of the chinese hamster, *J. Gerontol.,* 28, 452, 1973.

62. **Chlebovsky, D., Praslicka, M., and Horak, J.,** Chromosome aberrations: increased incidence in bone marrow of continuously irradiated rats, *Science,* 153, 195, 1966.
63. **Curtis, H. and Tilley, J.,** The life-span of dividing mammalian cells *in vivo, J. Gerontol.,* 26, 1, 1971.
64. **Liniecki, J., Bajerska, A., and Andryszek, C.,** Chromosomal aberrations in human lymphocytes irradiated *in vitro* from donors (male and female) of varying age, *Int. J. Radiat. Biol.,* 4, 349, 1971.
65. **Bochkov, N. P.,** Spontaneous chromosome aberrations in human somatic cells, *Humangenetik,* 16, 159, 1972.
66. **Galloway, S. M. and Buckton, K. E.,** Aneuploidy and ageing: chromosome studies on a random sample of the population using G-banding, *Cytogenet. Cell. Genet.,* 20, 78, 1978.
67. **Ayme, S., Mattei, J. F., Mattel, M. G., Aurran, J., and Giraud, F.,** Nonrandom distribution of chromosome breaks in cultured lymphocytes of normal subjects, *Hum. Genet.,* 31, 161, 1976.
68. **Jarvik, L. and Kato, T.,** Chromosome examinations in aged twins, *Am. J. Human Genet.,* 22, 562, 1970.
69. **Mattevi, M. S. and Salzano, F. M.,** Senescence & human chromosome changes, *Humangenetik,* 27, 1, 1975.
70. **Jacobs, P. A., Court Brown, W. M., and Doll, R.,** Distribution of human chromosome counts in relation to age, *Nature (London),* 191, 1178, 1961.
71. **Court-Brown, W. M., Buckton, K. E., Jacobs, P. A., Tough, I. M., Kuenssberg, E. V., and Knox, J. D. E.,** Chromosome studies on adults, *Eugene. Lab. Mem.,* 42, 1, 1966.
72. **Hamerton, J. L., Taylor, A. I., Angell, R., and McGuire, V. M.,** Chromosome investigations of a small isolated human population: Chromosome abnormalities and distribution of chromosome counts according to age and sex among the population of Tristan da Cunha, *Nature (London),* 206, 1232, 1965.
73. **Sandberg, A. A., Cohen, M. M., Rimm, A. A., and Levin, M. L.,** Aneuploidy and age in a population survey, *Am. J. Hum. Genet.,* 19, 633, 1967.
74. **Cadotte, M. and Fraser, D.,** Etude de l'aneuploidie observee dans les cultures de sang et de moelle en fonction du mombre et de longeur des chromosomes de chaque groups et de l'age et du sexe des sujets, *Union Med. Can.,* 99, 2003, 1970.
75. **Pierre, R. V. and Hoagland, H. C.,** 45, X cell lines in adult men: loss of Y chromosome, a normal aging phenomenon? *Mayo Clin. Proc.,* 46, 52, 1971.
76. **Pierre, R. V. and Hoagland, H. C.,** Age-associated aneuploidy: loss of Y chromosome from human bone marrow cells with aging, *Cancer,* 30, 889, 1972.
77. **Fang, J. S., Jagiello, G., Ducayen, M., and Graffeo, J.,** Aging and X chromosome loss in the human ovary, *Obstet. Gynecol.,* 45, 455, 1975.
80. **Nielsen, J.,** Chromosomes in senile, presenile, and arteriosclerotic dementia, *J. Gerontol.,* 25, 312, 1970.
81. **Kadontani, T., Ohama, K., Nakoyama, T., Takahara, H., and Makino, S.,** Chromosome aberrations in leukocytes of normal adults from 49 couples, *Proc. Jpn. Acad.,* 47, 724, 1971.
82. **Jacobs, P. A., Brunton, M., Court Brown, W. M., Doll, R., and Goldstein, H.,** Change in human chromosome count distributions with age: evidence of a sex difference, *Nature (London),* 197, 1080, 1963.
83. **Tas, S., Tam, C. F., and Walford, R. L.,** Disulfide bonds and the structure of the chromatin complex in relation to aging, *Mech. Ageing Dev.,* 12, 65, 1980.
84. **McFee, A. F., Banner, M. W., and Sherrill, M. N.,** Influence of animal age on radiation-induced chromosome aberrations in swine leukocytes, *Radiat. Res.,* 41, 425, 1970.
85. **Kurtz, D. I. and Sinex, F. M.,** Age-related differences in the association of brain DNA and nuclear protein, *Biochem. Biophys. Acta,* 145, 840, 1967.
86. **Bochkov, N. P. and Kuleshov, N. P.,** Age sensitivity of human chromosomes to alkylating agents, *Mutat. Res.,* 14, 345, 1972.
87. **Ivanov, B., Praskova, L., Mileva, M., Bulanova, M., and Georgieva, I.,** Spontaneous chromosomal aberration levels in human peripheral lymphocytes, *Mutat. Res.,* 52, 421, 1978.
88. **Schneider, E. L., Kram, D., Nakanishi, Y., and Monticone, R. E.,** The effect of aging on sister chromatid exchange, *Mech. Age Dev.,* 9, 303, 1979.
89. **Dzhemilev, Z. A., Mochavariani, M. G., and Bologovskaya, Z. H.,** Study of spontaneous chromosome aberration rates in monkey cells depending on age and sex of the animals, *Tsitol. Genet. (Acad. Nauk Ukn. SSR),* 2, 424, 1973.
90. **Rowley, J. D.,** Chromosomes in malignancies, in *Human Genetics,* Armendares, S. and Lister, R., Eds., Excerpta Medica, Oxford, 1976, 69.
91. **Harnden, D. G.,** The relationship between induced chromosome aberrations and chromosome abnormality in tumor cells, in *Human Genetics,* Armendares, S. and Lister, R., Eds., Excerpta Medica, Oxford, 1976, 355.

92. **Harnden, D. G.**, Cytogenetics of human neoplasia, in *Genetics of Human Cancer,* Mulvihill, J. J., Miller, R. W., and Fraumeni, J. F., Jr., Eds., Raven Press, New York, 1977, 87.
93. **Jarvik, L. F., Yen, F. S., Fu, T. K., and Matsuyama, S. S.**, Chromosomes in old age: a six year longitudinal study, *Hum. Genet.,* 33, 17, 1976.
94. **Court Brown, W. M., Buckton, K. E., Longlands, A. O., and Woodcock, G. E.**, The identification of lymphocyte clones, with chromosome structural aberrations in irradiated men and women, *Int. J. Rad. Biol.,* 13, 155, 1967.
95. **Lawler, S. D., Millard, R. E., and Kay, H. E. M.**, Further cytogenetical studies in polycythemia vera, *Eur. J. Cancer,* 6, 223, 1970.
96. **Nielsen, J.**, Chromosomes in senile dementia, *Br. J. Psychiatr.,* 114, 303, 1968.
97. **Nielsen, J.**, Chromosomes in senile, presenile, and arteriosclerotic dementia, *J. Gerontol.,* 25, 312, 1970.
98. **Jarvik, L. F., Altshuler, K. Z., Kato, T., and Blumner, B.**, Organic brain syndrome and chromosome loss in aged twins, *Dis. Nerv. Sys.,* 32, 159, 1971.
99. **Cohen, D.**, A behavioral-chromosome relationship in the elderly: a critical review of a biobehavioral hypothesis, *Exp. Aging Res.,* 2, 271, 1976.
100. **Moshell, A. N., Barrett, S. F., Tarone, R. E., and Robbins, J. H.**, Radiosensitivity in Huntington's disease: implications for pathogenesis and presymptomatic diagnosis, *Lancet,* 9, 1980.
101. **Paterson, M. G. and Smith, P. G.**, Ataxia telangietasia: an inherited disorder involving hypersensitivity to ionizing radiation and related DNA-damaging chemicals, *Ann. Rev. Genet.,* 13, 291, 1979.
102. **Robbins, J. H., Moshell, A. N., Scarpinato, S. G., and Tarone, R. E.**, Cells from patients with olivopontocerebellar atrophy and familial dysautonomia are hypersensitive to ionizing radiation, *Clin. Res.,* 28, 290A, 1980.
103. **Moshell, A. N., Scarpinato, R. G., Tarone, R. E., and Robbins, J. H.**, Cells from a patient with tuberous sclerosis are abnormally sensitive to radiation (abs.), *Clin. Res.,* 28, 576A, 1980.
104. **Andrews, A. D., Barrett, S. F., and Robbins, J. H.**, Xeroderma pigmentosum neurological abnormalities correlate with colony-forming ability after ultraviolet radiation, *Proc. Natl. Acad. Sci. USA,* 75, 1984, 1978.
105. **Reed, W., Landing, B., Sugarman, G., et. al.**, Xeroderma pigmentosum: clinical and laboratory investigation of its basic defect, *JAMA,* 207, 2073, 1969.
106. **Hokkanen, E., Iivanainen, M., and Waltimo, O.**, Zu den neurologischen Manifestation des Xeroderma pigmentosum, *Deutsch. Z. Nervenhielk.,* 196, 208, 1969.
107. **Heston, L. L.**, Alzheimer's disease and senile dementia: genetic relationships to Down's syndrome and hematologic cancer, in *Congenital and Acquired Cognitive Disorders,* Katzman, R., Ed., Raven Press, New York, 1979, 167.
108. **Yunis, J. J., Ed.**, *New Chromosomal Syndromes,* Academic Press, New York, 1977.
109. **Berkowitz, E. M., Sanborn, A. C., and Riggs, E. A.**, Chromosomal aging changes in neuronal and neuroglial cell nuclei (abs.), *The Gerontologist,* 20, 5, 1980.
110. **Hart, R. W., D'Ambrosio, S., Ng, K. J., and Modak, S. P.**, Longevity, stability and DNA repair, *Mech. Ageing Dev.,* 9, 203, 1979.
111. **Orgel, L. E.**, The maintenance of the accuracy of protein synthesis and the relevance to aging, *Proc. Natl. Acad. Sci. USA,* 49, 517, 1963.
112. **Burnet, Macfarlane**, *Intrinsic Mutagenesis: A Genetic Approach to Ageing,* John Wiley & Sons, New York, 1974.
113. **Martin, R.**, A possible genetic mechanism of aging, rejuvenation, and recombination in germinal cells, in *Molecular Human Cytogenetics,* Sparkes, R. S., Comings, D. E., and Fox, C. F., Eds., Academic Press, N.Y., 1977, 355.
114. **Amacher, D. E. and Lieberman, M. W.**, Removal of acetylaminoflourene from the DNA of control and repair deficient human fibroblasts, *Biochem. Biophys. Res. Comm.,* 74, 285, 1977.
115. **Robbins, J. H.**, Yearly review: new forms of disease with DNA repair defects, *Photochem. Photobiol.,* 30, 739, 1979.
116. **Robbins, J**, Significance of repair of human DNA: evidence from studies of xeroderma pigmentosum, *J. Natl. Canc. Inst.,* 61, 645, 1978.
117. **Friedberg, E. C., Ehmann, U. K., and Williams, J. E.**, Human diseases associated with defective DNA repair, *Adv. Radiat. Biol.,* 8, 85, 1979.
118. **Weichselbaum, R. R. and Little, J. B.**, Familial retinoblastoma and ataxia telangietasia: human models for the study of DNA damage and repair, *Cancer,* 45, 775, 1980.
119. **Setlow, R. B.**, Repair deficient human disorders and cancer, *Nature (London),* 271, 713, 1978.
120. **Scudiero, D. A. and Robbins, J. H.**, Fibroblasts from Huntington's Disease and other neurodegenerations are hypersensitive to killing by N-methyl-N′-nitrosoguanidine (abs.), *Clin. Res.,* 28, 290A, 1980.
121. **Arlett, C. F. and Lehmann, A. R.**, Human disorders showing increased sensitivity to the induction of genetic damage, *Ann. Rev. Genet.,* 12, 95, 1978.

122. **Hoar, D. I. and Waghorne, C.**, DNA repair in Cockayne's syndrome, *Am. J. Human Genet.*, 30, 590, 1978.
123. **Pero, R. W., Bryngelsson, C., Mitelman, F., Thulin, T., and Norden, A.**, High blood pressure related to carcinogen-induced unscheduled DNA synthesis. DNA carcinogen binding, and chromosomal aberrations in human lymphocytes, *Proc. Natl. Acad. Sci. USA*, 73, 2496, 1976.
124. **Swift, M.**, Malignant neoplasms in heterozygous carriers of genes for certain autosomal recessive syndromes, in *Genetics of Human Cancer*, Mulvihill, J. J., Miller, R. W., and Fraumeni, J. F., Eds., Raven Press, New York, 1977, 209.
125. **Rudiger, H. W., Marxen, J., Kohl, F. V., Melderis, H., and Von Wichert, P.**, Metabolism and formation of DNA adducts of benzo(a)pyrene in human diploid fibroblasts, *Cancer Res.*, 39, 1083, 1979.
126. **Hart, R. W. and Setlow, R. P.**, Correlation between deoxyribonucleic acid excision-repair and lifespan in a number of mammalian species, *Proc. Natl. Acad. Sci. USA*, 71, 2169, 1974.
127. **Hart, R. W., Sacher, G. A., and Hoskins, T. L.**, DNA repair in a short and a long lived rodent species, *J. Gerontol.*, 34, 808, 1979.
128. **Kato, H., Harada, M., Tsuchuya, K., and Moriwaki, K.**, Absence of correlation between DNA repair in ultraviolet irradiated mammalian cells and lifespan of the donor species, *Jpn. J. Genet.*, 55, 99, 1980.
129. **Paffenholz, V.**, Correlation between DNA repair of embryonic fibroblasts and different life spans of three inbred mouse strains, *Aktuel Gerontol.*, 8, 419, 1978.
130. **Hanawalt, P. C., Cooper, P. K., Ganesan, A. K., and Smith, C. A.**, DNA repair in bacteria & mammalian cells, *Ann. Rev. Biochem.*, 48, 783, 1979.
131. **Schwartz, A. G. and Moore, C. J.**, Inverse correlation between species life span and capacity of cultured fibroblasts to bind 7, 12, dimethylbenz(a)anthracene to DNA, *Exp. Cell Res.*, 109, 448, 1977.
132. **Schwartz, A. G.**, Correlation between species life span and capacity to activate 7, 12-dimethylbenz(a)anthracene to a form mutagenic to mammalian cells, *Exp. Cell Res.*, 94, 445, 1975.
133. **Moore, C. J. and Schwartz, A. G.**, Inverse correlation between species lifespan and capacity of cultured fibroblasts to convert benzo(a)pyrene to water soluble metabolites, *Exp. Cell Res.*, 116, 359, 1978.
134. **Grover, P. L., Ed.**, *Chemical Carcinogens and DNA*, CRC Press, Boca Raton, Fla., 1979.
135. **McCaw, B. A., Dipple, A., Young, S., and Roberts, J. J.**, Excision of hydrocarbon — DNA adducts and consequent cell survival in normal and repair defective human cells, *Chem. Biol. Interact.*, 22, 139, 1978.
136. **DeBoni, U., Seger, M., and Crapper, D.**, Interaction of aluminum and chromatin in human cells *in vitro* as assessed by DNA repair, *Age*, 2, 125, 1979.
137. **Wattenberg, L. W.**, Inhibitors of chemical carcinogenesis, *Adv. Cancer Res.*, 26, 197, 1978.
138. **Smith, P. J. and Paterson, M. C.**, Defective DNA repair and increased lethality in ataxia telangiectasia cells exposed to 4-nitroquinoline-1-oxide, *Nature (London)*, 287, 747, 1980.
139. **Sandberg, A. A.**, *The Chromosomes in Human Cancer and Leukemia*, Elsevier, New York, 1980.
140. **Polani, P. E.**, DNA repair defects and chromosome instability disorders, *Ciba Found Symp.*, 66, 81, 1979.
141. **Kuhnlein, U., Penjart, E. E., and Linn, S.**, An altered apurinic DNA endonuclease activity in group A and group D xeroderma pigmentosum fibroblasts, *Proc. Natl. Acad. Sci. USA*, 73, 1169, 1976.
142. **Emanuel, I., Sever, L. E., Milham, S., and Thuline, H. C.**, Accelerated aging in young mothers of children with Down's Syndrome, *Lancet*, 361, 1972.
143. **Movchan, O. T., Kossichenko, L. P., Karkaryan, D. S., and Avdzhyan, V. M.**, A comparative analysis of the spontaneous chromosomal aberration rate in monkeys and some small laboratory animals, *Tsitologiya*, 9, 864, 1967.
144. **Kopelovich, L. and Sirlin, S.**, Human skin fibroblasts from individuals genetically predisposed to cancer are sensitive to an SV40-induced T antigen display and transformation, *Cancer*, 45, 1108, 1980.
145. **Lambert, B., Ringborg, V., and Swanbeck, G.**, Ultraviolet-induced DNA repair synthesis in lymphocytes from patients with actinic keratosis, *J. Invest. Derm.*, 67, 594, 1976.
146. **Carter, D. B. and Chae, C. B.**, Composition of liver histones in aging rat and mouse, *J. Gerontol.*, 30, 28, 1975.
147. **Liew, C. and Gornall, A.**, Covalent modification of nuclear proteins during aging, *Fed. Proc. Fed. Am. Soc. Exp. Biol.*, 34, 186, 1975.
148. **O'Meara, A. R. and Pochron, S. F.**, Age-related effects on the incorporation of acetate into rat liver histones, *Biochem. Biophys. Acta*, 586, 391, 1979.
149. **Medvedev, Z., Medvedeva, M., and Robson, L.**, Age-related changes of the pattern of non-histone chromatin proteins from cat and mouse liver, *Gerontology*, 25, 219, 1979.

150. **Cornelis, J. J, Rommelaere, J., Urbain, J., and Errera, M.,** A sensitive method for measuring pyrimidine dimers *in situ, Photochem. Photobiol.,* 26, 241, 1977.
151. **Abo-Darub, J. M., Mackie, R., and Pitts, J. D.,** DNA repair deficiency in lymphocytes from patients with actinic keratosis, *Bull. Cancer,* 65, 357, 1978.
152. **Sbano, E. L., Andreassi, M., Fimiani, M., Valentino, A., and Barochi, R.,** DNA repair after UV-irradiation in skin fibroblasts from patients with actinic keratosis, *Arch. Dermatol. Res.,* 262, 55, 1978.
153. **Terry, R. D.,** Structural changes in senile dementia of the Alzheimer type, in *Aging of the Brain and Dementia,* Vol. 13 Amaducci, L., Davison, A. N., and Antuono, P., Eds., Raven Press, New York, 1980, 23.
154. **Weksler, M. E.,** The immune system and the aging process in man, *Proc. Soc. Exp. Biol. Med.,* 165, 200, 1980.
155. **Smerdon, M. J., Tilsty, T. D., and Lieberman, M. W.,** Distribution of ultraviolet-induced DNA repair synthesis in nuclease sensitive and resistant regions of human chromatin, *Biochem.,* 17, 2399, 1978.
156. **Wilkins, R. J. and Hart, R. W.,** Preferential DNA repair in human cells, *Nature (London),* 247, 35, 1974.
157. **Tice, R. R.,** Aging and DNA-repair capability, in *The Genetics of Aging,* Schneider, E. L. Ed., Plenum Press, New York, 1978, 53.
158. **Shaham, M., Becker, Y., and Cohen, M. M.,** A diffusable clastogenic factor in ataxia telangiectasia, *Cytogenet. Cell Genet.,* 27, 155, 1980.
159. **Tice, R. R., Rory, J. M., and Bender, M. A.,** An investigation of DNA repair potential in Bloom's syndrome, in *DNA Repair Mechanisms,* (ICN-UCLA Symposia on Molecular and Cellular Biology 9) Hanawalt, P. C., Friedburg, E. C., and Fox, C. F., Eds., Academic Press, New York, 1978, 659.
160. **Goldstein, S.,** Human genetic disorders that feature premature onset and accelerated progression of biological aging, in *The Genetics of Aging,* Schneider, E. L., Ed., Plenum Press, New York, 1978, 171
161. **Herron, D. C. and Shank, R. C.,** Methylated purines in human liver DNA after probable dimethylnitrosamine poisoning, *Cancer Res.,* 40, 3116, 1980.
162. **Jaggi, W., Lutz, W. K., and Schlatter, C.,** Covalent binding of ethinylestradiol and estrone to rat liver DNA *in vivo, Chem. Biol. Interact.,* 23, 13, 1978.
163. **Dewitt, R. C., Pelkonen, O., Okey, A. B., and Nebert, D. W.,** Genetic differences in metabolism of polycyclic aromatic carcinogens and aromatic amines by mouse liver microsomes. Detection by DNA binding of metabolites and by mutagenicity in histidine-dependent Salmonella typhimurium *in vitro, J. Natl. Cancer Inst.,* 62, 947, 1979.
164. **Cook, P. R., Brazell, I. A., Pawsey, S. A., and Gianelli, F.,** Changes induced by ultraviolet light in the superhelical DNA of lymphocytes from subjects with xeroderma pigmentosum and normal controls, *J. Cell. Sci.,* 29, 117, 1978.
165. **Burch, P. R. J.,** *An Inquiry Concerning Growth, Disease, and Aging,* Oliver and Boyd, Edinburgh, 1968.
166. **Curtis, H. J.,** Biological mechanisms underlying the aging process, *Science,* 141, 686, 1963.
167. **Dean, R. G. and Cutler, R. C.,** Absence of significant age-dependent increase of single-stranded DNA extracted from mouse liver nuclei, *Exp. Gerontol.,* 13, 287, 1978.

Chapter 4

# TESTING THE FREE RADICAL THEORY OF AGING

**Arthur K. Balin**

## TABLE OF CONTENTS

## I. INTRODUCTION

Free radicals are ubiquitous in living systems. It is increasingly evident that many intracellular biochemical reactions occur by one electron steps and free radical mechanisms. Further, many environmentally induced stresses such as exposure to ultraviolet and ionizing irradiation, oxygen, ozone, and petrochemical pollutants induce cellular damage via free radical mechanisms. Much free radical damage is random and irreversible and could account for many of the deteriorative processes that accompany the aging process.

This chapter explores the role of free radicals in biological systems and reviews some of the experimental approaches that have been undertaken to test the free radical theory of aging.

## II. THE FREE RADICAL THEORY OF AGING

The free radical theory of aging was one of the first aging theories subject to direct experimental analysis. Denham Harman proposed in 1956, that the degenerative changes associated with aging might be related to deleterious side reactions of free radicals which are normally produced during cellular metabolism.[1,2] He suggested that the aging process might be the accumulative result of the random free radical reactions that are continuously occurring throughout our cells and tissues. Additionally, he hypothesized that DNA damage induced by free radical reactions could lead to mutation and, thereby, be responsible for neoplasia. These random free radical reactions would, therefore, cause death and mutations, assuring evolution.[3,4]

The aging process is a complex incompletely understood phenomena that appears to involve both environmental and intrinsically programmed components.[5] Free radical damage could contribute to the aging process via several mechanisms. Macromolecular cross-links of connective tissue could impede nutrient diffusion and impair tissue viability with age.[6] DNA mutation and cross-links could lead to somatic mutations and lack of expression of essential enzymes with age. Membrane lipid peroxidation could result in loss of integrity of subcellular organelles and/or accumulation of intracellular peroxidized lipoprotein debris (lipofuscin), which might impair cell function.[7] Continual oxidative stress on a cell might necessitate diversion of energy and reducing equivalents that are normally needed for biosynthetic processes, to repair reactions that reduce oxidized cellular components. Oxidation of unique oxygen sensitive sulfhydryl groups could cause cellular damage through loss of critical specific cellular function (such as assembly and disassembly of mitotic and cytoplasmic microtubules).

**Table 1**
**FREE RADICAL REACTIONS**

| | Reaction | | |
|---|---|---|---|
| Initiation | $RH \xrightarrow{\text{initiator}} R\cdot$ | | (1) |
| Propagation | $R\cdot + O_2 \longrightarrow ROO\cdot$ | | (2) |
| | $ROO\cdot + RH \longrightarrow ROOH + R\cdot$ | | (3) |
| | $Q\cdot + RH \longrightarrow RH + R\cdot$ | Atom (or group) transfer | (4) |
| | $Q\cdot + R_2C{=}CH_2 \longrightarrow R_2\dot{C}{-}CH_2{-}Q$ | Addition | (5) |
| | $Q{-}C(R)(X){-}O\cdot \longrightarrow R\cdot + Q{-}C({=}O){-}X$ | β-scission | (6) |
| | $e(H_2O)^{-}n + ArR \longrightarrow nH_2O + ArR\cdot$ | Electron transfer | (7) |
| | $Ar_3C{-}\dot{C}H_2 \longrightarrow Ar_2\dot{C}{-}CH_2Ar$ | Rearrangements | (8) |
| Termination | | | |
| | $2R\cdot \longrightarrow R{-}R$ | | (9) |
| | $R\cdot + ROO\cdot \longrightarrow ROOR$ | | (10) |
| | $2ROO\cdot \longrightarrow ROOR + O_2$ | | (11) |
| | $AntiOxH + ROO\cdot \longrightarrow ROOH + [Anti\ Ox\cdot]$ | | (12) |

## III. PEROXIDATIVE THREAT TO BIOLOGIC SYSTEMS

A brief review of the peroxidative threat to biologic systems will facilitate critical evaluation and design of experiments testing the free radical theory of aging. Recent comprehensive reviews of oxygen toxicity,[8,9] cellular antioxidant defense systems,[10] hydroperoxide metabolism,[11] lipid peroxidation,[12] and free radicals in biology,[13] are recommended for the reader who wishes more detail.

### A. Free Radical Reactions

A free radical is any chemical species with an odd number of electrons. The unpaired electrons can be detected by electron paramagnetic resonance spectroscopy.[14] Typical free radical reactions are summarized in Table 1.[15]

Free radicals are produced in the cell by a number of initiation mechanisms, which include the following: (1) oxygen, (2) unimolecular homolysis of molecules with weak bonds, (3) radiolysis, (4) photolysis, (5) one electron transfer from transition metal ions to organic species, (6) exposure to pollutants or drugs such as ozone, $NO_2$, singlet oxygen, adriamycin or paraquat,[11] and (7) enzymatic processes which produce and release radicals in vivo.[15]

### B. Oxygen

Oxygen is the molecule that most commonly generates free radicals in biologic systems.[16] Toxic effects of oxygen have been known to occur in many systems.[9,17,18,19] Rueckert and Mueller found that HeLa cell division was depressed if the cells were incubated under 40% oxygen.[20] Others have reported inhibition of cell division or decreased nucleic acid synthesis in cells incubated under 95% oxygen.[21-26]

High partial pressures of oxygen have been shown to inhibit the activity of many enzymes, particularly those containing essential sulfhydryl groups.[18,27,28,29] Exposure to hyperbaric oxygen inactivates sensitive enzymes rapidly (20 to 180 min).[27,28,30-32] Dickens found that a 3-hr exposure to 2.9 atmospheres of 100% $O_2$ substantially and irreversibly decreased the respiratory rate and glucose utilization and inhibited the production of lactate in rat brain slices and homogenates.[27,28] Horn and Hargaard found that 1 atmosphere of 100% $O_2$ inhibited glucose metabolism within 20 min in rat heart homogenates, probably by inactivating glyceraldehyde-3-phosphate dehydrogenase.[30] Clearly, elevated oxygen tensions can irreversibly damage enzymes involved in metabolism. Additionally, as Dickens noted,[27] the finer a tissue is divided the greater is its sensitivity to oxygen. However, the results of studies in which sliced, minced, or homogenized tissues are exposed to high partial pressures of oxygen may not be relevant to the metabolic events of oxygen poisoning in intact tissue.[17]

Molecular oxygen has two unpaired electrons in the ground state which have parallel spins. These parallel spins prevent the direct entry of paired electrons. In order to add spin-paired electrons to ground state molecular oxygen, one electronic spin must be inverted so two parallel spins would not be placed in one orbital. The inversion of electronic spin is slow relative to the collisional complex lifetime. As a result, ground state oxygen tends to react by univalent reduction pathways.[33,34] Oxygen's reduction intermediates include superoxide anion ($O_2$ ), hydrogen peroxide ($H_2O_2$), and hydroxyl radical ($\cdot$OH) and are discused in the following pages.

Molecular oxygen's bond energy (O=O) is stronger that of just one covalent bond, but oxygen is also capable of behaving as a diradical ($\dot{O}-\dot{O}$). This diradical property gives oxygen the ability for initiation and/or addition reactions (Table 1).

Oxygen reacts with olefins to produce lipid hydroperoxides (see Equation 13). The oxidation is initiated by allylic H$\cdot$ abstraction followed by oxygen attack on the carbon radical.[12]

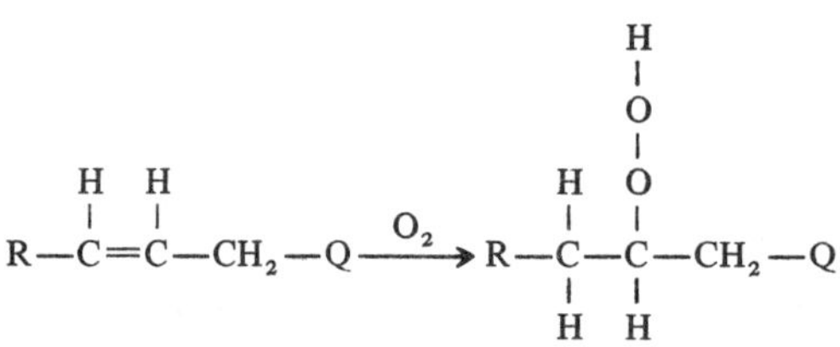

(13)

The mechanism of the initial allylic H$\cdot$ abstraction may vary depending on specific reaction conditions, but hydroxyl radical has been shown to initiate some peroxidation reactions.[35]

Lipid peroxidation occurs via Reactions 2 and 3, while termination occurs via Reactions 9, 10, and 11 (Table 1).

### C. Singlet Oxygen

Singlet oxygen (${}^1O_2$) is the electronic excited state of oxygen. ${}^1O_2$ has two excited states: ${}^1\Sigma_g^+O_2$ has an energy of 37 K cal/mole, a lifetime of $10^{-11}$ sec in solution and is due to oxygen's two outer electrons occupying separate orbitals but with opposite spins. ${}^1\Delta_gO_2$ has an energy of 22 K cal/mole, a lifetime of $2 \times 10^{-6}$ and is due to oxygen's two outer electrons occupying the same orbital with opposite spins. The lower energy state ${}^1\Delta_gO_2$ is thought to be the singlet oxygen species that reacts in solution.[36,37] Some of the reactions capable of generating ${}^1O_2$ include:[37-40]

$$O_2^{\cdot -} + H_2O_2 \xrightarrow{\text{metal}} {}^1O_2 + OH^- + \cdot OH \qquad (14)$$

$$OCl^- + H_2O_2 \longrightarrow {}^1O_2 + Cl^- + H_2O \quad (15)$$

$$O_2^{\overline{\cdot}} + \cdot OH \longrightarrow {}^1O_2 + OH^- \quad (16)$$

$$2O_2^{\overline{\cdot}} + RC(=O){-}O{-}O{-}C(=O){-}R \longrightarrow 2{}^1O_2 + 2RCO_2^- \quad (17)$$

Excited $NO_2$ can lead to singlet oxygen formation in the gas phase and is responsible for large quantities of $^1O_2$ formation in polluted atmospheres. Singlet oxygen is electrophilic and thus exhibits specificity by only reacting with fairly heavily substituted double bonds or electron rich moieties.[36] Methionine, histidine, tryptophan, tyrosine, and cysteine are the amino acids particularly susceptible to singlet oxygen and selective destruction of these amino acids leads to inactivation of many enzymes. Tocopherol is a good quencher of singlet oxygen.[36]

### D. Superoxide Anion

Superoxide radical ($O_2^{\overline{\cdot}}$) is univalently reduced oxygen. Since oxygen is usually reduced in one electron steps, $O_2^{\overline{\cdot}}$ is frequently formed in the cell. Many enzymes, such as cytochrome C oxidase, bind the oxygen reduction intermediates very tightly and release $H_2O$ (other enzymes release $H_2O_2$) as the first detectable product of oxygen reduction.[41] This is one way the cell reduces the threat from these toxic oxygen intermediates. However, other oxidative enzymes have been shown to produce and release substantial amounts of $O_2^{\overline{\cdot}}$. Among them are xanthine oxidase,[42,43,44] aldehyde oxidase,[45,46] dihydroorotic dehydrogenase,[47] flavin dehydrogenase,[48] galactose oxidase, indoleamine dioxygenase, 2-nitropropane dioxygenase,[49] and ribulose-1.5-diphosphate carboxylase.[50] The autooxidations of hydroquinones, thiols, catecholamines, leukoflavins, and tetrahydropterins have all been shown to generate $O_2^{\overline{\cdot}}$.[49] Mitochondrial membranes produce about 24 n mol $O_2^{\overline{\cdot}}$/min/g of tissue in the liver and are one of the main physiological sources of superoxide anions.[11] Most of the superoxide anions are rapidly converted to $H_2O_2$ by superoxide dismutase resulting in an estimated intramitochondrial steady state $O_2^{\overline{\cdot}}$ concentration of $8 \times 10^{-12}$ *M*.[51]

$O_2^{\overline{\cdot}}$ has been shown to induce lipid peroxidation, damage membranes, inactivate virus, kill cells,[49] cause single strand breaks in DNA, cause depolymerization of acid mucopolysaccharides,[52] and kill bacteria.[53]

$O_2^{\overline{\cdot}}$ does not seem to directly cause these effects, but reacts with $H_2O_2$ to produce hydroxyl radical,[54] (and possibly singlet oxygen),[37,40] which initiates radical chain reactions. The reaction of $O_2^{\overline{\cdot}}$ and $H_2O_2$ probably occurs via a Fenton type reaction with metal catalysis (see Equations 18, 19, and 20), since the direct Haber Weiss reaction (Equation 21) has been shown to occur too slowly in biologic systems to account for significant $\cdot$OH production.[55,56,57]

$$O_2^{\overline{\cdot}} + H_2O_2 \xrightarrow{Fe} \cdot OH + OH^- + {}^1O_2 \quad (18)$$

$$O_2^{\overline{\cdot}} + Fe^{3+} \longrightarrow Fe^{2+} + {}^1O_2 \quad (19)$$

$$Fe^{2+} + H_2O_2 \longrightarrow Fe^{3+} + OH^- + \cdot OH \qquad K = 76\ M^{-1}S^{-1} \quad (20)$$

$$O_2^{\overline{\cdot}} + H_2O_2 \longrightarrow \cdot OH + OH^- + O_2 \qquad K = 0.13\ M^{-1}S^{-1} \quad (21)$$

### E. Hydrogen Peroxide

Hydrogen peroxide is formed by the dismutation of $O_2$ (see Equation 22) or by the two electron reduction of $O_2$. Some enzymes, such as xanthine oxidase, produce both $H_2O_2$ and $O_2^{\overline{\cdot}}$.[44] $H_2O_2$ is the major product of oxygen reduction by a number of oxidases including D-amino acid oxidase, xanthine oxidase, uricase, and $\alpha$ hydroxy acid oxidase.[33] Mitochondria, microsomes, peroxisomes, and cytosolic enzymes are all $H_2O_2$ generators and contribute 15%, 45%, 35%, and 5%, respectively, to the cytosolic $H_2O_2$ level in rat liver at a $P_{O_2}$ of 158 mmHg.[11] $H_2O_2$ is produced at a rate of 380 n mol $H_2O_2$/min/g of liver in the rat, accounting for 10 to 15% of the total oxygen uptake.[11] The toxicity of $H_2O_2$ appears to be primarily due to its ability to react with $O_2^{\overline{\cdot}}$ and to generate $\cdot$OH.

### F. Hydroxyl Radical

Hydroxyl radical ($\cdot$OH) is the most potent oxidant known. It is formed by radiolysis of water and accounts for a large part of the effect of radiation in biological systems. As indicated in reaction Equations 17 to 19, hydroxyl radical is produced in biologic systems through the reactions of $O_2^{\overline{\cdot}}$ with its dismutation produce ($H_2O_2$) (see Equation 21) via a Fenton mechanism. $\cdot$OH is thought to account for most of the toxicity of oxygen and its reduction intermediates $O_2^{\overline{\cdot}}$ and $H_2O_2$.[33]

## IV. CELLULAR PROTECTIVE MECHANISMS

The cell is exposed to a continual oxidative and free radical stress. Multiple cellular defenses exist to prevent free radical destruction. These have been well reviewed recently and will, therefore, be summarized here. (For more detailed reviews note particularly those of Fridovich,[43,52,53] Chow,[10] Chance et al.,[11] Logani and Davies,[12] Kosower and Kosower,[51] Tappel,[58] and Witting.[59])

### A. Compartmentalization

One of the principal defense mechanisms against oxygen toxicity is structural. Ambient air has a $P_{O_2}$ of 158; tracheal air in the human, a $P_{O_2}$ of 149; alveolar air, a $P_{O_2}$ of 100; arterial blood, a $P_{O_2}$ of 95; and mixed venous blood, a $P_{O_2}$ of 40.[60] The $P_{O_2}$ venous blood overestimates the tissue $P_{O_2}$ because gradients on the order of tens of mmHg probably exist between the blood in the capillary systems and the sites of $O_2$ reduction.[61] Thus, the tissue is maintained at a relatively low oxygen tension by the barrier function of epidermal keratin and the steep tissue oxygen gradient from the microvasculature.[11] Additionally, cells are compartmentalized and most of the enzymes and antioxidants discussed in the following pages are located near the sites of generation of the peroxidative intermediates which they are best suited to nullify.

### B. Superoxide Dismutase

Superoxide dismutase (SOD), an enzyme ubiquitous in aerobic organisms, catalyzes the dismutation of $O_2^{\overline{\cdot}}$ (see Equation 22), thereby protecting oxygen metabolizing cells from the harmful effects of $O_2^{\overline{\cdot}}$.[53] SOD, among the most active enzymes known, speeds up the rate of spontaneous dismutation of $O_2^{\overline{\cdot}}$ which at pH 7.4 is $2 \times 10^5$ $m^{-1}$ $sec^{-1}$ (see Equations 23, 24, and 25).[48]

$$2H^+ + O_2^{\overline{\cdot}} + O_2^{\overline{\cdot}} \xrightarrow{SOD} O_2 + H_2O_2 \qquad K = 1.9 \times 10^9 m^{-1} sec^{-1} \qquad (22)$$

$$2H^+ + O_2^{\overline{\cdot}} + O_2^{\overline{\cdot}} \longrightarrow O_2 + H_2O_2 \qquad K = 1.0 \times 10^2 m^{-1} sec^{-1} \qquad (23)$$

$$H^+ + HO_2\cdot + O_2^{\overline{\cdot}} \longrightarrow O_2 + H_2O_2 \qquad K = 8.5 \times 10^7 m^{-1} sec^{-1} \qquad (24)$$

$$HO_2\cdot + HO_2\cdot \longrightarrow O_2 + H_2O_2 \qquad K = 7.6 \times 10^5 m^{-1} sec^{-1} \qquad (25)$$

At least three SOD enzymes have been found. A copper and zinc containing enzyme is in the cytosol and mitochondrial intermembrane space of eukaryotes and is sensitive to cyanide inhibition. Mitochondria contain a cyanide insensitive manganese enzyme in the matrix space. This is similar to the enzyme found in prokaryotes, except that the mitochondrial SOD contains four subunits while the prokaryotic enzyme contains two subunits. An iron containing enzyme has also been found in bacteria. The mechanism of the Cu/Zn SOD enzyme involves reduction and oxidation of the Cu moiety (see Equations 26 and 27).[33]

$$SOD - Cu^{2+} + O_2^{\cdot -} \longrightarrow SOD - Cu^{1+} + O_2 \quad (26)$$

$$SOD - Cu^{1+} + O_2^{\cdot -} + 2H^+ \longrightarrow SOD - Cu^{2+} + H_2O_2 \quad (27)$$

Superoxide dismutase appears to be distributed in cellular compartments prone to $O_2^{\cdot -}$ formation, such as the mitochondria and the cytosol.[62] SOD activity is inducible by exposure to hyperoxia in prokaryotes,[63] and in rat lung.[64]

### C. Catalase

Catalase is present in almost all mammalian cells and is an important enzyme in the intracellular regulation of $H_2O_2$. Catalase is predominantly located in peroxisomes and microperoxisomes where high levels of $H_2O_2$ are generated. When the steady-state concentration of $H_2O_2$ is low, the enzyme acts as a peroxidase (see Equation 28); when the steady-state concentration of $H_2O_2$ is high, it acts as a catalase (see Equation 29). Catalase's active site contains a $Fe^{3+}$-protoporphyrin complex.[11]

$$H_2O_2 + AH_2 \xrightarrow{\text{catalase}} 2H_2O + A \quad \text{peroxidatic} \quad (28)$$

$$H_2O_2 + H_2O_2 \xrightarrow{\text{catalase}} 2H_2O + O_2 \quad \text{catatalic} \quad (29)$$

The catalatic action evolves $O_2$ in the triplet state with less than 0.5% released as singlet oxygen.[65] Cellular catalase content, as well as the number of peroxisomes in a cell is influenced by a number of hormonal, nutritional, and pharmacologic factors.[11] Reduction of the availability of $H_2O_2$ will decrease its rate of reaction with $O_2^{\cdot -}$, resulting in less hydroxyl radical formation.

### D. Glutathione Peroxidase

Glutathione peroxidase catalyzes the reduction of hydroperoxides and oxidizes glutathione (GSH: $\gamma$ glutamylcysteinlglycine) in the process (see Equation 30). The enzyme is specific for GSH but nonspecific for the hydroperoxide.

$$ROOH + 2GSH \xrightarrow{\text{GP}} ROH + GSSG + H_2O \quad (30)$$

Thus, glutathione peroxidase is capable of reducing $H_2O_2$, lipid hydroperoxides, nucleotide hydroperoxides, and others, while catalase can only reduce $H_2O_2$. Glutathione peroxidase contains selenium which is probably at its active site.[11] A nonselenium glutathione peroxidase also exists which is unable to reduce $H_2O_2$.[66] In the rat liver, 2/3 of glutathione peroxidase is in the cytoplasm and 1/3 is in the mitochondria.[11] There is no glutathione peroxidase in the peroxisomes; therefore, its distribution is complementary to catalase.[11] The activity of the selenium containing GSH peroxidase is related to the availability of dietary selenium.[67]

The ability of glutathione peroxidase to reduce hydroperoxides is dependent on the availability of glutathione. The oxidation reduction state of the reduced glutathione-oxidized glutathione couple is fundamental to cellular metabolism because it is the largest mobile thiol redox system in the cell.[11] Living cells normally contain GSH at about $1\text{-}50 \times 10^{-4}$ $M$ and GSSG at $6\text{-}200 \times 10^{-6}$ $M$.[51] About 30% of the total cellular glutathione is present as mixed disulfides, such as protein-S-S.[68]

GSSG is reduced by NADPH-dependent glutathione reductase. NADPH producing reactions occur with glucose-6-phosphate dehydrogenase, isocitrate dehydrogenase, and malic enzyme while NADPH is normally consumed in many biosynthetic processes such as lipogenesis and mono-oxygenations.

The activities of GSH peroxidase, GSH reductase, and glucose-6-phosphate dehydrogenase have been shown to increase after animals were fed lipid hydroperoxides,[69] or were made vitamin E deficient,[70] or were exposed to ozone.[71]

It seems, then, that peroxidative damage may exert a direct destructive effect on the cellular component that is peroxidized and may exert a more subtle, harmful effect on the cell by draining it of reducing equivalents normally needed for biosynthetic processes.

### E. Other Antioxidants

Vitamin E is one of the most important biological free radical quenchers because of its hydrophobic structure and its ability to intercalate into biological membranes where the unsaturated fatty acids are located.[72,73] Vitamin E is mainly found in the endoplasmic reticulum and mitochondrial membranes.[59] Oxidation of one mole of $\alpha$ tocopherol to the quinone will reduce two moles of free radicals.

Vitamin E absorption in humans decreases with increased intake from 50 to 80% absorption at a dose of 0.04 mg/day, to 20 to 50% at a dose of 20 mg/day, to 5% when the dose was 200 mg/day.[74] Oxidized vitamin E may be regenerated by interaction with vitamin C, as has been shown in an in vitro solution.[75]

Ascorbate is an effective scavenger of the superoxide radical in cell free systems,[76,77] and can protect against oxidant and free radical mediated injury.[78] Vitamin C's role is not completely unraveled yet, because low levels of ascorbate can induce lipid peroxidation in vitro while higher levels appear to prevent lipid peroxidation. This may be due to ascorbates' ability to reduce $Fe^{3+} \rightarrow Fe^{2+}$, which catalyzes the decomposition of $H_2O_2$ (see Equation 20) to produce $\cdot OH$. Higher ascorbate levels will quench free radicals first forming ascorbate free radical and then dehydroascorbate, which can be reoxidized to ascorbic acid.[79] Ascorbic acid may have a particularly important role in the lung where it is found in high concentration in the extracellular fluid of the respiratory epithelium, while the enzymatic defenses are intracellular.[80,81] Dietary ascorbic acid has been shown to reduce lipid peroxidation in the mouse and guinea pig.[82,83]

Caeruloplasmin is a copper containing protein abundant in tissue which is capable of oxidizing $Fe^{2+} \rightarrow Fe^{3+}$ and has been shown to be an effective inhibitor of Fe dependent lipid peroxidation and DNA degradation.[84]

## V. TESTING THE FREE RADICAL THEORY OF AGING IN VIVO

### A. The Effect of Free Radical Inhibitors of Life Span of Mammals

One of the most direct ways to test whether free radical reactions contribute to or cause aging is to feed animals antioxidant chemicals to see if their life span is lengthened. As we review a number of these experiments we will note that unequivocal interpretation of the existing data is difficult. In longevity studies it is critical to separate effects due to prevention of disease from those due to a modification of the basic aging rate. Life span extension (when looking for a basic aging mechanism) requires extension of the life span of the longest lived survivors of a species clearly beyond the max-

# Table 2
# DIETARY ANTIOXIDANT EFFECT ON LIFE SPAN OF MICE

| | AKR Male | | C3H Female | |
|---|---|---|---|---|
| Dietary additive | Months 50% survival (n)[a] | Months maximum | Months 50% survival (n) | Months maximum |
| Control | 7.5 ± 2.1 (26) | 16 (1)[b] | 14.5 ± 4.6 (22) | 16 (4)[b] |
| Cysteine HCl | | | | |
| (0.5% w) | 9.0 ± 2.4 (30) | 16 (1)[b] | 13.0 ± 3.6 (29) | 16 (7)[b] |
| (1.0% w) | 10.5 ± 2.9 (30) | 16 (3)[b] | 13.0 ± 3.4 (30) | 16 (7)[b] |
| Ascorbic acid | | | | |
| (2% w) | 7.5 ± 2.0 (29) | 15.5 (2)[b] | 12.5 ± 3.3 (29) | 15.5 (5)[b] |
| 2-Mercaptoethylamine HCl | | | | |
| (0.5% w) | 8.2 ± 2.2 (30) | 14 | 13.5 ± 3.6 (30) | 14 (9)[b] |
| (1.0% w) | 10.5 ± 3.1 (24) | 15 (1)[b] | 14.5 ± 4.0 (29) | 14 (9)[b] |
| 2,2′ Diaminodiethyl disulfide dihydrochloride | | | | |
| (0.5% w) | 10.6 ± 2.8 (30) | 15 (3)[b] | 14.0 ± 3.8 (29) | 15 (11)[b] |
| (1.0% w) | 7.8 ± 2.2 (25) | 15 (1)[b] | 14.5 ± 3.9 (29) | 15 (11)[b] |
| 2-Mercaptoethanol | | | | |
| (0.5% w) | 7.6 ± 2.0 (26) | 15.5 (1)[b] | 15.0 ± 4.5 (28) | 15.5 (10)[b] |

*Note:* see text for explanation.

[a] (n) = number of animals at start of experiment.

[b] Experiment discontinued at indicated number of months. The figure in parentheses indicates the number of surviving mice at the time the experiment was discontinued.

imum life span reported for the species under optimal conditions. Usually "squaring off the curve" or extending the mean life span of the population is attributed to prevention or curing of disease rather than to altering the basic aging rate.

Denham Harman has reported a number of experiments testing the effect of various free radical inhibitors on the longevity of various mice strains. In the experiment summarized in Table 2, AKR male and C3H female mice obtained shortly after weaning were fed a standard mouse diet with the indicated antioxidant additive throughout their lives.[2] The diet was given ad lib and the mice were kept in groups of 10 per cage. AKR mice fed cysteine HCl (1% w), 2-mercaptoethylamine hydrochloride (1% w), or 2,2′-diamino diethyl disulphide HCl (0.5% w) had a 50% survival of 10.5 months compared to 7.5 months for control animals; (35% prolongation, $p < 0.01$). Ascorbic acid (2% w) and 2-mercaptoethanol (0.5% w) did not prolong 50% survival. None of the compounds studied prolonged 50% survival in the C3H mice. None of the compounds extended the life span of the longest lived survivors of either AKR or C3H mice.

In interpreting this experiment, it is important to note that both AKR and C3H mice have short life spans (for mice). AKR mice usually die of lymphatic leukemia while C3H mice usually die of mammary carcinoma. In life extension studies investigating the mechanism of the aging process, it is critical to be able to distinguish an effect which retards or prevents disease (such as penicillin treatment of pneumococcal pneumonia) from an effect which retards or prevents aging. The former will "square up the mortality curve," i.e., prolong the mean or 50% survival of the population, while the latter will prolong the life span of the longest lived survivors. The antioxidant compounds in Harman's experiment did not affect the aging rate, although they may have delayed the development of leukemia in the AKR mice.

For an unequivocal demonstration of retardation of the aging process, the life span of the control mice should equal the maximally recorded life span of that species. Therefore, it is usually preferable to work with the healthiest and longest lived strains of a particular animal species.

A second experiment reported by Harman is summarized in Table 3.[3] The experimental procedure was similar to that in Table 1 and more long lived Swiss mice were used as well as the AKR and C3H mice. The 50% survival of the control AKR mice was about 20% longer in this experiment than that reported in Table 2, raising additional doubts about significance of the prolongation in that first experiment described. The statistically significant prolongation of mean survival in this second experiment was: (1) AKR — 17% prolongation with 2% hydroxylamine HCl ($p < 0.05$) and (2) C3H — 26% prolongation with (1% w) 2-mercaptoethylamine ($p < 0.01$). The MEA did not prolong C3H survival in the first experiment (Table 2) and none of the antioxidants prolonged survival in the Swiss mice. Unfortunately, maximum longevity was not determined in these experiments since there were a few remaining animals in most of the groups when the experiment was terminated. However, there is no indication from the available data that there was any maximum life span prolongation from any of the antioxidants in any of the mouse strains.

Harman has repeated the antioxidant feeding experiments using $LAF_1$ mice,[4] which is a low tumor incidence strain, in order to attempt to obviate the objection that any increase in mean life span of the AKR and C3H mice was due primarily to an influence preventing the development of neoplasia in those strains. The experimental design was similar to those discussed earlier and the data is presented in Table 4.[4] No difference was found in mean or maximal survival of $LAF_1$ mice fed a commercial diet with or without the antioxidant 2 MEA-HCl included. If, however, a period of poor animal care and early, nonage related deaths are excluded by setting the 100% survival at 15 months, 12.8% and 29.2% prolongation of the mean life span of the $LAF_1$ mice occurred for mice fed 2 MEA-HCl (0.5% w and 1% w respectively, $p < 0.01$).

The synthetic diet used for the major part of this study enhanced the mortality of the $LAF_1$ mice compared to the commercial diet. (Control: mean, 14.5 months vs. 20 months; maximum, 26 months vs. 42 months). The mean life spans of the synthetic diet fed mice that were fed 2 MEA-HCl (1% w) were $16.3 \pm 2.7$ months, or butylated-hydroxytoluene (BHT) (0.25% w, $17.0 \pm 5.0$ months; 0.50% w, $20.9 \pm 4.9$ months) were greater ($p < 0.01$) than those fed the control synthetic diet. None of the other antioxidants increased the animals' mean or maximum life spans. $LAF_1$ mice are genetically susceptible to the development of amyloidosis.[85] Twenty percent of the animals on the commercial diet died with amyloidosis while 60% of the animals on the synthetic diet died with the disease. The beneficial effect of 2 MEA and BHT on the mean life span of the mice fed the synthetic diet may have been due to an inhibition of the rate of amyloid formation. Harman has reported that the incidence of casein induced amyloidosis in C3HeB/FeJ male mice was decreased in Santoquin fed mice (0.25% w, 1,2-dehydro-6-ethoxy-2,2,4-trimethylquinoline, ethoxyquin).[86]

Overall, this experiment illustrates the difficulty in attributing the significance of small prolongation of mean population survival to the mechanism of the aging process, especially when the growth conditions are not optimal.

In Harman's experiments, there was little difference in the weight between treated and control animals. Before reviewing other life span experiments, the magnitude of the effect that caloric restriction can have on life span must be examined. This is crucial to the design and interpretation of experiments intended to examine whether an added dietary antioxidant (or other factor) can influence life span. It was shown by McCay et al.[87,88] and later confirmed by Ross,[89] Barrows,[90] and others that substantial caloric restriction can markedly extend the mean and maximum life span of a population.

## Table 3
## DIETARY ANTIOXIDANT ON LIFE SPAN OF MICE

| Dietary additive | AKR Male | | | C3H Female | | | Swiss Male | | |
|---|---|---|---|---|---|---|---|---|---|
| | Months 50% survival | (n)[a] | Months maximum | Months 50% survival | (n) | Months maximum | Months 50% survival | (n) | Months maximum |
| Control | 9.6 ± 1.7 | (60) | 16 (3)[c] | 14.5 ± 2.3 | (92) | 21 (13)[c] | 22.0 ± 4.4 | (60) | 29 (7) |
| 2 MEA · HCl[b] | | | | | | | | | |
| (1% w) | 9.3 ± 2.1 | (42) | 16 (5)[c] | 18.3 ± 3.9 | (49) | 21 (13)[c] | 18.0 ± 3.7 | (48) | 29 (3) |
| DDD · HCl[b] | | | | | | | | | |
| (1% w) | 9.8 ± 2.2 | (43) | 13 | 12.9 ± 2.6 | (48) | 15 | 15.5 ± 3.1 | (51) | 22 |
| Cysteine HCl | | | | | | | | | |
| (1% w) | 11.0 ± 2.3 | (47) | 16 (5)[c] | 13.0 ± 2.6 | (49) | 21 (3)[c] | 19.0 ± 4.0 | (46) | 29 (1) |
| $NH_2OH$ · HCl[b] | | | | | | | | | |
| (1% w) | 10.4 ± 2.4 | (38) | 16 (2)[c] | 15.5 ± 3.6 | (36) | 21 (7)[c] | 21.0 ± 4.9 | (51) | 29 (4) |
| (2% w) | 11.2 ± 2.4 | (40) | 16 (3)[c] | 13.0 ± 3.7 | (24) | 18 | 21.0 ± 4.9 | (37) | 29 (2) |

*Note:* see text for explanation.

[a] (n) = number of animals at start of the experiment.

[b] Abbreviations: 2 MEA · HCl = 2-Mercaptoethylamine hydrochloride
DDD · HCl = 2,2′-Diaminodiethyl Disulfide di hydrochloride
$NH_2OH$ · HCl = Hydroxylamine hydrochloride

[c] Experiment discontinued at indicated number of months. The figure in parenthesis indicates the number of surviving mice at the time the experiment was discontinued.

Table 4
**DIETARY ANTIOXIDANT EFFECT ON LIFE SPAN OF MICE**

| Dietary additive | N | Commercial diet $LAF_1$ male mice: 50% Survival (months) | Months maximum | Average weight (g) |
|---|---|---|---|---|
| Control | 120 | 20.0 ± 8.1 | 42 | 30.2 |
| 2 MEA · HCl (0.5% w) | 60 | 20.0 ± 9.7 | 39 | 29.1 |
| 2 MEA · HCl (1% w) | 60 | 22.9 ± 10.8 | 42 | 27.0 |
| 100% Survival set at 15 Months | | | | |
| Control | | 24.5 ± 6.7 | | |
| 2 MEA · HC (0.5% w) | | 27.6 ± 4.1 | | |
| 2 MEA · HCl (1.0% w) | | 31.6 ± 6.8 | | |
| | | **Synthetic diet $LAF_1$ male mice** | | |
| Control | 120 | 14.5 ± 4.6 | 26 | 31.6 |
| 2 MEA · HCl (0.5% w) | 60 | 14.9 ± 4.4 | 27.5 | 29.8 |
| 2 MEA · HCl (1% w) | 60 | 16.3 ± 2.7 | 25 | 27.7 |
| Cysteine HCl (0.5% w) | 60 | 13.2 ± 3.6 | —[a] | 31.3 |
| Cysteine HCl (1% w) | 60 | 14.1 ± 3.0 | —[a] | 31.2 |
| BHT (0.25% w) | 60 | 17.0 ± 5.0 | 30 | 30.2 |
| BHT (0.50% w) | 60 | 20.9 ± 4.7 | 30 | 29.2 |
| PG (0.25% w) | 60 | 15.6 ± 4.1 | —[a] | 31.1 |
| PG (0.50% w) | 60 | 14.8 ± 3.6 | —[a] | 30.4 |
| Di-t-BH (0.25% w) | 60 | 15.5 ± 4.0 | —[a] | 31.4 |
| Di-t-BH (0.50% w) | 60 | 14.0 ± 3.1 | —[a] | 30.0 |
| $NH_2OH \cdot HCl$ (1% w) | 60 | 14.0 ± 3.6 | —[a] | 29.5 |
| $NH_2OH \cdot HCl$ (2% w) | 60 | 12.5 ± 4.0 | —[a] | 27.5 |

*Note:* see text for explanation. Abbreviations: 2 MEA · HCl = 2 Mercapteothylamine hydrochloride; BHT = 2,6-Di-tert-butyl-4-methylphenol; PG = Propyl gallate; Di-t-BH = 2,6-Di-tert-butyl hydroquinone; $NH_2OH \cdot HCl$ = Hydroxylamine hydrochloride.

[a] data not available. The synthetic diet contained 200 mgm $\alpha$ tocopherol acetate per Kg diet.

Increased life span associated with underfeeding has been reported in Tokophrya Lemnarum,[91] Daphnia,[92] Rotifers,[93] Drosophilia,[94] fish,[95] rats,[87,88] hamsters, and mice.[96]

Table 5 reviews data obtained from an experiment conducted by McCay et al.[97] and will serve to illustrate the effect of caloric restriction on life span. All rats were given the same limited amount of a Basal diet daily. The control groups were allowed ad lib supplementation with one of four different compositions of food, as indicated in Table 5.[97] The rats were started on the diet at weaning. Retardation was not started until the rats weighed 50 g and retarded rats were allowed to increase their body weight by 5 g every 50 days. Their weight was increased by feeding them a supplement of fresh beef liver and fresh lettuce; the supplement was given in equal amounts to control animals. Some of the retarded animals were allowed to feed ad lib after 300 or 900 or 1100 days to test growth recovery. The mean life span of the animals whose diets were restricted 900 days was increased an average of 450 days or about 70% while the average maximum life span of animals on restricted diets for longer than 1100 days was increased by 410 days or about 45%. The restricted animals' growth was clearly stunted, as they weighed less than half of the unrestricted animals' weight, on the average.

## Table 5
## EFFECT OF CALORIC RESTRICTION ON LIFE SPAN OF RATS

| Group | No. | Sex | Life span: 50% Survival (days) | Life span: Maximum (average of 3 oldest in days) | Mean maximum weight (g) |
|---|---|---|---|---|---|
| Control | | | | | |
| 1. Basal[a] + AD LiB "Starch"[b] | 19 | F | 722 | 1095 | 277 |
| | 19 | M | 595 | 877 | 381 |
| 2. Basal + AD LiB "Sugar"[c] | 19 | F | 733 | 1077 | 303 |
| | 19 | M | 674 | 835 | 445 |
| 3. Basal + AD LiB "Milk"[d] | 19 | F | 610 | 771 | 330 |
| | 19 | M | 688 | 863 | 515 |
| 4. Basal + AD LiB "Liver"[e] | 19 | F | 683 | 900 | 324 |
| | 19 | M | 531 | 737 | 460 |
| Control average — groups 1-4 | 76 | F | 687 | 960 | 308 |
| | 76 | M | 622 | 828 | 450 |
| Retarded | | | | | |
| 1. Basal 300 days, then ad lib | 28 | F | 812 | 1170 | 270 |
| | 24 | M | 777 | 1042 | 351 |
| 2. Basal 900 days, then ad lib | 10 | F | 1124 | 1230 | 193 |
| | 10 | M | 1086 | 1179 | 248 |
| 3. Basal 1100 days (or more), then ad lib | | F | f | 1381 | 175 |
| | | M | f | 1269 | 197 |
| 4. Basal entire life | | F | f | 1362 | 159 |
| | | M | f | 1208 | 160 |

*Note:* see text for explanation.

[a] Basal: The basal diet consisted of a mixture containing: cooked starch 20 g, cellulose 2 g, cod liver oil 8 g, lard 7 g, sucrose 5 g, alfalfa leaf meal 1 g, salt mixture 6 g, dry yeast 14 g, crude casein 27 g, dry liver 10 g.
[b] Starch = lard 10 g, cooked starch 90 g.
[c] Sugar = lard 10 g, cooked starch 50 g, sugar 40 g.
[d] Milk = lard 10 g, cooked starch 60 g, dried whole milk 30 g.
[e] Liver = lard 10 g, cooked starch 60 g, dried pork liver 30 g.
[f] Not given.

Clearly, caloric restriction increases life span and is a fruitful area to investigate, but is not the subject of the current review. The discussion of McCay et al. work is relevant, however, because it illustrates the magnitude of the effect we would like to see in antioxidant experiments and because it is crucial to keep in mind when designing and interpreting longevity experiments involving feeding. A possible criticism of some antioxidant feeding experiments is that feeding animals the chemical simply makes them sick; consequently, they do not eat as much and so the animals live a little longer. The criticism is difficult to refute because many of the antioxidant induced changes are subtle (15 to 25% in mean extension on Harman's work), while the caloric restriction effect is of greater magnitude. It is known, for example, that the highest nontoxic level of butylated hydroxytoluene is about 0.2% of the diet.[83] Growth parameters of the animals, such as weight, become essential to record.

Comfort has examined the effect of ethoxyquin on the longevity of C3H mice,[98] (see Table 6). The mice were 3 months old at the start of the experiment. They were caged by tens and weighed monthly. Both groups were given a standard pellet diet ad lib;

**Table 6**
**THE EFFECT OF ETHOXYQUIN ON THE LONGEVITY OF C3H MICE**

| Group[a] | Sex | Mean survival (days) | Maximum (days) |
|---|---|---|---|
| Control | M | 552 ± 25 | 711 |
| Diet | F | 541 ± 33 | 722 |
| Ethoxyquin 0.5% | M | 652 ± 27 | 887 |
| + | | | |
| Control diet | F | 649 ± 27 | 907 |

*Note:* see text for explanation.

[a] n = 20 per group.

the treated groups' pellets were moistened with 0.5% w ethoxyquin. The ethoxyquin treated animals had a mean survival increase of about 100 days (~18%) and a maximum survival increase of about 180 days (~25%). However, the ethoxyquin treated mice grew into significantly lighter adults (about 20 to 25% lighter) and lost weight earlier than the control animals.

Kohn has investigated the effect of antioxidants on the life span of C57 BL female mice.[99] The animals were kept 20 to a cage and fed Wayne Mouse Breeder Blox food ad libitum. This diet contained $\alpha$ tocopherol at a concentration of 35.2 ppm. The antioxidant test chemicals were added to this diet and the animals were weighed weekly. When survival of the control mice was optimal (Experiment 1, Table 7), the antioxidants had no effect on either the 50% survival time or the maximum life span. When survival of the controls was less than optimal (Experiment 2, decreased control maximum life span; Experiment 3, decreased control 50% survival) the antioxidant additive caused lengthening of the life span. However, under no circumstance did the antioxidants increase the 50% survival time or maximum lifespan significantly beyond optimal values for control mice. The antioxidant fed rats were lighter than the control animals.

Clapp et al.[100] examined the effect of butylated hydroxytoluene (BHT) on the life span of barrier derived BALB/c mice. The mice were kept eight to a cage and were fed ad lib Purina laboratory chow with or without 0.75% BHT. The data summarized in Table 8,[100] reveals that the mean life span of the animals fed the antioxidant was prolonged but the maximum life span was not. The antioxidant fed animals were said to be generally heavier, although data was not provided. Clapp et al. observed that BHT treated animals had an increased liver size at autopsy. A different property of the BHT, aside from its antioxidant function, may be responsible for the mean life span prolongation since both BHT and ethoxyquin appear to be hepatic enzyme inducers.[98] Ross showed that liver enzyme concentrations correlated with increased rat life expectancy.[101] As Comfort suggested,[98] life span experiments with other enzyme inducers such as barbituates would be useful in clarifying the mechanism of this mean life span prolongation.

The antioxidant feeding experiments thus far discussed do not show a dramatic effect on the life span of the animals tested. Several facts should be remembered when trying to reconcile this data with the free radical theory of aging. Most of the antioxidants fed in these biologic experiments were developed for industrial uses such as stabilizing rubber or petroleum products. Vitamin E, a biologic antioxidant, has a long isoprenoid side chain which is responsible for its predominant distribution in the membrane lipids of the endoplasmic reticulum and the mitochondria which are near sites of free radical generation. The synthetic antioxidants, such as ethoxyquin or butylated

## Table 7
## THE EFFECT OF DIETARY ANTIOXIDANTS ON THE LIFE SPAN OF C57 BL FEMALE MICE

| Experiments | Life span (weeks) | | |
|---|---|---|---|
| | 50% Survival | Maximum | Maximum weight (g) |
| Experiment 1 | | | |
| (Begun at rate age 40 weeks) | | | |
| Control n = 60, | 121 | 148 | 42 |
| 1% MEA[a] n = 100, | 115 | 145 | 40 |
| BHT[b] n = 100, | 119 | 146 | 37 |
| Experiment 2 | | | |
| (Begun at rat age 40 weeks) | | | |
| Control n = 50, | 113 | 125 | 40 |
| 1% MEA[a] n = 50 | 113 | 147 | 35 |
| Experiment 3 | | | |
| (Begun at rat age 5 weeks) | | | |
| Control n = 100, | 90 | 146 | 40 |
| BHT[c] n = 100, | 113 | 151 | 34 |

*Note:* see text for explanation.

[a] MEA = 2-mercaptoethylamine HCl
[b] BHT = 2,6-di-tert-butyl-4-methylphenol: additive concentration varied due to early deaths — 1% wk 40-42; 0% wk 42-45; 0.2% wk 45-65; 0.5% wk 65-78; 0% wk 78-82; 0.5% wk 82-91; 0.2% wk 91-end.
[c] BHT = Additive concentration varied due to early deaths — 0.5% wk 5-10; 0% wk 10-12; 0.5% wk 12-22; 0.2% wk 22-26; 0.5% 2k 26-end.

## Table 8
## THE EFFECT OF BHT ON THE LIFE SPAN OF BALB/C MICE

| Treatment regimen | No. | Sex | Mean survival times (days) ± SE | Maximum (days) |
|---|---|---|---|---|
| 0.75% BHT[a](8-11 weeks) | 49 | F | 759 ± 21 | |
| | 47 | M | 726 ± 24 | |
| 0.75% BHT (11 weeks - lifetime) | 49 | F | 875 ± 21 | 1150 |
| | 49 | M | 890 ± 26 | 1120 |
| 0.75% BHT (8 weeks - lifetime) | 98 | F | 798 ± 20 | 1150 |
| | 89 | M | 832 ± 19 | 1070 |
| Control | 97 | F | 701 ± 19 | 1100 |
| | 100 | M | 684 ± 20 | 1100 |

*Note:* see text for explanation.

[a] Butylated Hydroxytoluene(2,6-di-tert-butyl-4-methylphenol).

hydroxytoluene are nonspecifically distributed in fat and are largely found in the cytosol (60%). Ethoxyquin is metabolized and eliminated much faster than vitamin E.[59] Many of the other compounds tested, such as cysteine, are water soluble and, therefore, not distributed near sites of free radical generation.

Furthermore, actual tissue levels of the antioxidants were not measured in the preceding experiments. As mentioned earlier, vitamin E absorption decreases rapidly with increasing dietary dose.[74] Many other antioxidants are poorly absorbed. Dietary concentrations of butylated hydroxytoluene greater than 0.2% give toxic manifestations of reduced growth in rats.[83] Rats fed 0.5% BHT have less than 1 ppm deposited in their livers.[100] Thus, the limited biologic effect demonstrated by antioxidant feeding experiments may be related to poor absorption, poor subcellular distribution, and rapid turnover of the synthetic antioxidants.

Several additional studies that focus on antioxidant fed animals and aging will be discussed in the following pages. Since succeeding studies also look at lipofuscin accumulation, a brief discussion of lipofuscin may be helpful in understanding the antioxidant studies.

### B. Lipid Peroxidation and Lipofuscin

Lipid peroxidation and lipofuscin have each been reviewed several times, notably by Toth,[103] Miquel et al.,[104] Barber and Bernheim,[105] and Logani and Davies.[12] Salient features of those reviews will be summarized because of their relationship to the free radical theory of aging. The mechanism of lipid peroxidation was discussed earlier (see Table 1, Equations 2 and 3). The final products of lipid peroxidation include ethane, propane, pentane, and malonaldehyde.[12] Detection of the hydrocarbon gases has been used as an in vivo measure of lipid peroxidation.[106,107]

Lipid peroxides are extremely toxic to animals as observed by Horgan et al.,[108] Olcott and Dolen,[109] Findlay et al.,[110] and Cortesi and Privett.[111] For example, the $LD_{50}$ for methyl linoleate hydroperoxide was 0.07 n mole/100 gram body weight for adult male rats. Lung toxicity is prominent, even when the hydroperoxide is given intraperitoneally or intravenously.[111] Many enzymes, especially sulfhydryl enzymes, are inactivated by lipid hydroperoxides.[112,113,105]

Cellular membranes contain polyunsaturated fatty acids subject to peroxidation. Subcellular organelles such as mitochondria and peroxisomes seem to be at particular risk because of their high content of oxidative enzymes. Oxidation of membrane polyunsaturated fatty acids will perturb the membrane microarchitecture due to the introduction of hydrophilic groups, even after reduction to the corresponding hydroxylipids. Membrane permeability and function may be affected by this peroxidation. Extensive oxidation can lead to rupture of membrane. If the particular organelle involved was a lysozome, release of lysozomal enzymes could be expected to have detrimental consequences for the cell.

The breakdown products of lipid peroxides include aldehydes, such as malonaldehyde, which can react to form lipofuscin. Intracellular lipofuscin accumulation is one of the strongest pieces of evidence that free radical processes occur in vivo. Lipofuscin or aging pigment accumulates in an age related manner in the postmitotic cells of virtually every animal examined including man, other mammals, insects, nematodes, fungi, protozoa, and cells in tissue culture.[103,104] It appears to accumulate particularly in metabolically active nondividing cells such as brain, skeletal and cardiac muscle, liver, kidney, thymus, pancreas, testes, prostate, uterus, adrenal and connective tissue.[104] Lipofuscin is a fluorescent pigment which originates as the peroxidation product of polyunsaturated membrane lipids and denatured proteins. Ceroid is formed similarly, but has a higher content of $Fe^{++}$ and $Ca^{++}$ and a lower content of $Zn^{++}$ than lipofuscin. Ceroid can be solubilized by chelating agents or ion exchange resins, but not lipofuscin.[114]

Free radical intermediates of lipid peroxidation react with proteins causing denaturation and polymerization. Malonaldehyde is a major product of the peroxidation of unsaturated lipids and it reacts with the amino groups of proteins, nucleic acids, and

**Table 9**
**DIETARY ADDITIVES IN EXPERIMENTAL DIETS USED IN TABLE 10**

| | Amount (mg/Kg Diet) | | |
|---|---|---|---|
| Additive | Diet 1 | Diet 2 | Diet 3 |
| Dl αtocopherol acetate | 65 | 1280 | 2740 |
| Ascorbic acid | 0 | 920 | 920 |
| DL methionine | 0 | 1470 | 2940 |
| Butylated hydroxytoluene | 0 | 44 | 2000 |
| Sodium selenite | 0 | 0 | 0.11 |

*Note:* see text for explanation.

phospholipids to cause cross-linking. The Schiff base product, RN = CH − CH = CH − NH − R, has fluorescent excitation maximum in the 360 to 390 nm range and emission maximum in the 450 to 470 nm region. Brain or heart lipofuscin has an excitation maximum of 365 nm and an absorption maximum of 470 nm.

Lipid peroxidation of lysozomes, mitochondria, and microsomes give absorption spectra characteristic of lipofuscin. Vitamin E deficient rats accumulate lipofuscin twice as fast as control animals.[115] The highly insoluble cross-linked lipofuscin is absorbed by lysozomes, but is not completely degraded and accumulates as inert material in the cell. Strehler et al.[116] have shown that lipofuscin accumulates in human myocardium linearly with age at a rate of 0.6% of the intracellular volume per decade.

Lipofuscin has also been shown to increase linearly with age in testes and brain of aging mice.[83] In old Drosophila, intracellular lipofuscin accumulates to more than 50% of the cellular volume.[114] Worker honey bee drones have a high rate of oxidative metabolism, a low level of vitamin E, no glutathione peroxidase, and live 6 weeks. They accumulate fluorescent pigment with age and have substantially more of the pigment than the queens or drones that are less metabolically active.[117]

These studies have clearly established the in vivo occurrence of lipid peroxidation by the peroxidized lipid protein product left as debris. Lipid peroxidation induced loss of membrane integrity and inactivation of enzymes clearly seem detrimental to the cell. Although lipofuscin has not been established as harmful to the cell, the loss of cytoplasmic organelles and the disruption of normal cellular anatomy is probably not beneficial. Since the organism's ability to deal with the consequences of lipid peroxidation could help account for species differences in life span, this area seems fruitful for further investigation.

### C. Dietary Antioxidant Effect on Lipid Peroxidation and Aging

Tappel et al.[83] have examined the effect of antioxidants on lipid peroxidation and aging parameters in mice. Male CD-1 retired breeder mice were begun on the experimental diet (diet 1: n = 100; diet 2: n = 50; diet 3: n = 50) at 9 months of age and were housed individually (see Table 9). A 0.2 g sample of tissue was homogenized and extracted with chloroform:methanol for fluorescence measurements at the indicated ages. The data show (see Table 10) that fluorescent products accumulate in the testes with age and that, on the average, diet 3 reduced this accumulation in the testes ($p < 0.02$). A large degree of individual variation was found in the mice. Tappel reported no difference in the weight or survival statistics of the antioxidant fed mice. The last available data point on the survival curve was at 1.75 years and showed that 50% of diet 1, 29% of diet 2, and 43% of diet 3 mice were still alive. The experiment indicated

### Table 10
### RELATIVE LIPOFUSCIN ACCUMULATION OF TISSUE EXTRACTS OF MICE FED ANTIOXIDANT CONTAINING DIETS

| Diet | Age | Heart | Testes |
|---|---|---|---|
| Diet 1 | 0.25 years | 27 ± 9 ( 8)[a] | 29 ± 9 ( 8) |
| Diet 1 | 0.83 years | 32 ± 9 ( 9) | 81 ± 39 ( 8) |
| 0.6 years, Diets 1 & 2 combined | 1.3 years | 40 ± 13 ( 7) | 162 ± 66 ( 7) |
| 0.6 years, Diet 3 | 1.3 years | 34 ± 4 ( 6) | 75 ± 27 ( 6) |
| Diet 1 | 1.9 years | 41 ± 14 (15) | 243 ± 102 (15) |
| 1.2 years, Diet 2 | 1.9 years | 38 ± 20 ( 9) | 171 ± 108 (10) |
| 1.2 years, Diet 3 | 1.9 years | 32 ± 4 (10) | 135 ± 103 ( 8) |

*note:* see text for explanation. Antioxidant composition of the experimental diets is presented in Table 9. Relative lipofuscin accumulation determined by fluorescent measurements of $CHCl_3$/$CH_3OH$ extracted tissue.

[a] (n) = number of determinations.

### Table 11
### EFFECT OF α TOCOPHEROL QUINONE ON NEMATODE LIFE SPAN

| Additive | Day added | Mean (days) | Maximum (days) |
|---|---|---|---|
| None | | 36 | 53 |
| α Tocopherol quinone | 1 | 49 | 73 |
| (400 μg/mℓ) | 10 | 41 | 62 |
| | 20 | 33 | 62 |
| | 30 | 35 | 62 |

*Note:* see text for explanation.

that added antioxidants can reduce fluorescent accumulation, although the effect was not dramatic. The experiment should be repeated using mice immediately after they have been weaned, (rather than at 9 months) and with enough mice to have an adequate mortality curve to establish maximum life span. It is also worthwhile to remember that vitamin E absorption falls off dramatically with increasing oral dose.[83]

## D. Antioxidants and Nematodes

Epstein and Gershon have examined the effect of the antioxidant α tocopherol quinone on the nematode, Caenorhabditis Briggsae.[118] The animals were grown axenically and survival was determined from groups of 100 isolated animals. The antioxidant α tocopherol quinone was used at 400 μg/mℓ in 0.1 mℓ ethanol and added to the medium. The 50% survival of the treated animals was prolonged from thirty-five ± 2 days (control) to 46 ± 2 days, while the maximum life span was prolonged from 56 ± 3 days (control) to 69 ± 4 days (treated) (see Table 11). When the antioxidant was added at hatching, and then removed (see Table 12), the antioxidant exhibited significant activity, although the effect was greatest when the antioxidant was never removed. Electron microscopic examination demonstrated that animals treated with the antioxidant have a marked delay in the appearance of lipofuscin pigment. Butylated hydroxytoluene had no effect on the life span of this nematode. This experiment, however,

Table 12
EFFECT OF WITHDRAWAL OF α-TOCOPHEROL QUINONE ON NEMATODE LIFE SPAN

| | Days | |
|---|---|---|
| α-Tocopherol quinone | Mean | Maximum |
| Never withdrawn | 46 | 70 |
| Withdrawn day 10 | 39 | 66 |
| Withdrawn day 6 | 36 | 63 |
| Never added | 31 | 57 |

*Note:* see text for explanation.

clearly demonstrated mean and maximal life span prolongation with α tocopherol quinone. An experiment analogous to caloric depletion has not been done with nematodes.

### E. Antioxidants and Fungi

Munkves has investigated a recessive mutant of Neurospora Crassa called "natural death."[119] This mutant fungus was induced by ultraviolet irradiation and showed a decreasing clonal growth potential and irreversible cessation of growth under all nutritional conditions. Clonal growth is the rate of extentional growth of the mycelial frontier on a minimal agar surface in horizontal "race" tubes. The mycelia is obtained from a single ascosporic clone heat shocked to induce germination. Cessation of growth was defined as extension less than 0.1 mm/hr. Wild type neurospora do not age. Under Munkves' conditions the onset of death was prolonged from 106 hr to 139 hr by the addition of antioxidant nordihydroguaiaretic acid. The specific activities of superoxide dismutase, glutathione peroxidase, and glutathione reductase were two to four times higher in the mycelia of the mutant than the wild type.[119] Antioxidants delayed the appearance of lipofuscin pigment in the natural death mutant.[120] Similar conclusions were drawn from analogous studies on the related fungus, Podospora Anserina.[121]

The results show that antioxidant additives can delay the time to cessation of mycelial extension in a postmitotic fungal mycelium. It has not been determined why wild fungi do not senesce.

### F. Reduced Metabolic Activity Decreases Lipofuscin and Increases Life Span in Houseflies

Sohal and Donato have experimentally altered the life span of the housefly by restricting the amount of flying activity permitted.[122,123] For maximum flight activity, 100 male and 20 female flies were put into a one cubic foot cage while for minimal activity, male flies were individually kept in 250 mℓ glass jars that had cardboard partitions. Both the mean and maximal survival of the low activity flies was significantly longer than the high activity flies (see Table 13). The concentration of fluorescent pigments increased linearly with age in both groups of flies, but increased 3.6 times faster in the high activity flies. Lipofuscin appears to be a measure of physiologic rather than chronological age in this system.

These studies have established some useful experimental systems for examining the relation between metabolically generated free radicals and aging.

### G. Effect of Unsaturated Fatty Acid Diets on the Life Span of Mice

Harman has examined the effect of the amount and degree of unsaturation of dietary fat on the mortality rate of mice and rats.[124] He fed groups of C3H female mice,

**Table 13**
**EFFECT OF ACTIVITY OF HOUSEFLIES ON THEIR LIFE SPAN**

| | Days | |
|---|---|---|
| **Amount of activity** | **50% Survival** | **Maximum** |
| High activity | 18 | 33 |
| Low activity | 46 | 70 |

*Note:* see text for explanation.

**Table 14**
**PER CENT FATTY ACID COMPOSITION OF DIETARY FATS USED IN THE EXPERIMENT PRESENTED IN TABLE 15**

| Fat | Saturated | 16:1 | 18:1 | 20:1 | 16:2 | 18:2 | 18:3 | 18:4 | 20:4 | Relative peroxidizability |
|---|---|---|---|---|---|---|---|---|---|---|
| Lard | 40 | | 48 | | | 11.0 | 0.6 | | | 15 |
| Olive oil | 15 | | 75 | | | 10.0 | | | | 12 |
| Corn oil | 12.4 | 1.2 | 30 | | | 54.1 | 0.6 | | | 56 |
| Safflower oil | 8.2 | | 15.4 | | | 76.4 | | | | 77 |
| Menhaden oil[a] | 42.3 | 7.9 | 13.4 | 0.9 | 0.8 | 1.1 | 0.9 | 1.9 | 1.2 | 131 |

*Note:* see text for explanation. This table presents the fatty acid composition and the relative peroxidizability of the fats used in the experimental diets presented in Table 15.

[a] Menhaden oil contains 8% 14:0; 10.2% 20:5; 1.6% 22:5; 12.8% 22:6.

**Table 15**
**EFFECT OF DIETARY FAT ON MEAN LIFE SPAN OF C3H FEMALE MICE**

| | Mean Life Span ± SD | | |
|---|---|---|---|
| **Dietary additive** | **5%** | **10%** | **20%** |
| Lard | 14.7 ± 4.8 | 14.4 ± 4.4 | 14.5 ± 4.5 |
| Olive oil | 15.7 ± 5.0 | 14.8 ± 3.6 | 13.9 ± 3.9 |
| Corn oil | 14.8 ± 4.3 | 14.4 ± 3.9 | 12.9 ± 3.6 |
| Safflower oil | 14.4 ± 4.7 | 13.8 ± 3.9 | 1.4 ± 3.9 |
| Menhaden oil | 13.6 ± 4.2 | 13.7 ± 3.3 | 13.3 ± 3.7 |

*Note:* see text for explanation. Fatty acid composition of the diet and relative peroxidizability given in Table 14. 50 animals per group.

Swiss male mice, and Sprague-Dawley male rats a semisynthetic diet containing 5%, 10%, or 20% by weight of lard or olive oil or corn oil or safflower oil or distilled triglycerides of Menhaden oil (See Table 14 for fatty acid composition and relative peroxidizability of the fats.)[124] The diets contained 20 mg of vitamin E per 100 g of finished diet. Statistical analysis of the data presented in Table 15 revealed that for C3H mice, the mean life span decreased ($p < 0.05$) with an increase in the degree of unsaturation and/or the amount of dietary fat. There was no effect on the maximum life span of the C3H mice. The degree of unsaturation or amount of dietary fat had no effect on the mean or maximum life span of the Swiss male mice or the Charles River male rats (data not shown).[124]

The results show very little effect from varying the dietary content of unsaturated lipids with adequate vitamin E in the diet. The study represents another approach used in attempting to establish the relation between free radical damage and aging.

There was no effect on the mortality curve of Portor rats when the percent of linoleic acid (18:2) was increased from 2% to 21% of the consumed dietary fat.[125]

### H. Changes in Antioxidant Protective Mechanisms with Age

Another approach taken to examine the free radical theory of aging has been to determine whether any age related changes occur in cellular antioxidant protective mechanisms. Superoxide dismutase activity has been examined by a number of investigators. Reiss and Gershon found an age related reduction in specific activity; age related accumulation of antigenetically cross-reacting material; and age related increased sensitivity to temperature inactivation, in superoxide dismutase that was isolated from rat liver.[126] However, Kelly and Fridovich found that the specific activity of total dismutase in extracts of the brain and liver of male CD Sprague-Dawley rats remained unchanged with age, although they found a 30% decrease in the mitochondrial enzyme.[127] Others have found no change in the level of erythrocyte superoxide dismutase, either immunochemically or by enzyme activity in humans of various ages,[128,129] although SOD activity has been reported to decrease by about 30% with aging of erythrocytes.[130] Superoxide dismutase activity has been found to be lower in short living vestigial strains of Drosophila compared to the wild type Drosophila.[131] SOD activity has been found to be lower in the brains and lungs of 9-month-old, long lived LP/J mice compared to 9-month-old, short lived (A/J) mice. No difference was found in SOD activity of heart, kidney, liver, or spleen of the animals at 9 months, nor was there difference in the specific activity of the brain SOD enzyme at 2, 5, or 12 months.[127] Superoxide dismutase activity does not correlate with passage level of human diploid fibroblasts in culture.[132]

Levels of mitochondrial catalase activity and selenium dependent glutathione peroxidase activity were found to be increased in 2-year-old male Wistar rats compared to 3-month-old rats. No differences in superoxide dismutase activity were detected.[133] Important to note is that this study compared young growing animals with adult animals, but did not compare adult animals with aged animals.

The serum mercaptan concentration has been reported to be decreased in older humans from 55 $\mu$ moles per deciliter in 20 to 40-year-old males to 40 $\mu$moles per deciliter in 80-year-old males.[134]

Hazelton and Lang have examined the glutathione content of C57RL/6J male mice with age.[135] They found that at all ages the total glutathione and GSH concentrations in the liver were three times higher than in the kidney and ten times higher than in the heart. The old animals (31 months, less than 25% still surviving) had 30% lower GSH in the liver, 34% lower GSH in the kidney, and 20% lower GSH in the heart (per gram of tissue) than mature animals of 17 to 23 months (see Table 14 for data on the liver). Oxidized glutathione concentration of the tissue did not vary with age and represented less than 3% of the total glutathione. Organ weight was constant from 10 to 36 months of age. The constant GSSG levels indicate that GSH is not simply getting oxidized. Decreased synthesis or increased degradation of GSH might be possible. An increase in the percentage of GSH bound as mixed disulfides (such as Protein S-SG) would also be possible and might reflect significant oxidation of vital protein components with age. This will be an important avenue to pursue in further research.

## VI. TESTING THE FREE RADICAL THEORY OF AGING IN VITRO

We have developed a system that allows examination of the effect of controlled defined partial pressures of oxygen on human diploid cells in culture. This can facili-

Table 16
GLUTATHIONE CONCENTRATIONS IN THE LIVER OF C57 BL/6J MICE DURING THEIR LIFE SPAN

| | | Glutathione (equivalent GSH/g tissue) | | |
|---|---|---|---|---|
| Age (months) | No. | GSH | GSSG | Total |
| 6 | 5 | 8.57 ± 0.32 | 0.167 ± 0.030 | 8.73 ± 0.30 |
| 17 | 4 | 7.85 ± 0.33 | 0.219 ± 0.033 | 8.05 ± 0.35 |
| 23 | 3 | 7.79 ± 0.36 | 0.212 ± 0.020 | 7.98 ± 0.34 |
| 25 | 4 | 7.39 ± 0.71 | 0.192 ± 0.028 | 7.59 ± 0.74 |
| 28 | 4 | 6.78 ± 0.39 | 0.187 ± 0.009 | 6.97 ± 0.39 |
| 31 | 6 | 5.47 ± 0.27 | 0.181 ± 0.014 | 5.67 ± 0.28 |

*Note:* see text for explanation.

tate unraveling the biochemical mechanism of oxygen toxicity, pinpoint sites sensitive to free radical damage, and explore the free radical theory of aging. Human diploid cells in culture have a finite life span in terms of the number of population doublings they can achieve.[136,137] The cultures can be serially subcultivated many times, but eventually growth slows, debris accumulates, and the population is lost. This degeneration has been interpreted as a manifestation of aging at the cellular level.

Several lines of evidence indicate that the aging changes observed in vitro may have relevance to those changes observed in vivo. For example, normal cells that are serially transplanted in vivo in syngeneic host animals also have a limited proliferative capacity.[138-142] In cultures derived from human donors of different ages, there appears to be an inverse relationship between the life span of the culture and the age of the donor.[136,143-147] Aging changes in fibroblasts that have terminally differentiated (phase 3) will be discussed below.

As cultures of WI-38 cells age, the number of lysosomes and amorphous insoluble deposits increases,[148,149] and intracellular fluorescent deposits associated with the lysosomes and most pronounced in the nondividing cells accumulate.[150] These deposits have been interpreted as being analogous to lipofuscin accumulation in the cells of aging animals and associated with lipid peroxidation.[7,150-153]

Methodological details of the experiments summarized below have been previously reported.[154-157] Briefly, the cells were grown under optimal conditions. Subcultivations were carried out weekly on confluent monolayers. The cells were released from the plastic by treatment with trypsin (0.25%) in $Ca^{++}$ and $Mg^{++}$ free Eagle's MEM. After suspension in medium containing 10% fetal calf serum (FBS), the cells were counted and seeded into appropriate vessels at a density of $1 \times 10^4$ cells/cm$^2$. All cell counts were done electronically, using a Coulter Counter.

If the cultures were not confluent after 7 days of growth, they were refed every 7 days until confluence was reached or until phase-out. Phase-out was defined as the inability to achieve confluence after four feedings over a 4-week period.

Population doublings were calculated in the standard way,[158] by comparing cell counts per vessel at seeding with counts at confluence. The percentage of labeled nuclei was determined autoradiographically by the method of Cristofalo and Sharf.[158]

The flasks were gassed to equilibrium both before and after the cells were seeded with analyzed certified standard gas mixtures. These included 5% $CO_2$, balance $N_2$; 5% $CO_2$, 5% $O_2$, balance $N_2$; 5% $CO_2$, 20% $O_2$, balance $N_2$; 5% $CO_2$, 50% $O_2$, balance $N_2$; 5% $CO_2$ and 95% $O_2$.

All vessels were incubated stationary at 37°C for 24 hr to allow the cells to attach; the flasks were then placed (unless indicated) on a horizontally moving platform on a

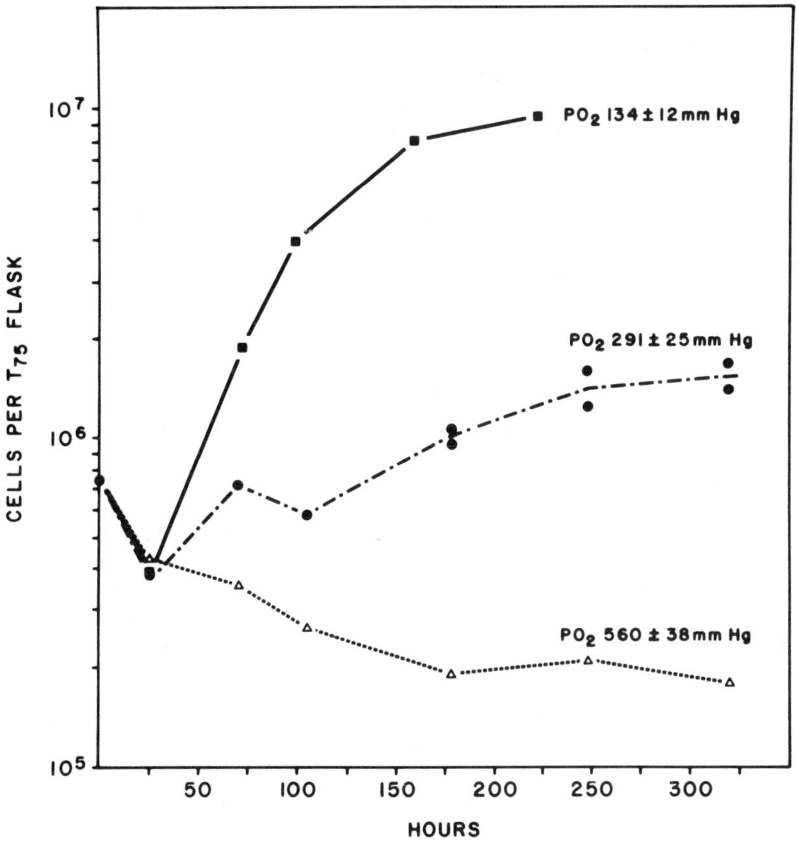


FIGURE 1. The growth of human diploid (WI-38) cells during exposure to various partial pressures of oxygen. The numbers associated with each curve represent the measured $P_{O_2}$ of the media at harvest. Cells were seeded at $1 \times 10^4$ cells/cm² and were grown in 75-cm² polystyrene vessels. (From Balin, A. K., Goodman, D. G., Rasmussen, H., and Cristofalo, V. J., *J. Cell Biol.*, 78, 390, 1978. With permission.)

model 6250 Eberbach Shaker adjusted to move through a 4 cm excursion cycle in 9 s. The gentle shaking insured that significant gas diffusion gradients would be minimized in the medium.

The oxygen tension of the medium of each flask used for growth curve experiments and at weekly intervals for life span experiments was measured as described previously,[154,155,156] using a Blood Gas Analyzer. At an atmospheric pressure of 760 mmHg, a 5.0% $CO_2$, 20.0% $O_2$, 75.0% $N_2$, gas mixture equilibrated in a flask with medium at 37°C would give a $P_{O_2}$ 47 mmHg, $P_{O_2}$ 35.6 mmHg, $P_{O_2}$ 142.6 mmHg and $P_{O_2}$ 534.8 mmHg.

### A. Effects of Changing Ambient Oxygen Tension on Cell Growth

Growth under normal atmospheric oxygen tension ($P_{O_2}$ 134 ± 12 mmHg) is illustrated in Figure 1. During the first 24 hr following inoculation, 25 to 50% of the inoculated cells failed to survive. Exponential growth began approximately 24 hr after inoculation and continued for 3 to 4 days yielding $10^7$ cells per vessel or about $1.5 \times 10^5$ cells/cm² (see Table 17). Comparison of cell growth at $P_{O_2}$ 7.8 mmHg with growth of sister cultures at $P_{O_2}$ 44 ± 7 mmHg or $P_{O_2}$ 134 ± 11 mmHg shows significant ($p < 0.001$) inhibition of growth in vessels incubated under $P_{O_2}$ 7.8. Furthermore, the population doubling time of the cells grown under $P_{O_2}$ 7.8 mmHg was significantly

**Table 17**
**THE POPULATION DOUBLING TIME AND CELL YIELD OF HUMAN DIPLOID (WI-38) CELLS INCUBATED UNDER VARIOUS PARTIAL PRESSURES OF OXYGEN**

| $P_{O_2}$ | Population doubling time (h) | Stationary phase cells $\times 10^4/cm^2$ |
|---|---|---|
| 7.8 ± 3.5[a] | 21.8 ± 2.9 (8)[b] stationary shaken | 6.5 ± 2.4 (17) |
| | | 7.3 ± 1.9 (16) |
| 26 ± 4 | 16.2 ± 1.7 (6) | 15.9 ± 1.6 (10) |
| 44 ± 7 | 16.6 ± 2.0 (14) | 15.2 ± 2.3 (30) |
| 134 ± 11 | 19.4 ± 1.7 (6) | 14.9 ± 2.4 (18) |
| 291 ± 25 | 72 ± 20 (3) | 2.3 ± 1.2 (12) |
| 291 → 50[c] | 28.7 ± 5.4 (3) | 8.0 ± 1.5 (8) |
| 389 ± 11 | N.G.[d] (5) | 0.83 ± 0.05 (5) |
| 560 ± 38 | N.G. (10) | 0.33 ± 0.14 (12) |
| 560 → 50[c] | 27.8 ± 9.5 (3) | 11.5 ± 3.2 (4) |
| 692 ± 19 | N.G. (3) | 0.33 ± 0.26 (4) |

*Note:* Results of representative experiments with cells of passage 20-27 (>90% labeled nuclei). $P_{O_2}$ measured in the media of each flask at harvest. Results obtained using glass and polystyrene vessels were similar and were combined by oxygen tension.

[a] ± standard deviation.
[b] (N) = number of determinations.
[c] Reequilibrated at 55 h.
[d] N.G. = no gain in cell number.

longer (21.8 hr vs. 16.6 hr, $p < 0.001$) than that of cells grown under $P_{O_2}$ 44 mmHg. Additionally, the growth inhibition at $P_{O_2}$ 7.8 mmHg was reversible, since flasks reequilibrated with $P_{O_2}$ 134 mmHg without changing the medium after 115 hr recovered and achieved saturation densities near those grown entirely at $P_{O_2}$ 134 mmHg (data not shown). Cells incubated at $P_{O_2}$ 26 or 44 mmHg displayed similar growth kinetics and confluent saturation densities (see Table 17). At $P_{O_2}$ from 25 to 50 mmHg, the population doubling time during exponential growth was 16.5 hr. Although the doubling time increased to 19.4 hr at a $P_{O_2}$ of 134 mmHg (16.6 hr vs. 19.4 hr, $p < 0.02$) there were no differences in the saturation densities achieved when cells were grown under various oxygen tensions ranging from 25 to 134 mmHg (see Table 17).

Striking effects upon cell growth and metabolism were observed when the $P_{O_2}$ was increased to 291 mmHg (Figure 1). The percentage of cells attached after 24 hr was identical to that obtained at lower oxygen tensions; however, with a $P_{O_2}$ of 291 ± 25 mmHg, the maximum cell number was only 10 to 20% ($p < 0.001$) of that achieved when cells were grown under $P_{O_2}$ from 25 to 140 mmHg (Table 17). This effect of increased $P_{O_2}$ on cell growth was reversible, at least in part since cells exposed to a $P_{O_2}$ of 291 mmHg for 55 hr and then reexposed to a $P_{O_2}$ of 50 mmHg entered a period of logarithmic growth that ceased after the cell sheet became confluent. The population at confluence was somewhat less ($p < 0.001$) than that achieved by control cells grown entirely under a $P_{O_2}$ of 50 mmHg (Table 17).

At $P_{O_2}$ 291 mmHg the doubling time was increased to 72 hr ($p < 0.001$), and at $P_{O_2}$ 389 ± 11, $P_{O_2}$ 560 ± 38 or $P_{O_2}$ 692 ± 19 mmHg the cell number did not increase ($p < 0.001$).

Cells seeded at a $P_{O_2}$ of 560 mmHg attached normally but did not proliferate (Figure 2). Cell growth resumed, however, in flasks that were reequilibrated with a $P_{O_2}$ of 50

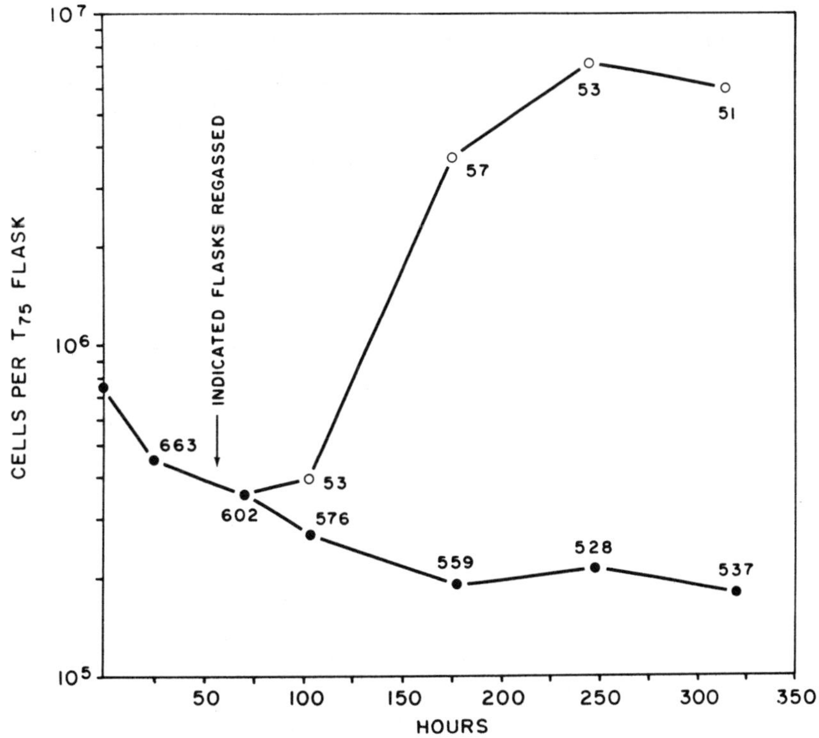


FIGURE 2. The growth of human diploid (WI-38) cells incubated at $P_{O_2}$ 560 ± 38 mmHg and recovery after reequilibration at $P_{O_2}$ 50 ± 5 mmHg. The numbers associated with each point represent the measured $P_{O_2}$ (in mmHg) of the media at harvest. The cells in 75 cm² polystyrene flasks were incubated stationary for 25 hr and then placed on a slow shaker at an average $P_{O_2}$ 560 ± 38 mmHg ( ● ); the indicated flask (O) were reequilibrated at an average $P_{O_2}$ 50 ± 5 mmHg at 55 hr. (From Balin, A. K., Goodman, D. G., Rasmussen, H., and Cristofalo, V. J., *J. Cell. Physiol.*, 89, 235, 1976. With permission.)

mmHg at 55 hr. After a 24 to 48 hr lag period, the cell number increased exponentially until the cell sheet achieved confluence. The population at confluence was about 80% of that achieved by control cells grown entirely under a $P_{O_2}$ of 50 mmHg (Table 17). Although there was no apparent growth under a $P_{O_2}$ of 560 mmHg, 55 to 70% of these cells excluded erythrocin B dye after 168 hr. Furthermore, cultures that were exposed to a $P_{O_2}$ of 560 mmHg for 168 to 192 hr and were then refed with fresh media and reequilibrated with a $P_{O_2}$ of 134 ± 11 mmHg gradually recovered, became confluent, and could be subcultivated weekly.

To test whether growth inhibition by oxygn was due to an effect on the media or an effect on the cells, flasks were incubated without cells at 37°C for 200 hr under 5% $CO_2$, 95% $N_2$ or 5% $CO_2$, 95% $O_2$. After this incubation, fresh glutamine was added (2 m*M*) and the atmosphere and media equilibrated with 5% $CO_2$ 5% $O_2$ 90% $N_2$ to a $P_{O_2}$ of 50 ± 5 mmHg. Cells were then seeded and subsequently over the next 250 hr displayed no difference in growth kinetics, saturation densities, or measured metabolic parameters when compared with cells grown on fresh media under $P_{O_2}$ 50 mmHg (data not shown). Additionally, media from flasks in which cells were inhibited by elevated oxygen tensions supported the growth of cells seeded at a $P_{O_2}$ of 134 mmHg (data not shown).

To exclude the possibility that the inhibition of growth was due either to glucose depletion or to lactate accumulation (see below), cells that had been grown under a $P_{O_2}$

**Table 18**
**THE EFFECT OF OXYGEN TENSION ON GLUCOSE AND OXYGEN CONSUMPTION AND LACTATE PRODUCTION DURING GROWTH OF HUMAN DIPLOID (WI-38) CELLS**

| $P_{O_2}$ | μm $O_2$ consumed/ h $10^6$ cells | μm glucose consumed/ h $10^6$ cells | μm lactate produced/ h $10^6$ cells |
|---|---|---|---|
| 7.8 ± 3.5[a] | 0.13 ± 0.19 (8)[b] | 0.42 ± 0.08 (8) | 0.72 ± 0.13 (8) |
| 26 ± 4 | | 0.31 ± 0.02 (4) | 0.53 ± 0.09 (4) |
| 44 ± 7 | 0.46 ± 0.14 (7) | 0.31 ± 0.05 (13) | 0.52 ± 0.10 (13) |
| 134 ± 11 | 0.54 ± 0.10 (4) | 0.23 ± 0.09 (7) | 0.38 ± 0.16 (7) |
| 291 ± 25 | | 1.47 ± 0.47 (4) | 2.12 ± 0.78 (4) |
| 291 → 50[c] | | 0.60 ± 0.17 (3) | 0.94 ± 0.27 (3) |
| 389 ± 11 | | 0.94 ± 0.10 (3) | 1.33 ± 0.20 (3) |
| 560 ± 38 | | 1.62 ± 0.21 (2) | 1.73 ± 0.11 (2) |
| 560 → 50[c] | | 0.38 ± 0.03 (2) | 0.50 ± 0.13 (2) |

*Note:* Results of representative experiments with cells of passage 20-27 (> 90% labeled nuclei). Average rate of growth parameters from 24 h after seeding to confluency were calculated: (confluent value - initial value)* $10^6$/(# h * ave. # cells). The average # cells was determined by the area under an arithmetically plotted growth curve. $P_{O_2}$ measured in the media of each flask at harvest. Results obtained using glass and polystyrene vessels were similar and were combined by oxygen tension. Oxygen consumption was not determined in polystyrene flasks because of the complications introduced by gas diffusion. The calculations for cells that did not become confluent were made over the same interval that was required for cells, which were exposed to lower oxygen tensions, to become confluent.

[a] ± standard deviation.
[b] (N) = number of determinations.
[c] Reequilibrated at 55 h.

of 291 mmHg for 220 hr were subcultivated into fresh medium at the usual seeding density of $1 \times 10^4$ cells/cm$^2$. Incubated under a $P_{O_2}$ of 134 mmHg, these cells grew to confluence and could be split weekly; incubated under a $P_{O_2}$ of 290 mmHg they did not proliferate, even after 3 weeks of weekly refeeding of fresh media. There was no difference in cell attachment at 24 hr between these conditions.

## B. Metabolic Effects of Altered Oxygen Tension

During log growth the cells incubated under $P_{O_2}$ 7.8 mmHg consumed more glucose ($p < 0.01$) and produced more lactate ($p < 0.01$) per cell than cells incubated under $P_{O_2}$ 44 mmHg (Table 18). No significant differences occurred in glucose consumption or lactate production per cell among cells grown under $P_{O_2}$ 26 mmHg, $P_{O_2}$ 44 mmHg or $P_{O_2}$ 134 mmHg (see Table 18).

Additionally, despite severely reduced growth at elevated oxygen tensions (Figure 1), both the cell population exposed entirely to a $P_{O_2}$ of 291 mmHg and the cell population whose atmosphere was changed from a $P_{O_2}$ of 291 to a $P_{O_2}$ of 50 mmHg at 55 hr utilized the available glucose and produced lactate. In fact, cells exposed to a $P_{O_2}$ of 291 mmHg consumed four to six times more glucose ($p < 0.01$) and produced four to six times more lactate ($p < 0.01$) per cell than cells grown entirely at $P_{O_2}$ 130 mmHg (Table 18) despite the reduced growth. Cells incubated under $P_{O_2}$ 389 mmHg or $P_{O_2}$ 560 mmHg showed four to six times the metabolic activity of cells incubated under $P_{O_2}$ 134 mmHg (Table 18). Cells exposed to a $P_{O_2}$ of 560 mmHg and then reequilibrated with a $P_{O_2}$ of 50 mmHg at 55 hr consumed glucose and produced lactate at the same rates, respectively, as cells grown entirely under a $P_{O_2}$ of 50 mmHg (Table 18).

Cellular oxygen consumption during exponential growth under $P_{O_2}$ 7.8 mmHg was only 25% of that present in cells grown at $P_{O_2}$ 44 mmHg ($p < 0.01$) (Table 18). Oxygen consumption during exponential growth at $P_{O_2}$ 44 mmHg and $P_{O_2}$ 134 mmHg was similar and averaged about 0.50 μmoles/(hours × $10^6$ cells) (Table 18).

Cellular oxygen consumption during stationary phase when growth was suppressed by a $P_{O_2}$ of 4.7 ± 1.1 mmHg was negligible at 0.016 ± 0.062 μ moles $O_2$/(hour × $10^6$ cells). Despite active glucose utilization growth continued during this period slowly, if at all (data not shown).[154] Comparisons of glucose utilization between oxygen tensions during stationary phase show decreased glucose utilization and lactate production accompany increased oxygen utilization.

Cellular oxygen consumption during stationary phase under a $P_{O_2}$ of 134 mmHg was 0.17 ± 0.05 μmoles/(hour × $10^6$ cells).[154] Thus, the oxygen utilization of exponentially growing cells at a $P_{O_2}$ of 134 mmHg was three times greater than that of stationary cells at the same oxygen tension.

The reversible depression in cellular growth under $P_{O_2}$ 7.8 mmHg demonstrates that WI-38 cell growth can be retarded by insufficient oxygen. During exponential cellular growth under $P_{O_2}$ 7.8 mmHg, oxygen consumption was decreased relative to cells grown at $P_{O_2}$ of 44 to 134 mmHg. Despite an increased glycolytic rate in the cells grown under the lower oxygen tension, their doubling time was prolonged. This growth inhibition was apparent despite adequate glucose present in the media and rapid glucose utilization and was accompanied by a lack of oxygen consumption. Furthermore, the inhibition was reversed without changing the media if the flasks were reequilibrated with a $P_{O_2}$ of 134 mmHg.

Kilburn et al.[24] reported a depression of growth in mouse LS cells grown in suspension culture at very low $P_{O_2}$ (1.2 mmHg). Others have found an inhibition of growth accompanied by an increased glycolytic rate under anaerobic conditions.[20,159-163] However, some investigators have reported equally good growth under aerobic and anaerobic conditions.[23,25,164,15] Harris,[164] for example, reported that over a 4-day period with daily changes of medium the growth rate and final population density was the same for cells grown under 5% $CO_2$ 95% $N_2$ and 5% $CO_2$ 95% $O_2$. He notes, using an oxygen electrode, that the medium was not entirely freed of oxygen by his gassing procedure but states that the small amount of oxygen remaining was rapidly consumed by the cells. Unfortunately, he did not investigate growth under 5% $CO_2$ 95% room air. If growth under 5% $CO_2$ 95% $N_2$ and 5% $CO_2$ 95% $O_2$ was similar to growth at 5% $CO_2$ 95% room air, the frequent changes of media which reintroduced small amounts of oxygen into the vessel probably supplied sufficient oxygen for cell growth. Other investigators who have reported equally good growth under aerobic and anaerobic conditions have not reported the $P_{O_2}$ of the media under their anaerobic environments.[23,25]

Although our study showed a 15% longer population doubling time at a $P_{O_2}$ of 134 mmHg compared to that at a $P_{O_2}$ of 44 mmHg ($p < 0.02$), there were no differences in the saturation density achieved or cellular rates of glucose consumption, oxygen utilization, or lactate production during exponential growth. This illustrates the broad range of oxygen tensions that can support normal growth, results that are in agreement with data obtained from widely different cell lines.[24,25] Furthermore, as noted earlier, other investigators have noted a more rapid doubling time when the percent of oxygen was decreased below that present in room air.[25,166-168]

Packer and Fuehr found that human diploid fibroblasts which were seeded at very low density (80 cells/$cm^2$) grew faster under 2% or 10% $O_2$ than under 20% $O_2$.[169] This difference disappeared, however, when the cells were seeded at 1 × $10^4$ cells per $cm^2$.[169] Others have shown increased clonal growth when the $O_2$ in the gas phase was lowered to 1%.[170,171]

Cristofalo and Kritchevsky have reported that the oxygen consumption by a suspension of trypsinized WI-38 cells under room air was independent of the glucose concentration of the incubation medium from 0 to 7.7 m*M*,[172,173] and averaged about 0.14 ± 0.06 μmoles/(hour × $10^6$ cells). Our results,[154] indicating that stationary phase cells at $P_{O_2}$ 119 mmHg consume 0.17 ± 0.05 μmoles/(hour × $10^6$ cells), agree with this previous measurement. However, we found a threefold greater oxygen consumption during exponential growth of cells under $P_{O_2}$ 44 to 134 mmHg [about 0.5 μmoles/(hour × $10^6$ cells)].[154]

The markedly increased glucose consumption and lactate production per cell at $P_{O_2}$ 291 mmHg (Table 18) and at $P_{O_2}$ 560 mmHg (Table 18) at a time when cell proliferation is inhibited (Figure 1), make it unlikely that the sulfhydryl groups in key glycolytic enzymes, e.g., glyceraldehyde-3-phosphate dehydrogenase are oxidized and the enzyme inactivated. Thus, in these intact cells failure of cell proliferation is not due simply to an inhibition of energy metabolism. These results are in agreement with those of Kilburn et al.[24] using mouse LS cells, Rueckert and Mueller,[20] using HeLa cells, and Allen et al.[17] using the toad bladder.

The contrast between a depressed rate of cellular proliferation and an increased rate of glycolysis may be an important clue to the mechanisms of growth inhibition. It is possible, for example, that the energy and reducing equivalents necessary for cell division are diverted and consumed in an attempt to compensate for increased oxidation of cellular components, particularly membrane lipids as proposed by Allen et al.[17]

### C. Effect of Oxygen on the Life Span Proliferative Capacity of Human Diploid Cells

Figure 3 illustrates the effect of oxygen tension on the life span of WI-38 cells. Cells serially subcultivated from population doubling level (PDL) 19 at $P_{O_2}$ of 24 mmHg, 49 mmHg, or 137 mmHg grew similarly and phased out after a similar number of population doublings, here 67-71. Cultures incubated at a $P_{O_2}$ of 608 mmHg did not proliferate. There were no differences in cell attachment between the various oxygen tensions throughout the cell life span.[154]

Table 19 summarizes the results of a series of replicate experiments performed with different sublines of WI-38 cells. These results show that, in every case, although elevated oxygen tensions (> atmospheric) poison WI-38 cells and markedly decrease their life span, there is no life span extension when cells are serially subcultivated at lower partial pressure (< atmospheric) of oxygen.

In a similar study, Packer and Fuehr found that human diploid cells grown under 10% $O_2$ underwent about 25% more population doublings than cells grown under 20% $O_2$.[169] However, they did not measure the partial pressure of oxygen to which their cells were exposed and they estimated PDL by adding two population doublings at each 1:4 split or one PDL at each 1:2 split rather than by direct cell count, comparing counts at seeding with counts at confluence.

To determine the effect of very low oxygen tensions on life span, the cells were grown in sealed glass vessels that were kept stationary to maximize any oxygen diffusion gradients. Cultures that were serially subcultivated at a $P_{O_2}$ of 5.6 mmHg grew more slowly (Table 17) and phased out after fewer population doublings than control cells grown at a $P_{O_2}$ of 119 mmHg (Table 20).

As we saw in Table 1, WI-38 cell growth was markedly inhibited at a $P_{O_2}$ of 7.8 ± 3.5 mmHg. This inhibition was accompanied by a markedly decreased $O_2$ consumption and both increased glucose consumption and lactate production. Serial cultivation of these cells at a $P_{O_2}$ of 5.6 ± 1.4 mmHg (Table 4) demonstrated some variability in the PDL at phase-out, but in no case did the life span equal or exceed that of control cells. These observations are of interest since Warburg hypothesized that hypoxia or any respiratory injury sufficient to decrease oxygen consumption and increase glycolytic metabolism was the basis for the etiology of neoplasia.[174] Although controversial,[175] this point of view has been proposed by others, including Goldblatt and Cameron,[176]

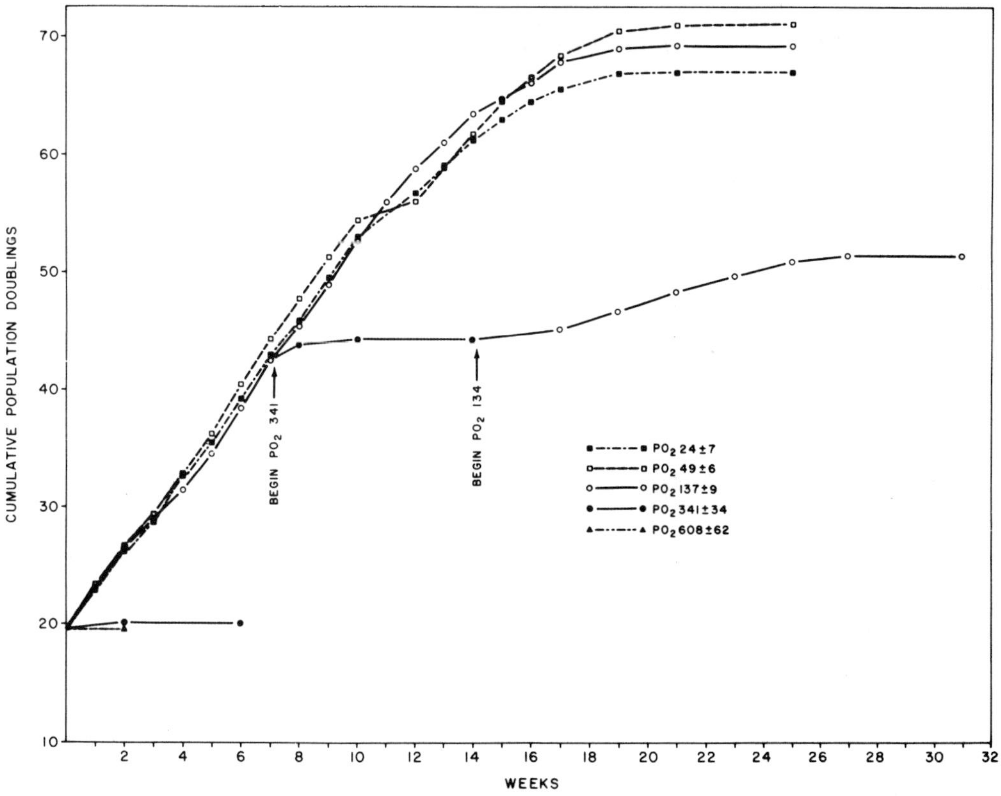


FIGURE 3. The effect of oxygen tension on the life span of human diploid cells. Cells were serially subcultivated as described in the text at the indicated oxygen tension. This figure is an accumulative representation of the data whose endpoints are expressed in Table 19, experiment 1 A and (for the recovery experiment) Table 21. (From Balin, A. K., Goodman, D. G., Rasmussen, H., and Cristfalo, V. J., *J. Cell Biol.*, 74, 58, 1977. With permission.)

who reported transformation of rat fibroblasts upon intermittent exposure to low oxygen tensions. In a subsequent publication, however, dealing with the malignant transformation of fibroblasts and epithelial cells exposed to hypoxic conditions, it was reported that both the cultures intermittently exposed to $N_2$ and the control cultures transformed.[177] Goldblatt et al.[177] explained this phenomenon by postulating that the control cells, which had free access to oxygen, transformed because of inadequate diffusion of atmospheric oxygen into the liquid medium of the stationary flask. In this regard, it is important to point out that, after more than 10 years of WI-38 cell cultivation, there have not been any published reports of a spontaneous transformation. In addition, Sanford was unable to induce malignant transformation of cells in vitro by intermittent anaerobiosis.[178] Furthermore, it should be emphasized that WI-38 cells, serially carried at a $P_{O_2}$ of 5.6 mmHg where oxygen consumption is minimal and glycolytic metabolism is markedly increased, do not acquire an indefinite life span in vitro.

### D. Recovery After Exposure to Elevated Oxygen Tensions

The cultures were exposed to a $P_{O_2}$ of 341 ± 34 mmHg for 7 days (week 1) and were then subcultivated and exposed to a $P_{O_2}$ of 137 ± 9 mmHg or to a $P_{O_2}$ of 341 mmHg for various numbers of weeks (refeeding at weekly intervals) before being equilibrated with a $P_{O_2}$ of 137 ± 9 mmHg serially for three additional weeks to allow recovery. Recovery was defined, in this experiment, as the ability to achieve enough cells in the

## Table 19
## THE EFFECT OF OXYGEN TENSION ON THE LIFE SPAN OF HUMAN DIPLOID (WI-38) CELLS

| | Experiment 1[a] PDL[e] | | Experiment 2 PDL | | Experiment 3 PDL | | Experiment 4 PDL | |
|---|---|---|---|---|---|---|---|---|
| 2 (mmHg)[b] | Begin | Phase out[d] A,B | Begin | Phase out | Begin | Phase out | Begin | Phase out |
| 24 ± 7[c] | 19 | 67, 69 | 25 | 62 | 24 | 66 | 28 | 74 |
| 49 ± 6 | 19 | 71, 72 | 25 | 59 | 24 | 74 | — | — |
| 37 ± 9 | 19 | 69, 73 | 25 | 62 | 24 | 72 | 28 | 69 |
| 41 ± 34 | 19.3 | 20.0, 20.1 | 25.0 | 25.4 | 34.5 | 35.5 | 28.5 | 29.4 ± 0.2 (N = 6) |
| 08 ± 62 | 19.3 | 19.3, 19.3 | 25.0 | 25.0 | 26.0 | 26.0 | 28.5 | 28.5 (N = 4) |
| | 32.8 | 32.8, 32.8 | | | | | | |

*Note:* The cells were serially subcultivated at the indicated oxygen tension and grown on a slowly shaking apparatus as described in the text.

[a] In Experiment 1, A and B represent the work of two independent investigators carrying cells from the same initial culture to phase-out. Experiment 1A is illustrated in Figure 3.
[b] Average $P_{O_2}$ during growth period.
[c] Standard deviation.
[d] Phase-out was defined as the inability to achieve confluence after four feedings over a 4-week period.
[e] PDL Population doubling level was determined by direct cell count.

## Table 20
## THE EFFECT OF LOW OXYGEN TENSION ON THE LIFE SPAN OF HUMAN DIPLOID (WI-38) CELLS

| | Population doubling level | | | | | |
|---|---|---|---|---|---|---|
| | Experiment 1 | | Experiment 2 | | Experiment 3 | |
| Oxygen tension | Begin | Phase-out[a] | Begin | Phase-out | Begin | Phase-out |
| mmHg[b] | | | | | | |
| 119 ± 9[c] | 27 | 61 | 26 | 54 | 24 | 65 |
| 5.6 ± 1.4[d] | 27 | 37 | 26 | 45 | 24 | 54 |
| 5.6 ± 1.4[d] | | | 26 | 35 | 24 | 55 |
| 5.6 ± 1.4[d] | | | 26 | 42 | 24 | 40 |
| 5.6 → 119[e] | | | | | 24 | 53 |

*Note:* The cells were serially subcultivated at the indicated oxygen tension and grown without shaking in sealed glass prescription bottles.

[a] Phase-out was defined as the inability to achieve confluence after four feedings over a 4-week period.
[b] Average $P_{O_2}$ during growth period.
[c] Standard deviation.
[d] Replicate experiments independently.
[e] Carried at $P_{O_2}$ 5.6 serially for 6 weeks (38 PDL), then subcultivated at $P_{O_2}$ 119 until phase-out.

flask to seed one daughter flask (at $1 \times 10^4$ cells per $cm^2$) and sufficient subsequent growth of the daughter flask to allow for subcultivation.

Cells incubated at a $P_{O_2}$ of 341 ± 34 mmHg for 1 week and then subsequently exposed to a $P_{O_2}$ of 137 ± 9 mmHg recovered and were subcultivated for nearly as long as control cells never exposed to the higher oxygen tension (Table 21).

## Table 21
## RECOVERY OF HUMAN DIPLOID (WI-38) CELL POPULATIONS AFTER PROLONGED EXPOSURE TO ELEVATED OXYGEN TENSIONS

| Treatment at $P_{O_2}$ 341 ± 34 mmHg | Recovery[a] | Life span of recovered cells PDL at phase-out experimental cultures (control)[b] |
|---|---|---|
| Weeks | No. recovered/no. of experiments | |
| 1 | 4/4 | 54 (60); 52 (54);51 (54);[c] |
| 2 | 3/4 | 45 (54);52 (60);[c] |
| 5-7 | 3/14 | 52[d] (70); 52 (69);[c] |

[a] Cultures were exposed to a $P_{O_2}$ of 341 mmHg for the indicated time. All cultures were refed with fresh medium weekly. After week 1, the cultures were subcultivated because they were confluent. They did not become confluent again at $P_{O_2}$ 341 mmHg. The ability of the culture to recover was tested by changing the atmosphere to $P_{O_2}$ 137 mmHg and allowing the cultures to incubate at the lower oxygen tension for 3 additional weeks. Recovery was defined as the ability to achieve enough cells to seed one daughter flask ($7.5 \times 10^5$ cells) and sufficient subsequent growth of the daughter flask to allow for subcultivation.

[b] Control: grown entirely at $P_{O_2}$ 137 ± 9 mmHg.

[c] In each case, one flask which met the criteria for recovery was lost to contamination during subsequent subcultivation procedure and before the lifespan was completed.

[d] Treatment begun at PDL 43 (the weekly cumulative PDL of this subline is shown in Figure 3; in all other experiments, treatment begun at PDL 23-26.

Recovery of the cell population from prolonged exposure to elevated partial pressures of oxygen, although variable, was sharply limited if the cells were exposed to a $P_{O_2}$ of 341 mmHg for more than 2 weeks. In addition, the life span of the cell populations that did recover after 5 to 7 weeks of exposure to $P_{O_2}$ 340 was shorter than that of sister cultures never exposed to this elevated oxygen tension (Table 21 and Figure 3).

Continuous label autoradiography experiments with a dose of [$^3$H]thymidine sufficient to prevent cell division established that substantial portions of the population were able to initiate DNA synthesis after exposure to elevated oxygen tensions and suggested that recovery was not simply due to a few resistant clones of cells.

### E. Effect of Vitamin E and Oxygen Tension on Cell Life Span

Vitamin E (d-1-α-tocopherol), an agent known to trap free radicals, has been reported to extend the life span of WI-38 cells in culture.[179]

Packer and Smith reported that the addition of 10 μg/mℓ or 100 μg/mℓ d-1-α-tocopherol to WI-38 cells at each subcultivation extended the in vitro life span of the cells from 65 to 115 PDL. Furthermore, they reported that a brief exposure to d-1-α-tocopherol (from the 45th to 73rd PDL) conferred the same effect as continual exposure. It should be noted that their experiments were begun with one lot of serum and that after their cells had gone 90-105 PDL, a new serum lot was started and the cells phased out. In subsequent studies,[180] they were unable to repeat this result and suggested that there was a unique property of their initial lot of serum that sustained cell growth when combined with vitamin E.

In our experiments, when vitamin E was first placed in the medium, about 14% (60 ± 11% vs. 74 ± 7%, N = 9, paired *t*-test, P <0.02) fewer cells attached at 20 hr in the vitamin E flasks than in controls that had an equivalent amount of homogenized medium added. This slightly decreased attachment was associated with a slight decrease in cell yield during the few weeks of cultivation under these conditions. However, cell attachment and cell yield equalized after 6 to 8 weeks of subcultivation under the two conditions.

Table 22 summarizes representative experiments that show the effects of d-1-$\alpha$-tocopherol on the life span of WI-38 cells at various oxygen tensions. Under our routine 5% $CO_2$ room air atmosphere, sister cultures carried serially in unsupplemented medium, or 10 $\mu$g, or 100 $\mu$g, of a d-1-$\alpha$-tocopherol per m$\ell$ showed no differences in life span. Similarly, cells carried serially under a $P_{O_2}$ of 49 mmHg or 137 mmHg showed no differences in the PDL at phase-out with or without vitamin E. Cells grown under a $P_{O_2}$ of 341 ± 34 mmHg were not protected by the addition of the antioxidant. Thus, in this series of experiments, vitamin E did not alter the life span of WI-38 cells in culture. The fact that the life span of WI-38 cells in vitro is not extended by serial cultivation of $P_{O_2}$ of 5.6 mmHg, 26 mmHg or 50 mmHg, suggests that neither oxygen toxicity nor free radical reactions play a significant role in delimiting the life span of human diploid WI-38 cells in vitro under ambient oxygen tensions.

The next section presents additional evidence that the loss of proliferative capacity of human diploid cells in culture and oxygen induced free radical toxicity occur by different mechanisms.

### F. Oxygen-Sensitive Phases in the Cell Cycle of WI-38 Cells Exposed to Elevated Oxygen Tension at Seeding

Cells grown for 72 hr under normal atmospheric oxygen tension ($P_{O_2}$ of 138 ± 5 mmHg) proliferated actively (see Figure 1); when cells were exposed to [$^3$H]dT from hour 71 to 72, 45% of the population was observed to be synthesizing DNA and 2.5% of the population was in mitosis (Figure 4a). The DNA content of the unlabeled interphase nuclei fell into two populations: 40% had a DNA content of 2C and 13% had a DNA content of 4C (Figure 4a). At a higher $P_{O_2}$ (373 ± 7 mmHg), cells grew very slowly over the 72-hr period; and from hour 71 to 72 only 13% of the population was engaged in DNA synthesis, while only 0.1% of the population was engaged in mitosis (Figure 4b, Table 23). However, a marked percentage of the population contained a 4C content of DNA (47% at 72 hr) while 35% of the cells were found to have a 2C DNA content. Cells exposed to a $P_{O_2}$ of 649 ± 33 mmHg do not proliferate (Figure 1). Only 1% of these cells synthesized DNA during the pulse from hour 71 to 72, and less than 0.1% were in mitosis (Table 23). After 72 hr, 70% of the population contained a 2C complement of DNA, only 10% contained a 4C complement of DNA, and 19% of the cells had an intermediate content of DNA, referred to as "3C." Occasionally, at all oxygen tensions, a few cells (<2%) were encountered with an 8C content of DNA (Figures 4b and c).

To illuminate these findings, we compared the time-course of the change in the distribution of cells through the cell cycle for the various oxygen tensions. Immediately after a confluent population (grown at a $P_{O_2}$ of 138 mmHg) was subcultivated (time 0) the population distribution was approximately 93% 2C, 5% 4C, 2% labeled (after a 1-hr [$^3$H]thymidine pulse), <0.1% mitosis (Figure 5); and the DNA content was 7.69 ± 1.9 $\mu$g DNA/$10^6$ cells (n = 19). The cells retained this distribution for 14 to 18 hr before the percentage of the population undergoing DNA synthesis began to increase. The population was parasynchronous for the first 36 hr at a $P_{O_2}$ of 138 mmHg, but became random by 48 hr (data now shown). A larger percentage of the population initiated DNA synthesis by 24 hr when cells were grown at a $P_{O_2}$ of 138 mmHg (57%) (Figures 4 and 5a) than when cells were grown at a $P_{O_2}$ of 365 mmHg (45%) (Figures 4b and 5b). This decrease at a $P_{O_2}$ of 365 mmHg indicates that the transition from the pre-DNA synthetic phase ($G_0$, $G_1$) to DNA synthesis (S) is slightly delayed or inhib-

Table 22
THE EFFECT OF VITAMIN E AND OXYGEN TENSION ON THE LIFE SPAN OF HUMAN DIPLOID (WI-38) CELLS

| | $P_{O_2}$ (mmHg) ⟶ | | 49 ± 6 | | 137 ± 9 | | 341 ± 34 | |
|---|---|---|---|---|---|---|---|---|
| | PDL[a] | | PDL | | PDL | | PDL | |
| Media supplement | Begin | Phase out[b] | Begin | Phase out | Begin | Phase out | Begin | Phase out |
| – | 18 | 67 | 19 | 61 | 19 | 63 | 16.0 | 17.5 |
| 4 mℓ homogenized media | 27 | 69 | 37 | 64 | 35 | 65 | 16.0 | 17.5 |
| 10 μg DL-α-tocopherol / mℓ | 24 | 66 | 37 | 63 | 35 | 64 | 16.0 | 17.3 |
| 100 μg DL-α-tocopherol / mℓ | 18 | 67 | 33 | 64 | 33 | 67 | 16.0 | 17.1 |

*Note:* The cells were serially subcultivated at the indicated oxygen tension.

[a] PDL Population doubling level was determined by direct cell count.
[b] Phase-out was defined as the inability to achieve confluence after four feedings over a 4-wk period.

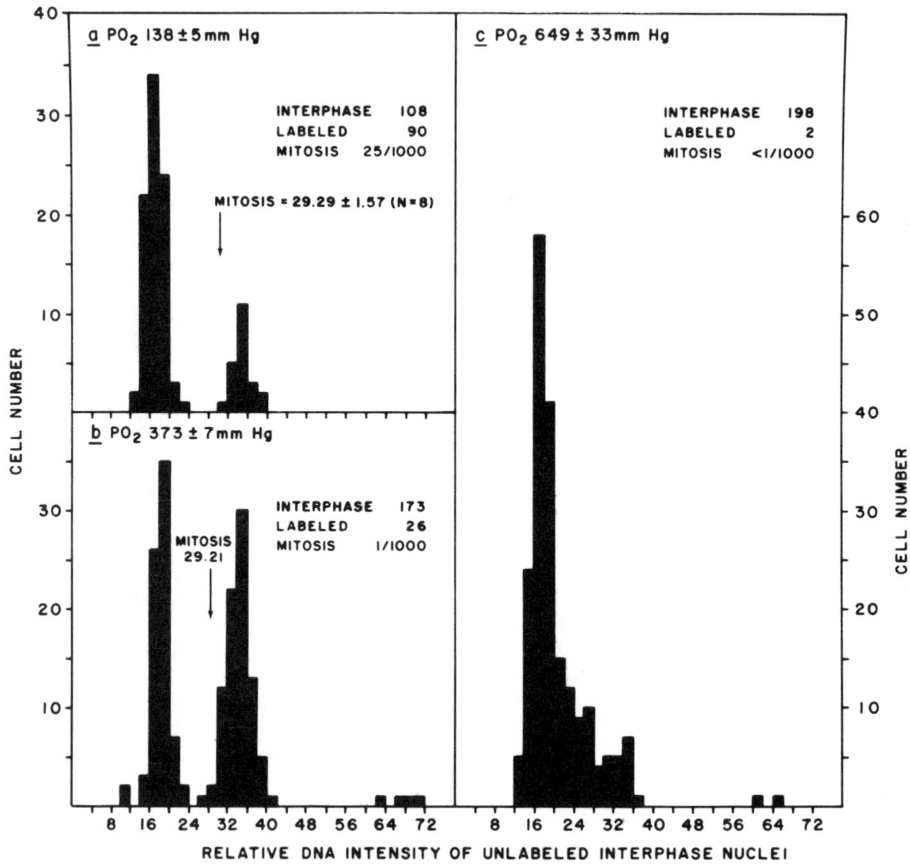


FIGURE 4. The distribution through the cell cycle of a cell population grown at various oxygen tensions for 72 hr. The scanning microdensitometer was used to determine the relative DNA content of the unlabeled interphase nuclei. Young confluent WI-38 cells were subcultivated and incubated at the indicated oxygen tensions at hour 0, pulsed with [$^3$H] thymidine from hour 71 to 72, fixed at hour 72, then Feulgen-stained and processed through autoradiography as described (see appropriate sections in text). Two hundred cells were randomly selected and scored as labeled (five grains over background), mitotic, or interphase cells. The relative DNA content of the unlabeled interphase nuclei is plotted in the histogram. The haploid content of DNA is referred to as "lC." Metaphase mitotic figures are used to indicate the 4C DNA peak. Absorption due to the condensed chromosomes of the metaphase mitotic cells usually falls at the lower end of the 4C distribution. Chick erythrocytes (2.4 pg/DNA nucleus) had a relative DNA intensity of 4.74 ± 0.56 (n = 6). (From Balin, A. K., Goodman, D. G., Rasmussen, H., and Cristofalo, V. J., *J. Cell Biol.*, 78, 390, 1978. With permission.)

ited at the higher oxygen tension. In addition, the percentage of cells synthesizing DNA decreased during the 72 hr incubation period under a $P_{O_2}$ of 365 mmHg from 45% at hour 24 to 13% by hour 72 (Figure 5b). Thus, it seems that the delay in initiation of DNA synthesis became more pronounced with increasing time of exposure to the elevated oxygen tension. The most striking finding, however, was the increasing proportion of the population with a 4C complement of DNA (47% by 72 hr) (Figure 5b). This indicates that at a $P_{O_2}$ of 365 mmHg, most of the population was delayed after completing DNA synthesis but before initiating mitosis.

The cell population exposed to a $P_{O_2}$ of 590 ± 35 mmHg immediately after subcultivation was markedly delayed in the initiation of DNA synthesis: 73% of the cells contained a 2C content of DNA and incorporated [$^3$H]thymidine from hour 23 to 24, whereas when cells were exposed to a $P_{O_2}$ of 138 mmHg for the same length of time, 35% contained a 2C content of DNA and 58% incorporated [$^3$H]thymidine (Figures

### Table 23
### THE TIME COURSE OF THE CHANGE IN MITOTIC INDEX DURING GROWTH AT VARIOUS OXYGEN TENSIONS

| | Mitosis (% of total population)[a] | | | |
|---|---|---|---|---|
| | Hours after subcultivation | | | |
| $P_{O_2}$ | 1 | 24 | 48 | 72 |
| 138 ± 5[b] | <0.1 (3)[c] | 1.3 ± .2 (2) | 1.9 ± 0.2 (2) | 2.2 ± 0.4 (4) |
| 365 ± 8 | <0.1 (3) | 0.2 ± 0.2 (2) | 0.4 ± 0.3 (3) | 0.1 ± 0.1 (4) |
| 590 ± 35 | <0.1 (3) | 0.2 ± 0.2 (2) | 0.1 (2) | <0.1 (4) |

[a] Mitotic index from experiment depicted in Figure 5. Index determined from counting > 1000 random cells per slide.
[b] Standard deviation.
[c] ( ) = number of replicate slides counted for this experiment.

5a and c). During continued exposure to a $P_{O_2}$ of 590 mmHg, there was no further initiation of DNA synthesis; at hours 48 and 72, 70% of the population retained a 2C DNA content (Figure 5c), and no increase in cell number was noted (Figure 1). Furthermore, the proportion of the population that was capable of initiating DNA synthesis (20%) aborted after an incomplete attempt, as shown by the progressive decline in the proportion of the population incorporating [$^3$H]thymidine and the corresponding increase in unlabeled 3C cells (Figure 5c). Unlabeled cells did not move through the cell cycle for there was no increase in 4C interphase cells (Figure 5c) or mitotic cells (Table 23). Thus, when confluent cells were subcultivated and exposed to a $P_{O_2}$ of 590 mmHg, initiation of effective DNA synthesis was inhibited.

## G. Oxygen-Sensitive Phases in the Cell Cycle of WI-38 Cells Exposed to Elevated Oxygen Tension After the Onset of DNA Synthesis

To examine the effect of oxygen on actively proliferating cells, a confluent population was subcultivated and grown at a $P_{O_2}$ of 138 mmHg for 24 hr before exposure to the experimental oxygen tensions. In this experiment, 50% of the exponentially growing cells kept at a $P_{O_2}$ of 138 mmHg incorporated [$^3$H]thymidine: 40% had a 2C content of DNA, and 10% had a 4C DNA content (Figure 6a). As in the previous experiment, there was a gradual accumulation of cells with a 4C DNA content when the atmosphere was changed to a $P_{O_2}$ of 353 mmHg (Figure 6a vs. 6b). When cells were allowed to begin DNA synthesis before exposure to a $P_{O_2}$ of 592 mmHg, the proportion of them engaged in DNA synthesis after the increase in $P_{O_2}$ to 592 mmHg increased from 0 to 16 hr, whereas at lower $O_2$ tensions the proportion of the population undergoing DNA synthesis declined gradually from hour 0 (Figures 6a-c). These data suggest that cells exposed to a $P_{O_2}$ of 592 mmHg needed more time to complete DNA synthesis than did cells at lower $P_{O_2}$. The absence of 3C cells at a $P_{O_2}$ of 592 mmHg indicates that cells initiating DNA synthesis eventually completed the process and accumulated as nonmitotic 4C cells (Figure 6c). The 4C accumulation (evidence of a delay in initiation of mitosis) was more pronounced at a $P_{O_2}$ of 592 mmHg than at a $P_{O_2}$ of 353 mmHg (Figure 6b vs. 6c). These findings show that when cells began DNA synthesis before being exposed to a $P_{O_2}$ of 592 mmHg, they were capable of completing DNA synthesis but were unable to initiate mitosis. In addition, after a 24-hr exposure to a $P_{O_2}$ of 592 mmHg, the proportion of the population incorporating [$^3$H]thymidine declined without a corresponding decline in 2C cells, indicating that the delay in the initiation of DNA synthesis was more pronounced with increasing time of exposure to the elevated oxygen tension.

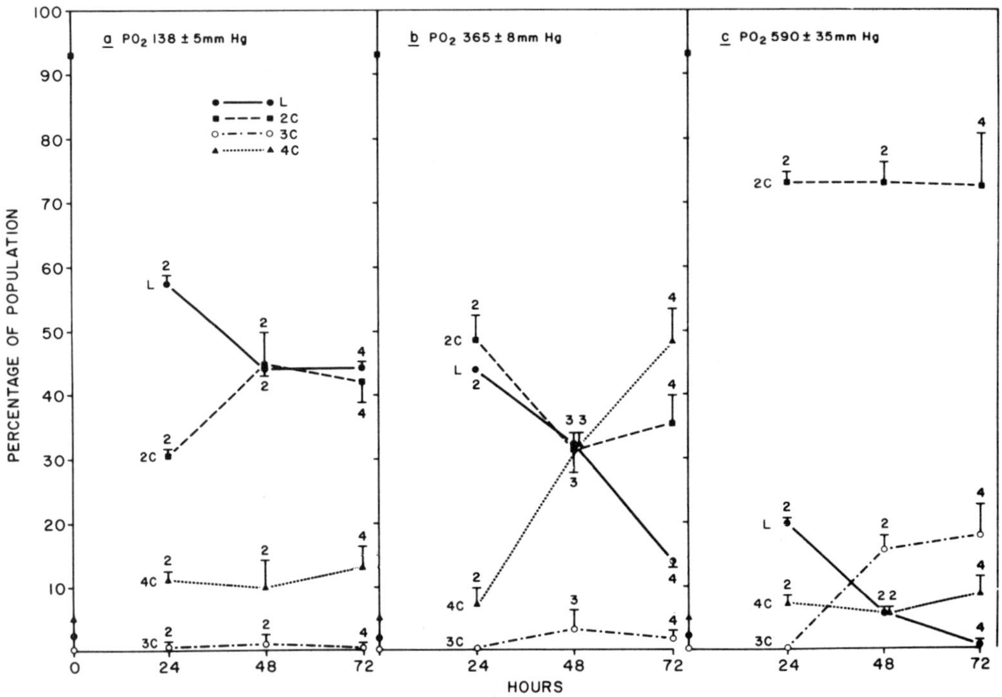


FIGURE 5. The time-course of the change in the interphase population distribution during growth of young WI-38 cells exposed to various oxygen tensions at seeding. Cells were seeded from confluent cultures and exposed to the indicated oxygen tension immediately upon subcultivation. The cells were pulsed with [$^3$H] thymidine for 1 hr immediately before fixation. The population distribution at time 0 represents the distribution of young confluent WI-38 cells for the first 14 to 18 hr after subcultivation. The number associated with each point is the number of replicate slides counted; error bars indicate standard deviation. The data in this figure were derived from histograms (e.g., Figure 4). The percentage of labeled nuclei (L) was determined from >100 random measurements. Cells with other DNA contents (such as 8C) represented <2% of the population in this experiment is presented in Table 23. (From Balin, A. K., Goodman, D. G., Rasmussen, H., and Cristofalo, V. J., *J. Cell Biol.*, 78, 390, 1978. With permission).

## H. Oxygen and the Rate of DNA Synthesis

Further evidence that elevated oxygen tension may decrease the rate of DNA synthesis is found in an analysis of the relative grain intensity of labeled cells. The relative grain intensity of labeled cells reflects the amount of [$^3$H] thymidine incorporated into DNA during the 1 hr pulse period. Analysis of histograms of the relative grain intensity of labeled cells reveals an inverse correlation between the rate of [$^3$H] thymidine incorporation and the oxygen tension (Figure 7). Furthermore, the decrease in the rate of [$^3$H] thymidine incorporation began shortly (by hour 5) after exposure to the elevated oxygen tension and was greatest when the oxygen tension was highest ($P_{O_2}$ 592 ± 55) (data not shown). Thus, in summary, three stages of the cell cycle were found in which oxygen-inhibited cells accumulate. The most striking data obtained showed that cells exposed to a $P_{O_2}$ of 350 mmHg at seeding were delayed primarily after DNA synthesis but before mitosis (Figures 4b, 5b, and Table 23). These findings indicate that the site most sensitive to oxygen causes a delay in $G_2$ (or early prophase). Another site, less sensitive to oxygen, delayed resting ($G_O$) cells from initiating DNA synthesis. Confluent cells that were subcultivated and exposed to a $P_{O_2}$ of 365 mmHg were partially delayed in entry to DNA synthesis since under this elevated $P_{O_2}$, the percentage of cells engaged in DNA synthesis at hour 24 (45%) was lower than the percentage of cells synthesizing DNA in the control group (57%) (Figures 5a and b). Furthermore, confluent cells that

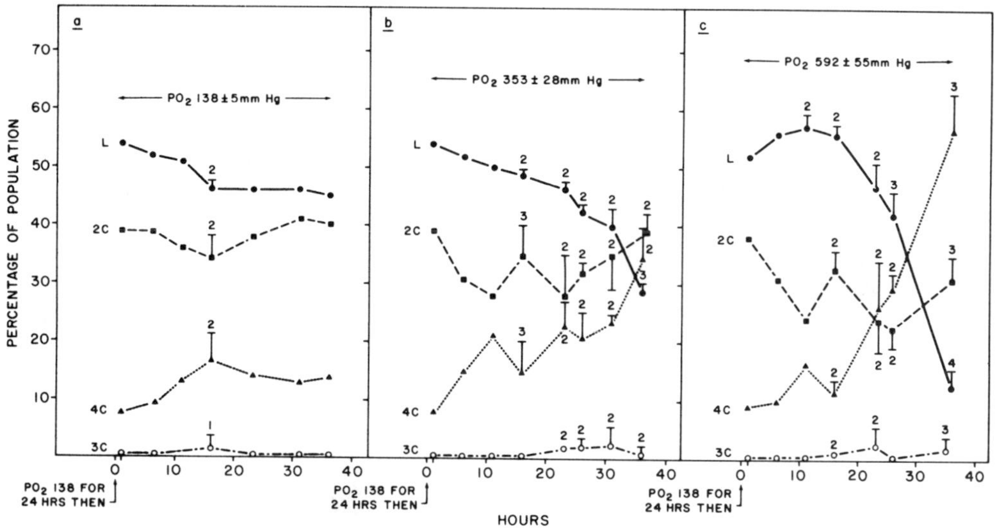


FIGURE 6. The time-course of the change in the interphase population distribution during growth of young WI-38 cells exposed to various oxygen tensions after the onset of exponential growth. Cells were seeded from confluent cultures and allowed to enter the cell cycle by incubation at a $P_{O_2}$ of 138 mmHg for 24 hr. The atmosphere was changed as indicated and designated time "0". The percentage of labeled nuclei was determined from 500 randomly selected cells, and the interphase cell distribution was determined from 100 random measurements. The data in this figure were derived from histograms (e.g., Figure 4). Cells with other DNA contents (such as 8C) represented <2% of the population and were not plotted on these graphs. The number associated with each point is the number of replicate slides counted; error bars indicate standard deviation. The mitotic index of the cel population in this experiment is not illustrated, but represented <4% of the population. (From Balin, A. K., Goodman, D. G., Rasmussen, H., and Cristofalo, V. J., *J. Cell Biol.*, 78, 390, 1978. With permission.)

were freshly subcultivated and exposed to a $P_{O_2}$ of 590 mmHg were primarily inhibited from entering DNA synthesis. It is unlikely that these results are related to selective detachment of cells from the substratum. Cell attachment at various $P_{O_2}$ levels has been reported in our previous work,[154] and has been shown to be independent of $P_{O_2}$.

A third site sensitive to oxygen inhibition reduced the rate of [$^3$H] thymidine incorporation into the DNA of cells that were exposed to elevated oxygen tensions during DNA synthesis (Figures 6c and 7). The reduction was due either to a decrease in thymidine transport and/or utilization, or to a decreased rate of DNA synthesis. On the basis of our results, it is not possible to completely resolve these alternative explanations. However, oxygen did not block thymidine transport and utilization completely (independent of the effect that slows the rate of DNA synthesis to zero), since no cells synthesized DNA and proceeded through the cell cycle without incorporating [$^3$H] thymidine. We know this because there were virtually no 3C cells in a population incubated under a $P_{O_2}$ of 365 mmHg (Figure 5b) and no increase in 4C cells under incubation at a $P_{O_2}$ of 592 mmHg (Figure 5c). On the other hand, the rate of DNA synthesis was slowed to zero for most cells exposed to a $P_{O_2}$ of 592 mmHg for 72 hr (Figure 5c). It should be noted that the stage of the cell cycle at which oxygen-inhibited cells accumulate is not necessarily the stage in which the oxygen-sensitive sites are located.

## I. The Limited Proliferative Capacity of Human Diploid Cells in Culture Is Not Due to Oxygen Toxicity

The experimental observations that the life span of WI-38 cells in vitro is not extended by serial cultivation at $P_{O_2}$ of 5.6 mmHg, 26 mmHg, or 50 mmHg, suggests

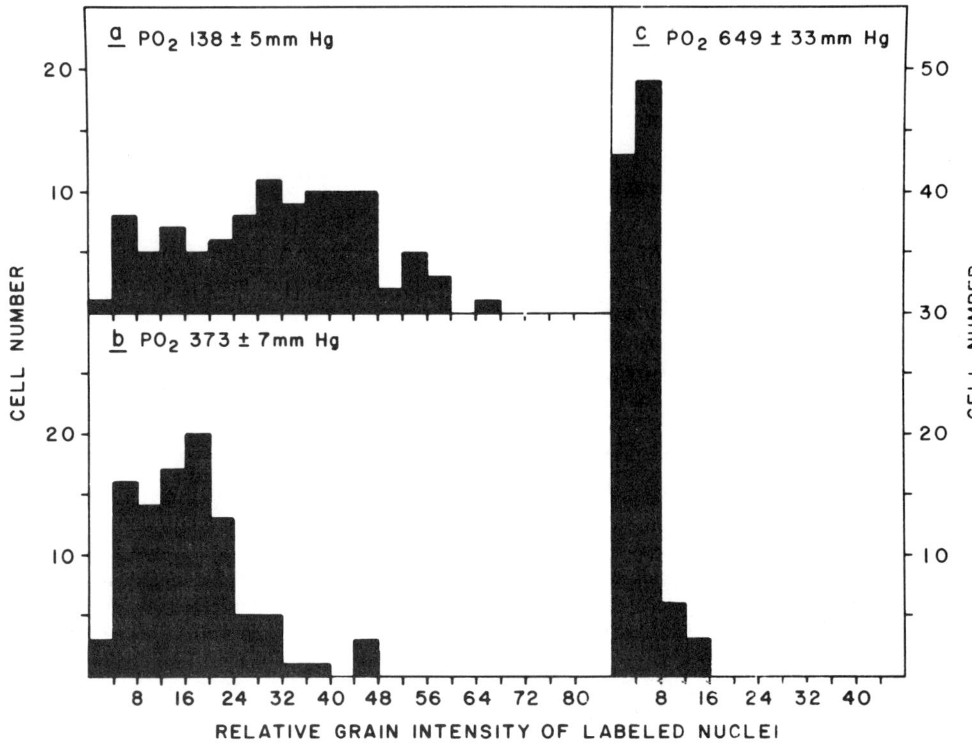


FIGURE 7. The relative grain intensity of a population of 101 randomly selected labeled nuclei after a 48 hr exposure to various oxygen tensions. Young confluent WI-38 cells were subcultivated and incubated at the indicated oxygen tensions at hour 0, pulsed with [$^3$H] thymidine from hour 47 to 48, fixed at hour 48, then Feulgen-stained and processed through autoradiography. The relative grain intensity of the labeled nuclei (at least five grains over background) was measured by the scanning microdensitometer. Unlabeled nuclei had a relative intensity of 1.9 ± 2.0 ($\eta$ <100). (From Balin, A. K., Goodman, D. G., Rasmussen, H., and Cristofalo, V. J., *J. Cell Biol.*, 78, 390, 1978. With permission.)

that neither oxygen toxicity nor free radical reactions play a significant role in limiting the proliferative capacity of human diploid cells in vitro under ambient oxygen tensions. This conclusion is further supported by the results showing that the addition of the free radical-trapping agent d-1-$\alpha$-tocopherol at each subcultivation did not prolong life span. Furthermore, recovery after growth arrest resulting from exposure to elevated partial pressures of oxygen suggests that oxygen inhibits growth by a mechanism different from that responsible for the ultimate limitation on the proliferative capacity of the cell population.

The above studies demonstrate that the site most sensitive to inhibition by elevated oxygen tension causes cells to accumulate with a 4C content of DNA. If oxygen toxicity and free radical reactions were limiting the proliferative capacity of human cell cultures, we would expect to see an accumulation of cells with a 4C DNA content ($G_2$) in the nonproliferative fraction of the older cell cultures. However, both confluence and loss of proliferative capacity in human diploid cell populations are associated with an accumulation of cells with a 2C content of DNA ($G_0$ or $G_1$).[181-183]

Furthermore, if accumulated peroxidative damage played a significant role in limiting the proliferative capacity of human diploid cells in culture, one would need to explain why similar damage does not limit the life span of tumor cell populations. It seems unlikely that the indefinite life span of HeLa or mouse LS cells could be due to a more efficient scavenging of free radicals since growth of these tumor cells is also very sensitive to inhibition by elevated partial pressures of oxygen.[20,24] Thus, it does not appear that oxygen toxicity is responsible for the loss of proliferative capacity of human diploid cells in culture under ambient oxygen tensions.

## J. Using Human Diploid Cells in Culture to Test the Free Radical Theory of Aging

A number of investigators have suggested that aging of cultures of human diploid cells proceeds by a two step process.[184,185] The first step is akin to the process of terminal differentiation and is responsible for the loss of proliferative capacity of the population. This view is supported by studies that show that when young and old cells are fused together the old phenotype is dominant and the product does not initiate DNA synthesis; but when transformed cells and old cells are fused, the transformed phenotype is dominant and the product does initiate DNA synthesis.[184] We have shown that oxygen induced free radical damage is not responsible for this first step loss of proliferative capacity.

The second step is the process responsible for the death of the cell after it has terminally differentiated. Most of the cells of the adult human exist in this state; for example, neurons, cardiac and skeletal muscle, or endocrine gland cells. Some cells, such as hepatocytes and fibroblasts, exist predominantly in the postmitotic state, although they retain the ability to divide. Other cells (skin, intestinal epithelium, and bone marrow) are continually proliferating and differentiating and it is the differentiated cell which eventually dies. We have found that although phase III human diploid cells lose their ability to proliferate, they can be kept alive (as measured by the ability to exclude erythrocin B dye) by weekly refeedings for months.[186] We believe that random free radical reactions could play a role in the demise of these nonmitotic cells. Indeed, Deamer and Gonzales have shown that it is the nondividing cells in aging human diploid cell cultures that accumulate the largest quantities of lipofuscin age pigments.[150]

Cultured human diploid cells can also be studied in a reversible nonmitotic state by cultivation in low serum (0.5% fetal calf serum) containing medium.[187] Thus, these cells are quite analogous to the nonreplicative cell populations of the adult human. This system facilitates exploration of the interrelated metabolic events triggered when intact human cells are subjected to an oxidative stress and should permit assessment of the threat produced by deleterious free radical reactions.

Specific questions, currently being addressed, will help test the free radical theory of aging. Do oxygen induced free radical reactions cause DNA damage and is the damage repaired properly? Are energy and reducing equivalents normally used by biosynthetic processes diverted and consumed by cellular reactions that are necessary to reduce oxidized cytoplasmic and nuclear cellular components? Is extranuclear damage, such as oxidation of membrane lipids or unique oxygen sensitive sulfhydryl groups responsible for cellular deterioration — either because of loss of membrane integrity or of critical specific enzyme function (such as assembly/disassembly of cytoplasmic and mitotic microtubles)? The regulation of cellular antioxidant defense mechanisms and the capability of the cell to respond to an oxidative stress can be explored. An additional strength of this system is that cells from patients with various genetic defects in DNA repair or in enzymes of intermediary metabolism such as glutathione synthetase, glutathione peroxidase, glucose-6-phosphate dehydrogenase, or catalase can be employed to determine the physiologic importance of the various repair systems that the cell employs to deal with free radical induced damage.

Finally, it will be important to determine whether the physiologic ability of postmitotic cells to respond to an oxidative stress correlates with the maximum life span potential of the species from which the cells were obtained.

It is clear that oxygen induced free radical reactions effect many cellular systems —

energy metabolism, lipid peroxidation, DNA synthesis, cell division. It is also clear that intact cells have multiple antioxidant defense systems and that simply because an enzyme or membrane is destroyed by oxygen in a homogenate does not mean it is relevant to the metabolic events of oxygen poisoning in intact tissues. One of the most expeditious ways to determine whether random free radical reactions play a major physiologic role in the degradation of living systems requires exploring the interrelated metabolic events that are triggered when intact cells are exposed to a carefully defined oxidative stress. The study of the type and extent of damage as well as capability for repair is facilitated using the cell culture system described.

## VII. SUMMARY

Oxygen related free radical reactions are pervasive in living systems. This chapter reviews the nature of the reactive intermediates, the various types of damage caused and the cellular antioxidant defense mechanisms. The theoretical basis for believing that random free radical reactions are a major factor in the degradation of living systems is discussed. Much of the existing experimental data purported to establish that free radical reactions cause the aging process is circumstantial or is subject to equivocal interpretation. It has not been established whether oxidative stress induced by free radical reactions and reaction products are a cause, a contributory cause or concomitant with the aging process.

An experimental system which is helping to test the free radical theory of aging has been reviewed. It employs both growing and nonmitotic human diploid cells cultured under defined partial pressures of oxygen to help unravel the interrelated metabolic pathways the cell uses to respond to an oxidative stress. We have already established that the limited proliferative capacity of cells in culture (thought to be analogous to a process of differentiation) is not due to oxygen induced free radical reactions. Determination of the extent of free radical induced damage as well as the cellular capacity for repair in intact nonmitotic cells should have physiologic relevance for differentiated cells of the aging human.

## REFERENCES

1. **Harman, D.,** A theory based on free radical and radiation chemistry, *J. Gerontol.,* 11, 298, 1956.
2. **Harman, D.,** Prolongation of the normal lifespan by radiation protection chemicals, *J. Gerontol.,* 12, 257, 1957.
3. **Harman, D.,** Prolongation of the normal lifespan and inhibition of spontaneous cancer by antioxidants, *J. Gerontol.,* 16, 247, 1961.
4. **Harman, D.,** Free radical theory of aging: effect of free radical reaction inhibitors on the mortality rate of male $LAF_1$ mice, *J. Gerontol.,* 23, 476, 1968.
5. **Cristofalo, V. J.,** Animal cell cultures as a model system for the study of aging, in *Advances in Gerontological Research,* Vol. 4, Strehler, B., Ed., Academic Press, New York, 1972, 45.
6. **Bjorksten, J.,** Crosslinkage and the aging process, in *Theoretical Aspects of Aging,* Rockstein, M., Ed., Academic Press, New York, 1974, 43.
7. **Tappel, A. L.,** Lipid peroxidation damage to cell components, *Fed. Proc. Fed. Am. Soc. Exp. Biol.,* 32, 1870, 1973.
8. **Frank, L. and Massaro, D.,** Oxygen toxicity, *Am. J. of Med.,* 69, 117, 1980.
9. **Haugaard, N.,** Cellular mechanisms of oxygen toxicity, *Physiol. Rev.,* 48, 311, 1968.
10. **Chow, C.,** Nutritional influence on cellular antioxidant defense systems, *Am. J. of Clin. Nutr.,* 32, 1066, 1979.

11. **Chance, B., Sies, H., and Boveris, A.,** Hydroperoxide metabolism in mammalian organs, *Physiol. Rev.,* 59, 527, 1979.
12. **Logani, M. K. and Davies, R. E.,** Lipid oxidation: biologic effects and antioxidants — a review, *Lipids,* 15, 485, 1980.
13. **Pryor, W., Ed.,** *Free Radicals in Biology,* Vol. 4, 1980, Academic Press, New York.
14. **Borg, D. C.,** Application of electron spin resonance in biology, in *Free Radicals in Biology,* Vol. 1, Pryor, W., Ed., Academic Press, New York, 1976, 69.
15. **Pryor, W.,** The role of free radical reactions in biological systems, in *Free Radicals in Biology,* Vol. 1, Pryor, W., Ed., Academic Press, New York, 1976, 1.
16. **Demopoulous, H. B.,** The basis of free radical pathology, *Fed. Proc. Fed. Am. Soc. Exp. Biol.,* 32, 1859, 1973.
17. **Allen, J. E., Goodman, D. B. P., Besarab, A., and Rasmussen, H.,** Studies on the biochemical basis of oxygen toxicity, *Biochim. Biophys. Acta,* 320, 708, 1973.
18. **Davies, H. C. and Davies, R. E.,** Biochemical aspects of oxygen poisoning, in *Handbook of Physiology, Respiration,* Section 3, Vol. II, Fenn, W. O., and Rahn, H., Eds., Am. Physiol. Soc., Washington, D.C., 1965, 1047.
19. **Swartz, H. M.,** Toxic oxygen effects, *Int. Rev. Cytol.,* 35, 321, 1973.
20. **Rueckert, R. R. and Mueller, G. C.,** Effect of oxygen tension on HeLa cell growth, *Cancer Res.,* 20, 944, 1960.
21. **Brosemer, R. W. and Rutter, W. J.,** The effect of oxygen tension on the growth and metabolism of a mammalian cell, *Exp. Cell Res.,* 25, 101, 1961.
22. **Drew, R. M., Painter, R. B., and Feinendegen, L. E.,** Oxygen inhibition of nucleic acid synthesis in HeLa S3 cells, *Exp. Cell Res.,* 36, 297, 1964.
23. **Jones, M. and Bonting, S. L.,** Some relationships between growth and carbohydrate metabolism in tissue cultures, *Exp. Cell Res.,* 10, 631, 1956.
24. **Kilburn, D. G., Lilly, M. D., Self, D. A., and Webb, F. C.,** The effect of dissolved oxygen partial pressure on the growth and carbohydrate metabolism of mouse LS cells, *J. Cell Sci.,* 4, 25, 1969.
25. **Pace, D. M., Thompson, J. R., and Van Camp, W. A.,** Effects of oxygen on growth in several established cell lines, *J. Natl. Cancer Inst.,* 28, 897, 1962.
26. **Stephenson, N. G.,** Effects of increased partial pressures of oxygen, nitrogen and helium on cells in culture, *Cell Tissue Kinet.,* 2, 225, 1969.
27. **Dickens, F.,** The toxic effects of oxygen on brain metabolism and on tissue enzymes. I. Brain metabolism, *Biochem. J.,* 40, 145, 1946.
28. **Dickens, F.,** The toxic effects of oxygen on brain metabolism and on tissue enzymes. II. Tissue enzymes, *Biochem. J.,* 40, 171, 1946.
29. **Mann, P. J. G. and Quastel, J. M.,** Toxic effects of oxygen and hydrogen peroxide on brain metabolism, *Biochem. J.,* 40, 139, 1946.
30. **Horn, R. S. and Haugaard, N.,** Inhibition of carbohydrate metabolism by oxygen and N-ethylmaleimideimide in rat homogenates, *J. Biol. Chem.,* 241, 3078, 1966.
31. **Stadie, W. C. and Haugaard, N.,** Oxygen poisoning. V. The effect of high oxygen pressure upon enzymes: succinic dehydrogenase and cytochrome oxidase, *J. Biol. Chem.,* 161, 153, 1945.
32. **Stadie, W. C. and Haugaard, N.,** Oxygen poisoning. VII. The effect of high oxygen pressure upon enzymes: uricase, xanthine oxidase, and *d*-amino acid oxidase, *J. Biol. Chem.,* 161, 181, 1945.
33. **Fridovich, I.,** Oxygen radicals, hydrogen peroxide, and oxygen toxicity, in *Free Radicals in Biology,* Vol. 1, Pryor, W., Ed., Academic Press, New York, 1976, 239.
34. **Taube, H.,** *Oxygen: Chemistry, Structure and Excited States,* Little, Brown, Boston, 1965.
35. **Fong, K., McCoy, P., Poyer, J., Keele, B., and Misra, H.,** Evidence that peroxidation of lysosomal membranes is initiated by hydroxyl free radicals produced during flavin enzyme activity, *J. Biol. Chem.,* 248, 7792, 1973.
36. **Foote, C.,** Photosensitized oxidation and singlet oxygen: consequences in biological systems, in *Free Radicals in Biology,* Vol. 2, Pryor, W., Ed., Academic Press, New York, 1976, 85.
37. **Badwey, J. A. and Karnovsky, M. L.,** Active oxygen species and the functions of the phagocytic leukocytes, *Ann. Rev. Biochem.,* 49, 695, 1980.
38. **Harrison, J. E. and Schultz, J.,** Studies on the chlorinating activity of myeloperoxidase, *J. Biol. Chem.,* 251, 1371, 1976.
39. **Danen, W. C. and Arudi, R. L.,** Generation of singlet oxygen in the reaction of superoxide anion radical with diacyl peroxides, *J. Am. Chem. Soc.,* 100, 3944, 1978.
40. **Kellog, E. W. and Fridovitch, I.,** Superoxide, hydrogen peroxide, and singlet oxygen in lipid peroxidation by a xanthine oxidase system, *J. Biol. Chem.,* 250, 8812, 1975.
41. **Malkin, R. and Malmstrom, B. G.,** The state and function of copper in biological systems, *Adv. Enzymol.,* 33, 177, 1970.
42. **Fridovich, K. and Handler, P.,** Xanthine oxidase. V. Differential inhibition on the reduction of various electron acceptors, *J. Biol. Chem.,* 237, 916, 1962.

43. **McCord, J. M. and Fridovich, I.,** The reduction of cytochrome c by milk xanthine oxidase, *J. Biol. Chem.*, 243, 5753, 1968.
44. **Fridovich, I.,** Quantitative aspects of the production of superoxide anion radical by milk xanthine oxidase, *J. Biol. Chem.*, 245, 4053, 1970.
45. **Rajagopalan, K. V., Fridovich, I., and Handler, P.,** Hepatic aldehyde oxidase. I. Purification and properties, *J. Biol. Chem.*, 237, 922, 1962.
46. **Rajagopalan, K. V., Fridovich, I., and Handler, P.,** Differential inhibition of electron transfer to various electron acceptors, *J. Biol. Chem.*, 239, 2022, 1964.
47. **Aleman, V. and Handler, P.,** Dihydroorotate dehydrogenase. I. General properties, *J. Biol. Chem.*, 242, 4087, 1967.
48. **Fridovich, I.,** Superoxide dismutase, *Annu. Rev. Biochem.*, 44, 147, 1975.
49. **Fridovich, I.,** The biology of oxygen radicals, *Science*, 201, 875, 1978.
50. **Bhagwat, A. S. and Sane, P. V.,** Evidence for the involvement of superoxide anions in the oxygenase reaction of ribulose-1,5-diphosphate carboxylase *Biochem. Biophys. Res. Commun.*, 84, 865, 1978.
51. **Kosower, N. S. and Kosower, E. M.,** The glutathione-glutathione disulfide system, in *Free Radicals in Biology*, Vol. 2, Pryor, W., Ed., Academic Press, New York, 1976, 55.
52. **Fridovich, I.,** Superoxide dismutases, in *Advances in Enzymology*, Vol. 41, Meister, A., Ed., John Wiley & Sons, New York, 1974, 35.
53. **Fridovich, I.,** Superoxide radicals, superoxide dismutases and the aerobic lifestyle, *Photochem. Photobiol.*, 28, 733, 1978.
54. **Beauchamp, C. and Fridovich, I.,** A mechanism for the production of ethylene from methional. The generation of hydroxyl radicals by xanthine oxidase, *J. Biol. Chem.*, 245, 4641, 1970.
55. **Walling, C.,** Fentons' reagent revisited, *Accounts Chem. Res.*, 8, 125, 1975.
56. **Bors, W., Michel, C., and Saran, M.,** Superoxide anions do not react with hydroperoxides, *FEBS Lett.*, 107, 403, 1979.
57. **Weinstein, J. and Bielski, B. H.,** Kinetics of the interaction of $HO_2$ and $O_2^{\cdot}$ radicals with hydrogen peroxide. The Haber-Weiss reaction, *J. Am. Chem. Soc.*, 101, 58, 1979.
58. **Tappel, A. L.,** Measurement of and protection from in vivo lipid peroxidation, in *Free Radicals in Biology*, Vol. 4, Pryor, W., Ed., Academic Press, New York, 1980, 1.
59. **Witting, L. A.,** Vitamin E and lipid antioxidants, in *Free Radicals in Biology*, Vol. 4, Pryor, W., Ed., Academic Press, New York, 1980, 295.
60. **Lambertson, C.,** The atmosphere and gas exchanges with the lungs and blood, in *Medical Physiology*, 13th ed., Mountcastle, V., Ed., C. V. Mosby, St. Louis, 1372, 1974.
61. **Forster, R. E.,** Oxygenation of the tissue cell, *Ann. N.Y. Acad. Sci.*, 117, 730, 1965.
62. **Tyler, D. D.,** Polarographic assay and intracellular distribution of superoxide dismutase in rat liver, *Biochem. J.*, 147, 493, 1975.
63. **Gregory, E. M. and Fridovich, I.,** Induction of superoxide dismutase by molecular oxygen, *J. Bacteriol.*, 114, 543, 1973.
64. **Crapo, J. D. and Tierney, D. F.,** Superoxide dismutase and pulmonary oxygen toxicity, *Am. J. of Physiol.*, 226, 1401, 1974.
65. **Porter, D. J. T. and Ingraham, L. L.,** Concerning the formation of singlet $O_2$ during the decomposition of $H_2O_2$ by catalase, *Biochim. Biophys. Acta*, 334, 97, 1974.
66. **Lawrence, R. A. and Burk, R. F.,** Species, tissue and subcellular distribution of non-selenium-dependent glutathione peroxidase activity, *J. Nutr.*, 108, 211, 1978.
67. **Chow, C. K. and Tappel, A. L.,** Response of glutathione peroxidase to dietary selenium in rats, *J. Nutr.*, 104, 444, 1974.
68. **Harrap, K. R., Jackson, R. C., Riches, P. G., Smith, C. A., and Hill, B. T.,** The occurrence of protein bound mixed disulfides in rat tissues, *Biochim. Biophys. Acta*, 310, 104, 1973.
69. **Reddy, K. and Tappel, A. L.,** Effect of dietary selenium and autooxidized lipids on the glutathione peroxidase system of gastrointestinal tract and other tissues in the rat, *J. Nutr.*, 104, 1069, 1974.
70. **Chow, C. K., Reddy, K., and Tappel, A. L.,** Effect of dietary Vitamin E on the activities of the glutathione peroxidase system in rat tissues, *J. Nutr.*, 103, 618, 1973.
71. **Chow, C. K. and Tappel, A. L.,** Increased activities of pentose shunt and glycolytic enzymes in lungs of ozone exposed rats, *Arch. Environ. Health*, 26, 205, 1973.
72. **Tappel, A. L.,** Vitamin E and free radical peroxidation of lipids, *Ann. N.Y. Acad. Sci.*, 203, 12, 1972.
73. **Green, J.,** Vitamin E and the biological antioxidant theory, *Ann. N.Y. Acad. Sci.*, 203, 29, 1972.
74. **Cosowsky, M. S., Kelleher, J., Walker, B. E., Davies, T., and Smith, C. L.,** Intake and absorption of tocopherol, *Ann. N.Y. Acad. Sci.*, 203, 212, 1972.
75. **Packer, J. E., Slater, T. F., and Willson, R. L.,** Direct observation of a free radical interaction between vitamin E and vitamin C, *Nature (London)*, 278, 737, 1979.
76. **Halliwell, B. and Foyer, C.,** Ascorbic acid, metal ions and the superoxide radical, *Biochem. J.*, 155, 697, 1976.

77. **Nishikimi, M.,** Oxidation of ascorbic acid with superoxide anion generated by the xanthine-xanthine oxidase system, *Biochem. Biophys. Res. Commun.,* 63, 463, 1975.
78. **DiLuzio, N. R.,** Antioxidants, lipid peroxidation and chemical induced liver injury, *Fed. Proc. Fed. Am. Soc. Exp. Biol.,* 32, 1875, 1973.
79. **Leibovitz, B. E. and Siegal, B.,** Aspects of free radical reactions in biological systems: aging, *J. Gerontol.,* 35, 45, 1980.
80. **Willis, R. J. and Kratzing, C. C.,** Ascorbic acid in the rat lung, *Biochem. Biophys. Res. Commun.,* 59, 1250, 1974.
81. **Willis, R. J. and Kratzing, C. C.,** Extracellular ascorbic acid in lung, *Biochim. Biophys. Acta,* 444, 108, 1976.
82. **Chen, L. H. and Chang, M. L.,** Effect of dietary vitamin E and vitamin C on respiration and swelling of guinea pig liver mitochondria, *J. Nutr.,* 108, 1616, 1978.
83. **Tappel, A. L., Fletcher, B., and Deamer, D.,** Effect of antioxidants and nutrients on lipid peroxidation, fluorescent products and aging parameters in the mouse, *J. Gerontol.,* 28, 415, 1973.
84. **Gutteridge, J. M. C., Richmond, R. and Halliwell, B.,** Oxygen free radicals and lipid peroxidation: inhibition by the protein caeruloplasmin, *FEBS Lett.,* 112, 269, 1980.
85. **Heston, W. E. and Deringer, M. K.,** Hereditary renal disease and amyloidosis in mice, *Arch. Pathol.,* 46, 49, 1948.
86. **Harman, D., Eddy, D., and Noffsinger, J.,** Free radical theory of aging: inhibition of amyloidosis in mice by antioxidants: possible mechanism, *J. Am. Geriatr. Soc.,* 24, 203, 1976.
87. **McKay, C. M., Crowell, M. F., and Maynard, L. A.,** The effect of retarded growth upon the length of lifespan and upon the ultimate body size, *J. Nutr.,* 10, 63, 1935.
88. **McKay, C. M., Maynard, L. A., Sperling, G., and Barnes, L. L.,** Retarded growth, lifespan, ultimate body size and age changes in the albino rat after feeding diets restricted in calories, *J. Nutr.,* 18, 1, 1939.
89. **Ross, M. H.,** Length of life and nutrition in the rat, *J. Nutr.,* 75, 197, 1961.
90. **Barrows, C. H. and Roeder, L. M.,** The effect of reduced dietary intake on enzymatic activities and lifespan of rats, *J. Gerontol.,* 20, 69, 1965.
91. **MacKeen, P. C. and Mitchell, R. B.,** Cytophotometric determination of cytoplasmic azure B RNA levels throughout the lifespan of Tokophyra Lemnarum, *The Gerontologist,* 15, 27, 1975.
92. **Ingle, E., Wood, T. R., and Banta, A. M.,** A study of longevity, growth reproduction and heart rate in Daphnia Longispina as influenced by limitations in quantity of food, *J. Exp. Zool.,* 76, 325, 1937.
93. **Fanestil, D. D. and Barrows, C. H.,** Aging in the rotifer, *J. Gerontol.,* 20, 462, 1965.
94. **Loeb, J. and Northrop, J. H.,** On the influence of food and temperature upon the duration of life, *J. Biol. Chem.,* 32, 103, 1917.
95. **Comfort, A.,** Effect of delayed and resumed growth on the longevity of a fish (Lebistes reticulatus, Peters) in captivity, *Gerontologia,* 8, 150, 1963.
96. **Barrows, C. and Kokkonen, G.,** Diet and life extension in animal model systems, *Age,* 6, 130, 1978.
97. **McCay, C. M., Sperling, G., and Barnes, L. L.,** Growth, aging, chronic diseases and lifespan in rats, *Arch. Biochem.,* 2, 469, 1943.
98. **Comfort, A., Youhotsky-Gore, I., and Pathmanathan, K.,** Effect of ethoxyquin on the longevity of C3H mice, *Nature (London),* 229, 254, 1971.
99. **Kohn, R.,** Effect of antioxidants on lifespan of C57 BL mice, *J. Gerontol.,* 26, 378, 1971.
100. **Clapp, N. K., Satterfield, L., and Bowles, N.,** Effects of the antioxidant butylated hydroxytoluene (BHT) on mortality in BALB/C mice, *J. Gerontol.,* 34, 497, 1979.
101. **Ross, M. H.,** Aging, nutrition and hepatic enzyme patterns in the rat, *J. Nutr.,* 97, 565, 1969.
102. **Daniel, J. W. and Gage, J. C.,** The absorption and excretion of butylated hydroxytoluene (BHT) in the rat, *Food Cosmet. Toxicol.,* 3, 405, 1965.
103. **Toth, S. E.,** The origin of lipofuscin age pigments, *J. Exp. Gerontol.,* 3, 19, 1968.
104. **Miguel, J., Oro, J., Bensch, K. G., and Johnson, J. E., Jr.,** Lipofuscin: fine-structured and biochemical studies, in *Free Radicals in Biology,* Vol. 3, Pryor, W., Ed., Academic Press, New York, 1977, 133.
105. **Barber, A. and Bernheim, F.,** Lipid peroxidation: its measurement, occurrence and significance in animal tissues, in *Advances in Gerontologic Research,* Vol. 2, Strehler, B., Ed., Academic Press, New York, 1967, 355.
106. **Riley, C. A., Cohen, G., and Lieberman, M.,** Ethane evolution: a new index of lipid peroxidation, *Science,* 183, 208, 1974.
107. **Dillard, C. J., Dunnelin, E. E., and Tappel, A. L.,** Effect of dietary vitamin E on expiration of pentane and ethane by the rat, *Lipids,* 12, 109, 1977.
108. **Horgan, V. J., Philpot, J. S. L., Porter, B. W., and Roodyn, D. B.,** Toxicity of autooxidized squaline and linoleic acid, and of simpler peroxides, in relation to toxicity of radiation, *Biochem. J.,* 67, 551, 1957.

109. **Olcott, H. S., and Dolen, A.,** Toxicity of fatty acid ester hydroperoxides, *Proc. Soc. Exp. Biol. Med.,* 114, 820, 1963.
110. **Findlay, G. M., Draper, H. H., and Bergan, J. G.,** Metabolism of 1-$^{14}$C methyl linoleate hydroperoxide in the rabbit, *Lipids,* 5, 970, 1970.
111. **Cortesi, R. and Privett, D. S.,** Toxicity of fatty $O_2$ ozonides and peroxides, *Lipids,* 7, 715, 1972.
112. **Green, R. C., Little, C., and O'Brien, P. J.,** The inactivation of isocitrate dehydrogenase by lipid peroxide, *Arch. Biochim. Biophys.,* 142, 598, 1971.
113. **O'Brien, P. J. and Green, R. C.,** The effects of lipid peroxide on intracellular metabolism, *Biochem. J.,* 103, 1, 1967.
114. **Miguel, J., Tappel, A. L., Dillard, C., Herman, M., and Bensch, K.,** Fluorescent products and lysosomal components in aging *Drosophila melanogaster, J. Gerontol.,* 29, 622, 1974.
115. **Reddy, K., Fletcher, B. L., Tappel, A., and Tappel, A. L.,** Measurement and spectral characteristics of fluorescent pigments in tissues of rats as a function of dietary polyunsaturated fats and vitamin E, *J. Nutr.,* 103, 908, 1973.
116. **Strehler, B., Mark, D. D., Mildvan, A. L., and Gee, M. V.,** Rate and magnitude of age pigment accumulation in the human myocardium, *J. Gerontol.,* 14, 430, 1959.
117. **Young, R. G. and Tappel, A. L.,** Fluorescent pigment and pentane production by lipid peroxidation in honey bees, *Apis mellifera, Exp. Gerontol.,* 13, 457, 1978.
118. **Epstein, J. and Gershon, D.,** Studies on aging in nematodes. IV. The effect of antioxidants on cellular damage and lifespan, *Mech. Aging Dev.,* 6, 257, 1972.
119. **Munkves, K. D. and Minssen, M.,** Aging of *Neurospora crassa,* I. Evidence for the free radical theory of aging from studies of a natural death mutant, *Mech. Aging Dev.,* 5, 79, 1976.
120. **Munkves, K. D. and Rana, R.,** Aging of *Neurospora crassa,* VII. Accumulation of fluorescent pigment (lipofuscin) and inhibition of the accumulation by nordihydroguiaretic acid, *Mech. Aging Dev.,* 7, 399, 1978.
121. **Munkves, K. D. and Rana, R.,** Antioxidants prolong lifespan and inhibit the senescence dependent accumulation of fluorescent pigment (lipofuscin) in clones of *Podospora anserinas, Mech. Aging Dev.,* 7, 407, 1978.
122. **Schal, R. S. and Donato, H.,** Effects of experimentally altered lifespans on the accumulation of fluorescent age pigment in the housefly, *Musca domestica, Exp. Gerontol.,* 13, 335, 1978.
123. **Schal, R. S. and Donato, H.,** Effect of prolongation of lifespan on lipofuscin content and lysosomal enzyme activity in the brain of the housefly, *Musca domestica, J. Gerontol.,* 34, 489, 1979.
124. **Harman, D.,** Free radical theory of aging: effect of the amount and degree of unsaturation of dietary fat on mortality rate, *J. Gerontol.,* 26, 451, 1971.
125. **Horn, P., Laver, J., Foggerty, A., and Johnson, A.,** Effects of lifespan feeding of ruminant-derived human diets to rats, *J. Nutr.,* 109, 1234, 1979.
126. **Reiss, U. and Gershon, D.,** Rat-liver superoxide dismutase. Purification and age-related modifications, *Eur. J. Biochem.,* 63, 617, 1976.
127. **Kellogg, E. W., III and Fridovich, I.,** Superoxide dismutase in the rat and mouse as a function of age and longevity, *J. Gerontol.,* 31, 405, 1976.
128. **Ueda, K. and Ogata, M.,** Levels of erythrocyte superoxide dismutase activity in Japanese people, *Acta Med. Okayama,* 32, 393, 1978.
129. **Joenje, H., Frants, R. R., Arwert, F., and Eriksson, A. W.,** Specific activity of human erythrocyte superoxide dismutase as a function of donor age. A brief note, *Mech. Aging Dev.,* 8, 265, 1978.
130. **Bartosz, G., Tannert, Ch., Fried, R., and Leyko, W.,** Superoxide dismutase activity decreases during erythrocyte aging, *Experientia,* 34, 11, 1978.
131. **Bartosz, G., Leyko, W., and Fried, R.,** Superoxide dismutase and lifespan of *Drosophila melanogaster, Experientia,* 35, 1193, 1979.
132. **Yamanaka, N. and Deamer, D.,** Superoxide dismutase activity in WI-38 cell cultures: Effects of age, trypsinization and SV-40 transformation, *Physiol. Chem. Phys.,* 6, 95, 1974.
133. **Nohl, H., Hegner, D., and Summer, K.-H.,** Responses of mitochoncrial superoxide dismutase, catalase and glutathione peroxidase activities to aging, *Mech. Aging Dev.,* 11, 145, 1979.
134. **Harman, D.,** The free radical theory of aging: effect of age on serum mercaptan levels, *J. Gerontol.,* 15, 38, 1960.
135. **Hazelton, G. and Lang, C.,** Glutathione contents of tissues in the aging mouse, *Biochem. J.,* 188, 25, 1980.
136. **Hayflick, L. and Moorhead, P. S.,** The serial cultivation of human diploid cell strains, *Exp. Cell Res.,* 25, 585, 1961.
137. **Hayflick, L.,** The limited *in vitro* lifetime of human diploid cell strains, *Exp. Cell Res.,* 37, 614, 1965.
138. **Daniel, C. W., Deome, K. B., Young, J. T., Blair, P. B., and Faulkin, L. J., Jr.,** The *in vivo* lifespan of normal and preneoplastic mouse mammary glands: a serial transplantation study, *Proc. Natl. Acad. Sci. USA,* 61, 53, 1968.

139. **Daniel, C. W. and Young, L. J. T.**, Influence of cell division on aging process. Lifespan of mouse mammary epithelium during serial propagation *in vivo*, *Exp. Cell Res.*, 65, 27, 1971.
140. **Krohn, P. L.**, Heterochronic transplantation in the study of aging, *Proc. R. Soc. Ser. B.*, 157, 128, 1962.
141. **Siminovitch, L., Till, J. E., and McCulloch, E. A.**, Decline in colony-forming ability of marrow cells subjected to serial transplantation into irradiated mice, *J. Cell. Comp. Physiol.*, 64, 23, 1974.
142. **Williamson, A. R. and Askonas, B. A.**, Senescence of an antibody-forming cell clone, *Nature (London)*, 238, 337, 1972.
143. **Goldstein, S. J., Littlefield, W., and Soeldner, J. S.**, Diabetes mellitus and aging: diminished plating efficiency of cultured human fibroblasts, *Proc. Natl. Acad. Sci. USA*, 64, 155, 1969.
144. **Leguilly, Y., Simon, M., Lenoir, P., and Bourel, M.**, Long-term culture of human adult liver cells: morphological changes related to *in vitro* senescence and effect of donor's age on growth potential, *Gerontologia*, 19, 303, 1973.
145. **Martin, G. M., Sprague, C. A., and Epstein, C. J.**, Replicative lifespan of cultivated human cells, *Lab. Invest.*, 23, 86, 1970.
146. **Rheinwald, J. G. and Green, H.**, Serial cultivation of strains of human epidermal keratinocytes: the formation of keratinizing colonies from single cells, *Cell*, 6, 331, 1975.
147. **Schneider, E. L. and Mitsui, Y.**, Examination of the relationship between *in vitro* cellular aging and *in vivo* human age, *Proc. Natl. Acad. Sci. USA*, 73, 3584, 1976.
148. **Lipetz, J. and Cristofalo, V. J.**, Ultrastructural changes accompanying the aging of human diploid cells in culture, *J. Ultrastruct. Res.*, 39, 43, 1972.
149. **Robbins, E., Levine, E. M., and Eagle, H.**, Morphological changes accompanying senescence of cultured human diploid cells, *J. Exp. Med.*, 131, 1211, 1970.
150. **Deamer, D. W. and Gonzales, J.**, Autofluorescent structures in cultured WI-38 cells, *Arch. Biochem. Biophys.*, 165, 421, 1974.
151. **Chio, K. S., Reiss, U., Fletcher, B., and Tappel, A. L.**, Peroxidation of subcellular organelles: formation of lipofuscinlike fluorescent pigments, *Science*, 166, 1535, 1969.
152. **Hendley, D. D., Mildvan, A. S., Reporter, M. C., and Strehler, B. L.**, The properties of isolated human cardiac age pigment. II. Chemical and enzymatic properties, *J. Gerontol.*, 18, 250, 1963.
153. **Tappel, A. L.**, Will antioxidant nutrients slow aging processes? *Geriatrics*, 23, 97, 1968.
154. **Balin, A. K., Goodman, D. G., Rasmussen, H., and Cristofalo, V. J.**, The effect of oxygen tension on the growth and metabolism of WI-38 cells, *J. Cell. Physiol.*, 89, 235, 1976.
155. **Balin, A. K., Goodman, D. G., Rasmussen, H., and Cristofalo, V. J.**, Atmospheric stability in cell culture vessels, *In Vitro (Rockville)*, 12, 687, 1976.
156. **Balin, A. K., Goodman, D. G., Rasmussen, H., and Cristofalo, V. J.**, The effect of oxygen tension and Vitamin E on the lifespan of human diploid WI-38 cells, *J. Cell Biol.*, 74, 58, 1977.
157. **Balin, A. K., Goodman, D. G., Rasmussen, H., and Cristofalo, V. J.**, Oxygen sensitive stages of the cell cycle of human diploid cells, *J. Cell Biol.*, 78, 390, 1978.
158. **Cristofalo, V. J. and Sharf, B. B.**, Cellular senescence and DNA synthesis, *Exp. Cell Res.*, 76, 419, 1973.
159. **Clark, M. E.**, Growth and morphology of adult mouse fibroblasts under anaerobic conditions and at limiting oxygen tensions, *Exp. Cell Res.*, 36, 548, 1964.
160. **Dales, S.**, Effects of anaerobiosis on the rates of multiplication of mammalian cells cultured *in vitro*, *Can. J. Biochem. Physiol.*, 38, 871, 1960.
161. **Dales, S. and Fisher, K. C.**, The effect of carbon monoxide on oxygen consumption, glucose utilization, and growth in mammalian cells *in vitro*, *Can. J. Biochem. Physiol.*, 37, 623, 1959.
162. **Sanford, K. K. and Westfall, B. B.**, Growth and glucose metabolism of high and low tumor-producing clones under aerobic and anaerobic conditions *in vitro*, *J. Natl. Cancer Inst.*, 42, 953, 1969.
163. **Sanford, K. K., Westfall, B. B., and Jackson, J. L.**, Glucolysis during culture of neoplastic and nonneoplastic murine cell lines under aerobic and anaerobic conditions, *J. Natl. Cancer Inst.*, 44, 611, 1970.
164. **Harris, H.**, The relationship between the respiration and multiplication of rate connective tissue cells *in vitro*, *Br. J. Exp. Pathol.*, 37, 512, 1956.
165. **Pomerat, C. M. and Willmer, E. N.**, Studies on the growth of tissues in vitro. VII. Carbohydrate metabolism and mitosis, *J. Exp. Biol.*, 16, 232, 1939.
166. **Cooper, P. D., Burt, A. M., and Wilson, J. N.**, Critical effect of oxygen tension on rate of growth of animal cells in continuous suspended culture, *Nature (London)*, 182, 1508, 1958.
167. **Cooper, P. D., Wilson, J. N., and Burt, A. M.**, The bulk growth of animal cells in continuous suspension culture, *J. Gen. Microbiol.*, 21, 702, 1959.
168. **Zwartouw, H. T. and Westwood, J. C. N.**, Factors affecting growth and glycolosis in tissue culture, *Br. J. Exp. Pathol.*, 39, 529, 1958.
169. **Packer, L. and Fuehr, K.**, Low oxygen concentration extends the lifespan of cultured human diploid cells, *Nature (London)*, 267, 423, 1977.

170. **Taylor, W. G., Richter, A., Evans, V. J., and Sanford, K.**, Influence of oxygen and pH on plating efficiency and colony development of WI-38 cells and vero cells, *Exp. Cell Res.*, 86, 152, 1974.
171. **Richter, A., Sanford, K. K., and Evans, V. J.**, Influence of oxygen and culture media on plating efficiency of some mammalian tissue cells, *J. Natl. Cancer Inst.*, 49, 1705, 1972.
172. **Cristofalo, V. J. and Kritchevsky, D.**, Growth and glycolosis in the human diploid cell strain WI-38, *Proc. Soc. Exp. Biol. Med.*, 118, 1109, 1965.
173. **Cristofalo, V. J. and Kritchevsky, D.**, Respiration and glycolosis in the human diploid cell strain WI-38, *J. Cell. Physiol.*, 67, 125, 1966.
174. **Warburg, O.**, On the origin of cancer cells, *Science*, 123, 309, 1956.
175. **Weinhouse, S., Warburg, O., Burk, D., and Schade, A. C.**, On respiratory impairment in cancer cells, *Science*, 124, 267, 1956.
176. **Goldblatt, H. and Cameron, G.**, Induced malignancy in cells from rat myocardium subjected to intermittent anaerobiosis during long propagation *in vitro*, *J. Exp. Med.*, 97, 525, 1953.
177. **Goldblatt, H., Friedman, L., and Chechner, R. L.**, On the malignant transformation of cells during prolonged culture under hypoxic conditions *in vitro*, *Biochem. Med.*, 7, 241, 1973.
178. **Sanford, K. K.**, An attempt to induce malignant transformation of cells *in vitro* by intermittent anaerobiosis, *J. Natl. Cancer Inst.*, 35, 719, 1965.
179. **Packer, L. and Smith, J. R.**, Extension of the lifespan of cultured normal human cells by Vitamin E., *Proc. Natl. Acad. Sci. USA*, 71, 4763, 1974.
180. **Packer, L.**, Protection of environmentally stressed human cells in culture with the free radical scavenger, d-l-α-tocopherol, in *Aging Carcinogenesis and Radiation Biology*, Smith, K. C., Ed., Plenum Press, New York, 1976.
181. **Grove, G. L.**, A cytophotometric analysis of nuclear DNA contents of cultured diploid cells in log and in plateau phases of gowth, *Exp. Cell Res.*, 87, 386, 1974.
182. **Grove, G. L. and Mitchell, R. B.**, DNA microdensitometry as a measure of cycling-non-cycling activity in aged human diploid cells in culture, *Mech. Aging Dev.*, 3, 235, 1974.
183. **Yanishevsky, R., Mendelsohn, M. L., Mayall, B. H., and Cristofalo, V. J.**, Proliferative capacity and DNA content of aging human diploid cells in culture: a cytophotometric and autoradiographic analysis, *J. Cell Physiol.*, 84, 165, 1974.
184. **Martin, G. M., Sprague, C. A., Norwood, T. H., Pendergrass, W. R., Bornstern, P., Hoehn, H. and Arend, W. P.**, Do hyperplastoid cell lines "differentiate themselves to death," in *Cell Impairment in Aging and Development*, Cristofalo, V. J. and Holeckova, E., Eds., Plenum Press, New York, 1975, 67.
185. **Bell, E., Marek, L., Sher, S., Merrill, C., Levinstone, D., Young, I.**, Do diploid fibroblasts in culture age, *Int. Rev. of Cytol.*, 10, 1, 1979.
186. **Dell'Orco, R. T.**, Maintenance of human diploid fibroblasts as arrested populations, *Fed. Proc. Fed. Am. Soc. Exp. Biol.*, 33, 1969, 1974.

Chapter 5

# ERROR THEORIES AND FIDELITY IN AGING AND CANCER*

**Gerald P. Hirsch**

## TABLE OF CONTENTS



* This chapter was supported in part by V. A. Medical Research Funds.

## I. INTRODUCTION

The error theory of aging is among the most extensively studied molecular theories of aging.[1-4] Yet this simple idea, that aging and perhaps cancer result from a nonmutational decline in the fidelity of all biological components, remains as a possible explanation for the pervasive loss of function and control that accompanies aging. The error theory has had a popular following for two reasons, first is the general nature of turnover of cellular components, where nearly all intracellular structural and functional proteins and RNAs are randomly degraded, each with a characteristic half-life, and regularly replaced,[5-7] and second, that a feedback of errors in the system producing new components involved in the fidelity of replacements would result in an exponential increase in errors. This increase might explain the exponential increase in mortality which occurs among most higher animals maintained in the laboratory or cared for in zoos, and of course, for human populations around the world.

Errors are distinguished from mutations because they are not inherited from cell to cell or individual to progeny, and in some systems errors are reversible. Mutations, once induced, can only decrease when the cell affected is either killed or grows slowly because of selective disadvantage. If the frequency of accumulated mutations is low then it will not contribute to fidelity changes. The potential for mutation to be mistaken for errors should be kept in mind, especially when assays are conducted on populations of cells, because a mutation in one cell is equivalent to errors of the same kind in as many as 100,000 cells. For most assays, base substitution mutations and protein synthesis errors would produce the same populations of altered proteins. Mutations can be induced in cell cultures to a level of 1 in 10,000 cells.[8] This could correspond to a level of errors of one incorrect amino acid per million correct ones for a protein of 100 amino acids if every alteration resulted in a variant that demonstrated resistance to the selection procedure, or as much as 10 per million ($10^{-5}$) if only 10% of the total mutations induced resulted in a phenotype that conferred resistance to the selection procedure.

Amino acid substitutions represent the most common type of error and these are likely to play a central role in error cascades because enzymes are the catalysts for most reactions in cells and act as regulators and as structurally specific receptors for many hormones. If there is an overall degeneration of fidelity it should occur primarily through increases in the frequency of replacement of amino acids for one another. The simple view that errors will feedback to produce an error catastrophe has been modified since the demonstration of a steady state and reversible induction of errors in replicating bacteria by streptomycin treatment.[9-12] Comparable studies with nondividing mammalian cells have not been undertaken.

## II. GLOBAL EFFECTS OF ERRORS

The error theories are concerned primarily with those components that informationally feedback new errors within systems responsible for fidelity. But the general concept of errors extends to all components of cells and all reactions. The results of error accumulation should be pervasive for the elements that are regularly renewed, or stable elements which can be somehow modified. The spectrum of changes expected runs from the potential abnormal modification of macromolecules,[13] such as the attachment of methyl groups to RNAs where they would not normally occur, to loss of specificity of hormone receptors. Enzymes that catalyze single substrates would begin to catalyze similar reactions of analogous substrates. Errors could cause the production of molecules that were otherwise not antigenic and stimulate autoimmunity.

Among the fidelity components, errors are expected to result in elevated mutations through replication mistakes and by misrepair (a lower frequency of correction during the repair process). A variety of bacterial polymerase mutants have been described with decreased or increased fidelity.[14-17] Transfer RNAs and ribosomal RNAs might suffer abnormal base modifications including hypo- and hypermodification, and proteins associated with the translational apparatus might have reduced specificity resulting from previously incorporated amino acid substitutions which cause different interactions with RNAs. Amino acyl tRNA ligases should make more mistakes and and further stimulate misincorporation. In bacteria, fidelity may be regulated (by ppGpp).[18]

Altered membrane proteins may change the stability and selectivity of membranes,[19] and alterations in energy production components could result in "uncoupling" of ATP production and oxygen consumption. Similar arguments can be extended to other aspects of cell function, but as will be discussed in detail, many of these ideas have not been tested in experimental settings.

## III. AMINO ACID MISINCORPORATION

The presence of an amino acid at a position in a protein where the DNA normally codes for a different amino acid can represent errors or mutations. It is generally believed that the frequency of mutations is much lower than the frequency of errors. In bacteria, the frequency of mutation has been estimated to be about 10 per billion ($10^{-8}$) for each base copied for each cycle of replication.[20] In mammals, for example, after 100 cell divisions during development the accumulated frequency of mutations could rise to one per million at each position in the DNA if the fidelity of mammalian polymerases is the same as those of bacteria. At this rate the frequency of errors in proteins would be three substitutions per million per position because any one of the three bases is likely to change the coding of the amino acids. This level is 2 to 10-fold below the average level of errors measured in mammalian proteins[21-24] but higher than some substitutions measured by sequencing procedures.[22,25]

Amino acid misincorporation is thus likely to measure errors, whether detected as a single charge change that results from mistakes involving a charged amino acid and a neutral one or by quantitation of an amino acid that is not coded for in a particular protein. If other animal systems behave as one bacterial model, errors could be distinguished from mutations by the reversibility of the induction, where an elevated level of errors will decline after the agent used to induce the errors is withdrawn. Changes in misincorporation due to mutations would not decline in nonreplicating cells. Mutations induced in genes coding for fidelity components might yield a reduced rate of errors in dividing cell systems if there exists a distinct growth disadvantage for these cells.

## IV. THE ERROR THEORY

The error theory of aging was first explicitly proposed by Orgel.[26] He was not the first person to suggest that aging results from a loss of information fidelity, as pointed out in a recent review by Medvedev.[3] Orgel, however, clearly stated that the source of fidelity loss was through the information feedback that occurs during the replication of components involved in fidelity, especially proteins and RNAs that confer specificity to the process of protein synthesis. The theory proposed that the fidelity of newly made proteins was less than the fidelity of proteins used in their manufacture. In other words, the components of transcription and translation could not make new components with the same accuracy that existed within them. As long as a constant increase occurs in the level of mistakes, error catastrophe is inevitable. What determines the error rate increase is the proportionality constant relating the frequency of mistakes in the existing system to the level of the immediate replacements and the number of times that the system was replaced during the life span of the species (the rate of turnover of rRNAs, tRNAs, ligases, etc). Later, Orgel[27] amended his theory to allow for the constant of proportionality to be less than 1. Under this circumstance errors would not increase exponentially.

More complex mathematical models have been derived which describe an inherent stability for the accuracy of protein synthesis but predict that transient disturbances can push a cell beyond the region of stability and into error catastrophe.[28-31] Recent experiments with streptomycin induced errors in replicating bacteria have provided information on the proportionality constant for these induced errors between one round and subsequent rounds of growth replication. These data provide some of the coefficients of equations that describe the relationship between preexisting errors and new errors that are produced by them.

The evolutionary forces which affect the fidelity of protein synthesis and other errors have been discussed only briefly in the aging literature. The proponents of comparative gerontology have suggested that long-lived species should show a lower level of errors because there is a much longer time period for errors to increase to catastrophe.[32] Others argue that a constant level of protein synthesis errors exists among species because of the selective advantage of lower numbers of defective offspring that a greater fidelity allows.[24,33]

## V. METHODS FOR THE DETECTION OF ERRORS

A detailed discussion of the methods used to measure errors is presented elsewhere[34] so only a general review is presented here.

### A. Misincorporation

The most direct method for the quantitation of errors is amino acid misincorporation. The frequency that one noncoded amino acid replaces the genetically coded amino acid at a particular position in a specific highly purified protein is one measure of errors. The overall error rate is the sum of all noncoded substitutions for each amino acid in the protein. Depending on the particular steps of the purification procedure, the measured error rate can be an underestimate, especially for charge changing substitutions that alter chromatographic properties and result in these forms being discarded. Using the same procedure for samples from young and old animals allows relative comparisons to be made. The values obtained for amino acid substitutions range between 5 to 30 substitutions per million for one amino acid for each position.[21,22,24,35] Extrapolating from these values to include other amino acid substitutions at each position for the other 18 different natural amino acid substitutions brings the total rate to between 50 and 600 per million (0.005% to 0.06%). Thus for an average protein of 100 amino acids in size, a total of 0.5% to 6% of the proteins would contain a single amino acid change, or 99.5% to 94% of all proteins would be "perfect" products as coded for in the DNA. As discussed earlier, any potential contribution of mutation to amino acid misincorporation can be distinguished by sequencing the purified protein and comparing error rates at various positions.

### B. Analog Incorporation

One of the steps in protein synthesis is aminoacylation, where specific ligases catalyze the attachment of one amino acid to one or more tRNAs that base-pair with the correct codon. This reaction has been shown to have great specificity for the proper attachment of amino acids.[36-44] The probability of attachment of the incorrect amino acid should be increased if the errors within the ligases are elevated. In these cases, where a change in fidelity occurs at the level of aminoacylation, comparable changes are expected in the incorporation of amino acid analogs. The argument is simple and straightforward. The loss in specificity of amino acid recognition will occur for the misincorporation of natural amino acids (such as isoleucine attachment to valine tRNA) to the same degree as ''unnatural'' amino acid analogs which are proportionally different in shape and charge from the proper amino acid (alpha amino isobutyric acid attachment to valine tRNA). Thus, amino acid analog incorporation should increase if the error frequency increases.

### C. Heat Labile Enzyme

Amino acid misincorporation causes structural changes in proteins such that stability is reduced. From genetic variant enzymes it has been shown that amino acid substitution often results in the mutant enzyme becoming more sensitive to denaturation by heating. Because only a fraction of the enzymes are expected to contain substitutions that result in sensitivity to denaturation by heating, estimates of the percentage of heat sensitive enzymes is made by extrapolating a time course of loss of enzyme activity to zero time, where the fraction of heat sensitive enzymes is represented by the difference between the extrapolated zero heating time value and 100%. Enzymes of young animals show little or no fraction that is more sensitive to heat that the bulk population (see Tables 1 and 2).

### D. Antigenic-Inactive Enzymes (Cross-Reacting Material)

Many amino acid substitutions result in catalytically inactive proteins, without changing the overall three-dimensional structure of the protein. This structural similarity to the native protein has been used to search for errors where the ratio of enzyme activity to antibody added for precipitation shows the presence of that fraction of proteins which bind antibody but do not catalyze their usual reactions.[2]

### E. Protein Turnover

Genetic variant enzymes often have shorter half-lives than the normal enzyme.[5] Proteins containing amino acid analogs also have increased rates of turnover. This behavior of abnormal enzymes has been used as a probe to measure errors where increased turnover resulting from degradation is detected or increased protein synthesis occurs. Because overall protein levels are maintained, any increase in turnover must be balanced by increased protein synthesis.[45]

## VI. ERRORS IN YOUNG AND OLD MAMMALS

### A. Enzyme Properties

The discovery of some altered proteins in tissues of aging mammals have been reported (Table 1). Gershon and Gershon[46] found that 50% more antibody was required to precipitate half of the enzyme activity of fructose-1,6-diphosphate aldolase from old mouse liver and 10% more antibody in old mouse muscle.[47] More antibody was required for the precipitation aldolase A obtained from human muscle of persons between the ages of 64 and 84 compared to enzyme of younger persons 24 to 47.[48] The specific activity of purified superoxide dismutase was found to be 60% lower in preparations from old rat livers and, correspondingly, precipitation of 50% of the enzyme activity required 40% more antibody.[49] Harding[50] reported a four-fold increase in the fraction of thermally sensitive (heat labile) glutathione reductase which occurs abruptly above the age of 40 in human lenses.

Heat sensitive, catalytically active enzymes consist of molecules with at least one error in the polypeptide chain.[1] It is likely that the frequency of errors is underestimated by this method because some errors would not result in heat lability. Loss of catalytic function in those proteins detected with antibody binding properties would also be underestimated if activity loss occurs primarily among enzymes that have substitutions near the binding site of the substrate. Nevertheless, a 50% loss in active enzyme represents 50% "perfect" molecules and 50% molecules with only one error. This level is equivalent to an eightfold increase in the background as measures by misincorporation. More important than the absolute values of errors are the physiological implications for the old animal where either the average cell has only half the functioning enzyme, a condition not usually found,[51] or where the old animal must make twice as much protein to achieve the same level of catalytic function within the cell.

Similar changes are expected for all enzymes when the origin of the observed effect is increased errors. But several enzymes examined with the same or similar methods were not different between young and old mammals (Table 2). The thermal stability and immunoprecipitation values for tyrosine aminotransferase were the same in livers of young and old rats,[52] as were these properties for creatine kinase obtained from human muscle biopsies.[48] In contrast to the heat labile glutathione reductase in human lenses from older humans, the thermal stability of glucose-6-phosphate dehydrogenase of the lens was not different from that present in lenses from younger persons.[50]

### B. Post-Transcriptional Modification

One explanation for the differential appearance of altered proteins is post-transcriptional modification. In human and bovine lens, enzymes from the nuclear area show different electrophoretic characteristics from those for the epithelial lens cells and other tissues sources.[53] Postsynthetic modifications have been observed in a variety of blood cell enzymes.[54]

Another potential source of enzyme difference is the redox potential of the cell where sulfhydryl-sensitive proteins would be more affected by the redox potential than others. Oxidation of cysteine occurs in the nucleus of cataractious lenses,[55] but the SH content of histone III is not changed during aging in rodents.[56]

### C. Amino Acid Analog Probes

Two amino analogs have been used to estimate the accuracy with which aminoacyl tRNA ligases can discriminate against molecules structurally similar to the natural cognate amino acid (Table 9). Ethionine replaced methionine in protein synthesis at a 1% rate and was more frequently incorporated in proteins in older mouse tissues.[57] The ratio of analog incorporation was different among ribosomal proteins of various sizes, suggesting that factors besides misincorporation (selective degradation) influence the amount of analog retained. Methylation reactions could also have influenced the amount of label incorporated or retained in the various size classes showing different levels of errors.

The amino acid analog alpha amino isobutyric acid is incorporated very infrequently into protein, only 70 times per million amino acids polymerized. In aging and in mutagen-treated old mice the ratio of analog incorporated relative to that of a reference natural amino acid was unchanged. The estimate of a maximum difference that could be statistically valid was less than a 60% increase among 24-month-old mice as compared to 12-month-old mice.[58] In very old mice, 31 months of age, particular tissue of individual animals showed changes in incorporation of label similar to those produced in young mice by chronic treatment with 5% dimethyl sulfoxide in the drinking water,[59] a procedure which was designed to induce errors.[60,61]

### D. Altered Proteins Detected by Electrophoresis

About 1/3 of all possible amino acid substitutions result in a change in the net charge of the protein. In a high resolution system of electrophoresis or with a high percentage of altered proteins, single charge changed molecules can be identified and quantitated.[62] Such altered molecules are seen after histidine starvation in cell cultures where other nonbasic amino acids replace histidine. However, when a similar procedure was applied to proteins of sympathetic ganglia from young and old mice, similar "sidebands" characteristic of single charge substitutions were not detected. No general differences were noted in constituent proteins seen in this two-dimensional electrophoresis system.[63] No unusual proteins were seen during aging in mouse brain tissue after high resolution electrophoresis of denatured proteins (sodium dodecyl sulfate electrophoresis) where derepressed gene products or prematurely chain terminated proteins would be expected to be seen if they occurred during aging.[64]

### E. Increased Turnover

The mechanisms controlling protein degradation are poorly understood.[65] In almost all cases examined in mammals, proteins and RNAs turnover and the destruction of proteins and RNAs is random, where a "young" or "old" protein has equal probability of being degraded.[4,66] Because many mutant forms of enzymes have shorter half-lives and because analog-containing proteins are degraded more rapidly than their normal counterparts, error containing proteins are also expected to have reduced half-lives.[45,67] Detecting a small population of rapidly degraded enzymes among a large number of normal ones requires that measurements be taken soon after labeling. Total body protein turnover using selenium-tagged methionine was not different between young and old animals.[68] The broad range of half-lives of cellular proteins in mammals makes it difficult to detect in homogenates a subpopulation of proteins with rapid turnover, and Comolli et al.[69] did not find statistically significant differences in turnover of rat liver mitochondrial, lysosomal, or microsomal proteins between 5, 12, and 23-month-old animals. No change was detected in the turnover of mitochondria as might be expected from errors in the mitochondrial or the cytoplasmic protein synthesizing systems.[7]

In the case of RNAs where only a few species occur as major products, the rapid degradation of transfer RNAs in liver and kidneys of old rats was found.[70] Nearly twice as much tRNA was rapidly degraded in these tissues obtained from old rats as was the fraction with a normal (constant) half-life. While it remains to be shown that the rapidly degraded molecules are altered forms of tRNAs rather than unmodified or immature species, this potential loss of function and the energy wasted in these tissues as a result of this subfraction must be significant. Corresponding rapid degradation of ribosomal RNA was not detected in old rat tissues.

### F. Protein Synthesis Components

The tRNAs in old rat liver and kidneys that are degraded 5 to 10 times faster than normal, if altered in structure, should affect the fidelity of protein synthesis (Table 8). However, Foot and Stulberg[71] were not able to detect any differential function of old tRNAs purified from mouse tissues as compared to young when these tRNAs were used in a tRNA-dependent system transcribing a viral message. Frazer and Yang[72] did not find any unusual tRNAs or tRNA ligase specificity when enzyme preparations from young and old donors were used to aminoacylate tRNAs from either young or old tissues. Most of the amino acids were examined by chromatography that separated subspecies of tRNAs, and no quantitative or qualitative differences were found.

Ribosomal contributions to accurate protein manufacture were compared using synthetic message, poly U, and correct (phenylalanine) and incorrect (leucine) aminoacyl tRNAs. While the overall fidelity of translation is less than that seen in vivo, old ribosomes did not show an effect of reduced fidelity.[73] Mitochondrial ribosomes have much lower fidelity with synthetic templates than cytoplasmic ribosomes but there is no evidence for error catastrophe in the mitochondria.[7,64,69]

### G. Amino Acid Substitutions

The measurement of amino acid substitutions in highly purified proteins from young and old mammals has been conducted in only three systems. For human donors between the ages of 20 and 50 years, the average frequency of isoleucine substitutions in hemoglobin was 30 per million per position and independent of age.[75] The criteria for adequate purification for hemoglobin in these samples was the constant level of errors in the separated alpha and beta chains and the globin prior to chain separation. The objection to using hemoglobin for error analysis is that a cell having a high level of errors would be at a growth disadvantage during the replication and maturation of the red cell precursors, and thus no increase in errors that may have occurred in the precursor population would be apparent. Elevated levels of isoleucine were found in blood samples for persons exposed to whole body radiation. While the elevated level of isoleucine substitutions is thought to result from isoleucine containing mutant cells that have cloned during the assay period, sequencing and chain separation procedures will be required to distinguish the error and mutation origins for the radiation-induced increase.

Fidelity measurements have been made for a protein of the rat seminal vesicle gland and for histone 1 from mouse liver. In both tissues the cell turnover rate is very low. No age difference was seen by Medvedev and Medvedeva[35] for the misincorporation of methionine into histone 1 where the average frequency of misincorporation was 5 per million per position. Comparing 4 and 13-month-old rats, Bradshaw, Popp, and Hirsch[76] found a constant level of fidelity cysteine misincorporation of 10 per million per position. Thus, by the most direct and sensitive measurement of errors, fidelity during aging is maintained, and the error theory seems to be invalid for mammalian aging.

## VII. ERRORS IN INVERTEBRATES

Insects and other invertebrates have been used in aging studies because of their very short life spans and low cost of maintenance. Fruit flies, primarily Drosophila species, are of special value because of the detailed understanding of their genetics and because of a variety of available mutant stocks. But predictions that might be made about mammalian aging from a knowledge and understanding of insect aging depends on the similarity of biochemical and cellular processes, especially on cellular and molecular kinetics. The error theory requires that components of the transcription and translation processes be regularly renewed and, moreover, that many cycles of replacement occur during the life span. In mice, about 200 replacement cycles occur for the rRNA and tRNA components in various nondividing cell types examined. If the half-life of these RNAs were the same in Drosophila only 12 cycles would occur in the 90 day maximum longevity among strains. In the absence of data showing a high degree of turnover of fidelity components, the observations to be discussed should not be applied to aging in dissimilar organisms.

One of the early observations concerning error accumulation in Drosophila was a twofold increase in protein synthesis in old flies.[77] As discussed earlier, when protein levels are maintained, increased protein synthesis is expected to occur when protein degradation speeds up from the rapid turnover of faulty proteins. What was surprising data in this same experiment was the large fraction (70%) of proteins that were made in young flies and had very long half-lives. As a practical matter, if any of these relatively stable proteins are enzymes involved in fidelity they would not be subject to error accumulation resulting from the potential feedback of errors in the protein synthetic apparatus.

Life shortening was obtained in Drosophila only when late larval stage organisms were treated with amino acid analogs.[78] Levels of treatment that resulted in increased turnover of analog containing proteins or a 50% reduction of protein synthesis rate for 2 days of treatment did not shorten the life span of these flies.[79] Late 3rd instar larval treatment caused a large fraction of adult flies to die about 6 days after eclosion, but those adults that did not die prematurely lived nearly a normal life span. The expected progression of errors during the adult period of life does not seem to occur (Table 6).

Proteins from old Drosophila were examined by electrophoresis, but the level of errors was below 1 in 10,000, and any change during aging could not be determined.[80]

## VIII. ERRORS IN HUMAN CELL CULTURES

When mammalian tissue fragments are placed in culture, fibroblasts grow out from the fragment, and these fibroblasts can be subcultivated many times. Unless a variant cell arises during propagation, the cell strain will eventually stop replicating. Although the cells do not die, they can only be stimulated to initiate DNA synthesis by such techniques as cell fusion. The loss of cell division capacity is thought to be the result of aging during subcultivation and that the mechanism(s) responsible for this cessation of growth will occur during aging in the intact animal. Fibroblasts do not regularly divide in mammals, but the model could be applied to other cell types that do undergo regular cell turnover.

Experiments designed to test the error theory in fibroblast cultures are equally divided between those that show a difference between early and late passage cultures and those that show the same level of fidelity during in vitro aging (Table 7). Late passage fibroblasts show many of the characteristic changes expected from error accumulation including an increased amount of heat labile enzyme,[81,82] increased incorporation of the amino acid analog, ethionine,[83] increased protein turnover,[84] and an increased number of mistakes during in vitro translation of synthetic templates.[85] Human liver cells, unlike fibroblasts, can sustain only about 13 cycles of replication in culture. Liver cells in the final phases of growth show a heat labile enzyme fraction in homogenates but not for the same enzyme when partially purified.[86] Reduced fidelity of DNA polymerase in leukemic cells was traced to viral enzymes rather than altered fidelity of tumor cell polymerases.[87,88]

## IX. CANCER AND ERRORS

Wheldon and Kirk[89] extended the error theory of aging to explain the origin of cancer. The exponential age-associated increases in tumors in higher organisms are thought to result from the same molecular or cellular changes that may cause other aging effects. Despite the potential common origin of mechanisms of aging and cancer, the search for the cause of cancer through an understanding of normal aging mechanisms has rarely been pursued. In the case of error theories proportionately more effort has been made by gerontologists than cancer researchers to discover the contribution of molecular fidelity to the process of aging and cancer (Table 7).

A few alterations in aminoacylation were found among mammary tumors[90] and small but significant differences were seen among tRNAs in myeloma cells.[91] But much more dramatic changes were found in tRNA methylases[92,93] in a variety of tumors, but only modest effects were seen methylase activities in Morris hepatomas.[94]

Post-transcriptional changes may contribute to altered functions in tumor cells which may affect enzyme activity and alter isoelectric points or proteins.[95,96] Virus transformed cells demonstrated a 2.5 higher amount of tRNA-mRNA mispairing with synthetic template[97] but such transformed cells were equally sensitive to growth inhibition by amino acid analogs.[98] Amino acid analogs were more readily incorporated in spontaneous hepatomas[99] but the effect was not apparent in transplanted hepatomas (unpublished results).

## X. MODELS FOR ERROR INDUCTION

A clear resolution of the role that errors play in aging and cancer is dependent on the development of a model system in mammals of induced errors. Thus far, ethionine and other analog feeding methods and consumption of dimethyl sulfoxide in the drinking water have been proposed as models. Streptomycin, which works well in bacteria by changing the reading fidelity on the ribosome, is not effective on mammalian ribosomes. Ethionine feeding results in the ethylation of RNA (and perhaps DNA) as well as causing structural changes by its misincorporation. Other amino acid analogs have not been shown to be incorporated in mammals to an extent that they may be expected to produce errors. Dimethyl sulfoxide, while producing changes expected to result from errors, may just as well operate by causing mutations. Only by distinguishing errors and mutations by sequencing or by independent mutational tests, or by showing the reversibility of errors can such model systems be validated. With a good model for errors the many methods which purport to measure errors can be compared, correlated and independently validated. This validation of experimental models for error production in mammals and other species would then allow a definitive resolution of the role that errors may play in tumor induction or progression. Other important questions concerning the potential interaction of mutagens and error could also be studied. Analog feeding that slows growth by 30 to 35% results in mutation increases ranging from 20 to 130 times normal in *Coprinus*[100] and 3 to 5 times normal in yeast.[101] The mutations are presumed to result from altered fidelity of polymerases, and a correlation is expected between the reduced fidelity and the induced mutations. Any contribution of errors to the frequency of spontaneous mutations will affect the arguments that the mutation rate remains high so as to provide new variants able to adapt to changing environmental conditions.

## Table 1
## ALTERATIONS IN PROTEINS DURING AGING

| Protein | Property | Change (O-Y)/Y | Species/tissue | Age comp.# | Ref. |
|---|---|---|---|---|---|
| Purified superoxide dismutase | Specific activity | −60% | Rat liver | 6 vs 27 | 49 |
| Purified superoxide dismutase | Antibody precipitation | 40% | Rat liver | 6 vs 27 | 49 |
| Glutathione reductase | Thermal stability | 400% | Human lens | <40 vs >40 | 50 |
| Fructose-1, 6-diphosphate aldolase | Immunoprecipitation | 10% | Mouse muscle | 2 vs 31 | 47 |
| Fructose-1, 6-diphosphate aldolase | Immunoprecipitation | 50% | Mouse liver | 3 vs 31 | 46 |
| Aldolase A | Immunoprecipitation | 13% | Human muscle | 24-47 vs 64-84 | 48 |
| Glucose-6-phosphate dehydrogenase | Heat lability | 500% | Mouse 5 tissues (average) | 5-6 vs 25-26 | 102 |

*Note:* # rat and mouse in months, humans in years.

## Table 2
## PROTEINS THAT SHOW SIMILAR PROPERTIES DURING AGING

| Protein | Property | Species/tissue | Age comp. | Ref. |
|---|---|---|---|---|
| Superoxide dismutase | Isoelectric point | Rat liver | 8 vs 32 | 103 |
| Glucose-6-phosphate dehydrogenase | Thermal stability | Human lens | Range 2 to 89 yr. | 50 |
| Chromatin proteins | SH redox potential | Rat | 3,8,18, 33 mo. | 56 |
| Tyrosine amino-transferase | Immunoprecipitation | Rat liver | 3-6 vs 27-31 | 52 |
| Tyrosine amino-transferase | Thermal stability | Rat liver | 3-6 vs 27-31 | 52 |
| Creatine kinase | Thermal stability | Human muscle | 24-47 vs 64—84 | 48 |
| Creatine kinase | Immunoprecipitation | Human muscle | 24-47 vs 64-84 | 48 |
| DNA polymerase (low mol. wt.) | Heat Lability | Mouse spleen | 3-8 vs 24-30 | 104 |

## Table 3
## EFFECTS OF ANALOGS ON ERRORS IN MAMMALS

| | |
|---|---|
| Low doses of analog (parafluorophenylalanine) cause a 15% lifeshortening in male mice | 105 |
| High doses of analog (parafluorophenylalanine) did not cause lifeshortening in mice | 105 |
| Ethionine feeding caused increase amino acid incorporation | 106 |

## Table 4
## CHANGES IN AGING HUMAN CELL CULTURES

| | Measurement | Passages/lines | | Ref |
|---|---|---|---|---|
| 1. | Threefold increase in mutations at 2 loci measured | 0-80 | HSC 172 | 8 |
| 2. | Increase (2.5 times) in heat labile glucose-6-phosphate dehydrogenase | 10-40 vs 53-68 | MRC-5 | 81 |
| 3. | Eightfold increase in ethionine analog incorporation | 25-35 vs 50 | MRC-5 | 83 |
| 4. | Threefold increase in turnover of protein (confluent cells) | 26 vs 61 | MRC-5 | 84 |
| 5. | Sixfold increase in heat labile glucose-6-phosphate dehydrogenase in crude extracts | 4-6 vs 13 | Human liver cells | 86 |
| 6. | Heat labile glucose-6-phosphate dehydrogenase (23%) in old cells | 22-25 vs 42-45 | WI-38 | 82 |
| 7. | Five percent increase per passage (doubling) of mutations at the glucose-6-phosphate dehydrogenase (high activity mutants) | 16 to 60 | MRC-5 | 107 |
| 8. | More than threefold increase in mistakes of 2 polymerases using synthetic templates | 19 vs 56 | MRC-5 | 85 |

## Table 5
## FIDELITY IN HUMAN CELL CULTURES

| | Measurement | Passages | Line | Ref. |
|---|---|---|---|---|
| 1. | No change in mutation rate of poliovirus grown in fibroblasts | 23 vs 61 | WI-38 | 108 |
| 2. | No difference in heat sensitivity of poliovirus grown in fibroblasts | 23 vs 61 | WI-38 | 108 |
| 3. | Lower error rate in late passage fibroblasts with in vitro mistranslation | <50% vs >90%# | N-1, N-2 N-3 | 62 |
| 4. | Immunoprecipitation of glucose-6-phosphate dehydrogenase unchanged | 4-22 vs 50-60 | Infant skin line | 109 |
| 5. | Heat stability of glucose-6-phosphate dehydrogenase unchanged | 4-23 vs 40-60 | Infant skin line | 109 |
| 6. | Constant enzyme/antigen ratio (CRM) for glucose-6-phosphate dehydrogenase, glucose isomerase, pyruvate kinase, and phospholglycerate isomerase | 4-6 vs 10-19 | Human liver cells | 86 |
| 7. | No difference in heat stability of 3 lysosomal enzymes | 22-25 vs 42-45 | WI-38 | 82 |
| 8. | No significant difference in heat stability for mitochondrial sulfite cytochrome-c-reductase | 22-25 vs 42-45 | WI-38 | 82 |
| 9. | Constant fidelity measured by histidine mistranslation | <50% vs >90%# | WI-38 MRC-5 3 others | 97 |
| 10. | Total population doublings not decreased by 7 day analog treatment | 29 to 50 | WI-38 | 98 |

*Note:* # percentage of total doublings.

## Table 6
## DROSOPHILA ERRORS

| | Measurement | Ref. |
|---|---|---|
| 1. | Larval amino acid analog treatment slightly shortens adult life span. Treatment time-lifeshortening not correlated. | 78 |
| 2. | Errors in old drosophila below the level of detection of electrophoresis (1/10,000) | 80 |
| 3. | Analog feeding to adults resulted in increased turnover of analogs in protein but no lifeshortening | 110 |
| 4. | No lifeshortening by 2-day analog feeding which reduced protein synthesis by 50% | 79 |
| 5. | Twofold increase in protein synthesis in old flies | 77 |

## Table 7
## FIDELITY CHANGES IN TUMOR CELLS

| | Observation | Ref. |
|---|---|---|
| 1. | Increase, 2.5-fold, in synthetic message stimulated amino acid misincorporation in virus transformed human fibroblasts | 97 |
| 2. | SV 40 transformed fibroblasts equally sensitive to growth inhibition by amino acid analogs as nontransformed cells | 98 |
| 3. | Only slight differences in methylated bases in Morris Hepatomas as compared to normal rat liver tRNAs | 111 |
| 4. | Protein modifying factors exist in leukemic cells which alter the electrophoretic mobility and/or enzyme activities | 96 |
| 5. | Small but significant differences occur in the species of tRNA in myeloma cells | 91 |
| 6. | Quantitative and qualitative differences in tRNAs in Morris Hepatomas compared to normal rat liver | 94 |
| 7. | Quantitative changes in methylation of tRNAs and in the kinetic properties of methyl transferases | 92 |
| 8. | Summary of 29 tumors with elevated tRNA methylase activity | 93 |
| 9. | Alteration of isoelectric point of X-linked glucose-6-phosphate dehydrogenase (post-transcriptional?) | 95 |
| 10. | Two tumor synthetases charge mammary tRNA to differerent extents. Four liver synthetases charge tumor tRNA differently than homologous enzymes | 90 |

## Table 8
## FIDELITY OF PROTEIN SYNTHESIS COMPONENTS

| Component | System | Result | Ages | Species tissue | Ref. |
|---|---|---|---|---|---|
| tRNA | Viral message — electrophoresis | No change | 12 vs 24 | Mouse 4 organs | 71 |
| Ribosomes | Poly U directed amino acid misincorporation | No change | 6 vs 32 | Rat brain | 112 |
| Ribosomes | Poly U directed amino acid misincorporation | Slight change | 2, 14, 27 31 | Mouse liver | 73 |
| tRNA and Ligases | Chromatographic profiles of aminoacyl tRNAs | No change | 5-9 vs 28-36 | Mouse brain & liver | 72 |

## Table 9
## ERRORS DETECTED BY ANALOG INCORPORATION

| Analog | Species/tissue | Changes | Age | Ref. |
|---|---|---|---|---|
| Ethionine | Mouse/liver | 20-50% increase only in large ribosomal proteins | 4 vs 20 | 57 |
| Alpha-amino isobutyric acid | Mouse/brain liver, kid spleen | 60% maximum estimate for increased error during aging | 12 vs 24 | 58 |
| Alpha-amino isobutyric acid | Mouse/brain kidney, liver | No difference in analog incorporated | 3 vs 33 | 59 |

## REFERENCES


1. **Gershon, D. and Gershon, H.,** An evaluation of the error catastrophe theory of aging in the light of recent experimental results, *Gerontology,* 22, 212, 1976.
2. **Gershon, D.,** Current status of age altered enzymes: alternative mechanisms, *Mech. Ageing Dev.,* 9, 189, 1979.
3. **Mevedev, Z. A.,** The role of infidelity of transfer of information for the accumulation of age changes in differentiated cells, *Mech. Age. Dev.,* in press.
4. **Medvedev, A.,** Error theories of aging, in *Alternstheorien,* D. Platt, D., Ed., Springer-Verlag, New York, in press.
5. **Menzies, R. A.,** Long-lived molecules and the hourglass hypothesis of aging, *Interdiscip. Top. Gerontol.,* 9, 41, 1976.
6. **Nordgren, R. A., Hirsch, G. P., Menzies, R. A., Hendley, D. D., Kutsky, R., and Strehler, B. L.,** Evidence for long-lived components in developing mouse tissues labelled with leucine, *Exp. Gerontol.,* 4, 7, 1969.
7. **Fletcher, M. J. and Sanadi, D. R.,** Turnover of rat liver mitochondria, *Biochim. Biophys. Acta,* 51, 356, 1961.
8. **Gupta, R. S.,** Senescence of cultured human diploid fibroblasts. Are mutations responsible? *J. Cell. Physiol.,* 103, 209, 1980.
9. **Edelmann, P. and Gallant, J.,** On the translational error theory of aging, *Proc. Natl. Acad. Sci. USA,* 74, 3396, 1977.
10. **Gallant, J. and Foley, D.,** On the causes and preventation of mistranslation, in *Ribosomes; Structure, Function and Genetics,* University Park Press, Baltimore, 1977, 615.
11. **Gallant, J. and Palmer, L.,** Error propagation in viable cells, *Mech. Ageing Dev.,* 10, 27, 1979.
12. **Gallant, J. A. and Prothero, J.,** Testing models of error propagation, *J. Theor. Biol.,* 83, 561, 1980.
13. **Reporter, M.,** Methylation of basic residues in structural proteins, *Mech. Age. Dev.,* 1, 367, 1973.
14. **Gillin, F. D. and Nossal, N. G.,** Control of mutation frequency by bacteriophage T4 DNA polymerase. I. The CB120 antimutator DNA polymerase is defective in strand displacement, *J. Biol. Chem.,* 251, 5219, 1976.
15. **Allen, E. F., Albrecht, I., and Drake, J. W.,** Properties of bacteriophage T4 mutants defective in DNA polymerase, *Genetics,* 65, 187, 1970.
16. **Gillin, F. D. and Nossal, N. G.,** Control of mutation frequency by bacteriophage T4 DNA polymerase. II. Accuracy of nucleotide selection by the L88 mutator, CB120 antimutator, and wild type phage T4 DNA polymerases, *J. Biol. Chem.,* 251, 5225, 1976.
17. **Muzyczka, N., Poland, R. L., and Bessman, M. J.,** Studies on the biochemical basis of spontaneous mutation. I. A comparison of the deoxyribonucleic acid polymerases of mutator, antimutator, and wild type strains of bacteriophage T4, *J. Biol. Chem.,* 247, 7116, 1972.
18. **O'Farrell, P. H.,** The suppression of defective translation by ppGpp and its role in the stringent response, *Cell,* 14, 545, 1978.
19. **Munkres, K. D.,** Ageing of Neurospora crassa. IV. Induction of senescence in wild type by dietary amino acid analogs and reversal by antioxidants and membrane stabilizers, *Mech. Ageing Dev.,* 5, 171, 1976.
20. **Hibner, U. and Alberts, B. M.,** Fidelity of DNA replication catalyzed in vitro on a natural DNA template by the T4 bacteriophage multi-enzyme complex, *Nature (London),* 285, 300, 1980.
21. **Loftfield, R. B. and Vanderjagt, D.,** The frequency of errors in protein biosynthesis, *Biochem. J.,* 128, 1353, 1972.
22. **Popp, R. A., Hirsch, G. P., and Bradshaw, B. S.,** Amino acid substitution: its use in detection and analysis of genetic varients, *Genetics,* 92, s39, 1979.
23. **Medvedev, Z. A. and Medvedeva, M. N.,** Use of H1 histone to test the fidelity of protein biosynthesis in mouse tissues, *Biochem. Soc. Trans.,* 6, 610, 1978.
24. **Hirsch, G. P., Popp, R. A., Francis, M. S., Bradshaw, B. S., and Bailiff, B. S.,** Species comparison of protein synthesis accuracy, in *Aging, Cancer, and Cell Membranes,* Stamatoyannopoulos, G. and Neinhuis, A. W., Eds., 1980, 142.
25. **Popp, R. A., Bailiff, E. G., Hirsch, G. P., and Conrad, R. A.,** Errors in human hemoglobin as a function of age, *Interdiscip. Top. Gerontol.,* 9, 209, 1976.
26. **Orgel, L. E.,** The maintenance of the accuracy of protein and its relevance to ageing, *Proc. Natl. Acad. Sci. USA,* 49, 517, 1963.
27. **Orgel, L. E.,** The maintenance of the accuracy of protein synthesis and its relevance to ageing: a correction, *Proc. Natl. Acad. Sci. USA,* 67, 1476, 1970.
28. **Weigel, D., Beier, W., and Brehme, K-H.,** Vitality and error rate in biological systems: some theoretical considerations, *Mech. Ageing Dev.,* 2, 107, 1973.
29. **Goel, N. S. and Ycas, M.,** The error catastrophy hypothesis with reference to aging and the evolution of the protein synthesizing machinery, *J. Theor. Biol.,* 54, 245, 1975.

30. **Kirkwood, T. B. L. and Holliday, R.**, Stability of the translation apparatus, *J. Mol. Biol.*, 97, 257, 1975.
31. **Hoffman, G. W.**, On the origin of the genetic code and the stability of the translation apparatus, *J. Mol. Biol.*, 86, 349, 1974.
32. **Kirkwood, T. B. L. and Holliday, R.**, The evolution of aging and longevity, *Proc. R. Soc. London B*, 205, 531, 1979.
33. **Hirsch, G. P.**, Spontaneous mutations balance reproductive selective advantage and genetically determine longevity, *Mech. Age. Dev.*, 9, 355, 1979.
34. **Hirsch, G. P.**, The detection of altered proteins, in *Methods in Aging Research*, CRC Press, Boca Raton, Fla., 1981.
35. **Medvedev, A. A. and Medvedeva, M. N.**, Use of H1 histone to test the fidelity of protein biosynthesis in mouse tissues, *Biochem. Soc. Trans.*, 6, 610, 1978.
36. **Hopfield, J. J.**, Kinetic proofreading: a new mechanism for reducing errors in biosynthetic processes requiring high specificy, *Proc. Natl. Acad. Sci. USA*, 71, 4135, 1974.
37. **Baldwin, A. N. and Berg, P.**, Transfer ribonucleic acid-induced hydrolysis of valyladenylate bound to isoleucyl ribonucleic acid synthetase, *J. Biol. Chem.*, 241, 839, 1966.
38. **Fersht, A. R.**, Editing mechanisms in protein synthesis. Rejection of valine by the isoleucyl-tRNA synthetase, *Biochemistry*, 16, 1025, 1977.
39. **Fersht, A. R. and Kaethner, M. M.**, Enzyme hyperspecificity. Rejection of threonine by the valyl-tRNA by misacylation and hydrolytic editing, *Biochemistry*, 15, 3342, 1976.
40. **von der Harr, F. and Cramer, F.**, Hydrolytic action of aminoacyl-tRNA synthetases from baker's yeast: "chemical proofreading" preventing acylation of tRNA(lle) with misactivated valine, *Biochemistry*, 15, 4131, 1976.
41. **Igloi, G. L., von der Harr, F., and Cramer, F.**, Hydrolytic action of aminoacyl-tRNA synthetases from bakers yeast. "Chemical proofreading" of Thr-tRNA(Val) by val-tRNA synthetase studied with modified tRNA(Val) and amino acid analogues, *Biochemistry*, 16, 1696, 1977.
42. **Mulvey, R. S. and Fersht, A. R.**, Editing mechanisms in aminoacylation of tRNA: ATP consumption and the binding of amino acyl-tRNA by elongation factor Tu, *Biochemistry*, 16, 4731, 1977.
43. **Thompson, R. C. and Stone, P. J.**, Proofreading of the codon-anticodon interaction on ribosomes, *Proc. Natl. Acad. Sci. USA*, 74, 198, 2977.
44. **Yarus, M.**, Phenylalanyl-tRNA synthetase and isoleucyl-tRNA(Phe): a possible verification mechanism for aminoacyl-tRNA, *Proc. Natl. Acad. USA*, 69, 1915, 1972.
45. **Goldschmidt, R.**, *In vivo* degradation of nonsense fragments in *E. coli*, *Nature (London)*, 228, 1151, 1970.
46. **Gershon, H. and Gershon, D.**, Inactive enzyme molecules in aging mice: liver aldolase, *Proc. Natl. Acad. Sci. USA*, 70, 909, 1973.
47. **Gershon, H. and Gershon, D.**, Altered enzyme molecules in senescent organisms: mouse muscle aldolase, *Mech. Ageing Dev.*, 2, 33, 1973.
48. **Steinhagen-Thiessen, E. and Hilz, H.**, The age-dependent decrease in creatine kinase and aldolase activities in human striated muscle is not caused by an accumulation of faulty proteins, *Mech. Ageing Dev.*, 5, 447, 1976.
49. **Reiss, U. and Gershon, D.**, Rat-liver superoxide dismutase, *Eur. J. Biochem.*, 63, 617, 1976.
50. **Harding, J. J.**, Altered heat-lability of a fraction of glutathione reductase in aging human lens, *Biochem. J.*, 134, 995, 1973.
51. **Finch, C. E.**, Enzyme activities, gene function and ageing in mammals, *Exp. Gerontol.*, 7, 53, 1972.
52. **Weber, A., Guguen-Guillouzo, C., Szajnert, M. F., Beck, G., and Schapira, F.**, Tyrosine aminotransferase in senesent rat liver, *Gerontology*, 26, 9, 1980.
53. **Skala-Rubinson, H., Vibert, M., and Dreyfus, J. C.**, Electrophoretic modifications of three enzymes in extracts of human and bovine lens, *Clin. Chim. Acta*, 70, 385, 1976.
54. **Rubinson, H., Kahn, A., Boivin, P., Schapira, F., Gregori, C., and Dreyfus, J.-C.**, Aging and accuracy of protein synthesis in man: Search of inactive enzymatic crossreacting material in granulocytes of aged people, *Gerontology*, 22, 438, 1976.
55. **Truscott, R. J. W. and Augusteyn, R. C.**, Oxidative changes in human lens proteins during senile nuclear cataract formation, *Biochim. Biophys. Acta*, 492, 43, 1977.
56. **Carter, D. B.**, No age-dependent oxidation of H3 histone, *Exp. Gerontol.*, 14, 101, 1979.
57. **Ogrodnik, J. P., Wulf, J. H., and Cutler, R. G.**, Altered protein hypothesis of mammalian ageing processes. II. Discrimination ratio of methionine versus ethionine in the synthesis of ribosomal protein and RNA of C57B1/6J mouse liver, *Exp. Gerontol.*, 10, 119, 1976.
58. **Hirsch, G. P., Grunder, P., and Popp, R. A.**, Error analysis by amino acid analog incorporation in tissues of aging mice, *Interdiscip. Top. Gerontol.*, 10, 1, 1976.
59. **Hirsch, G., Holland, J. M., and Popp, R. A.**, *Genetic Aspects of Aging*, Birth Defects: Original Article Series, 14, 421, 1978.

60. **Ritter, P. O., Kull, F. J., and Jacobsen, K. B.,** Effects of Tris and dimethylsulfoxide on the aminoacylation of *Escherichia coli* valine transfer RNA by *Neurospora crassa* phenylalanyl transfer RNA synthetase, *Biochim. Biophys. Acta,* 179, 524, 1969.
61. **Yarus, M.,** Why do organic solvents enhance mistakes in aminoacyl tRNA synthesis? *Arch. Biochem. Biophys.,* 174, 350, 1976.
62. **Wojtyk, R. I. and Goldstein, S.,** Fidelity of protein synthesis does not decline during aging of cultured human fibroblasts, *J. Cell. Physiol.,* 103, 299, 1980.
63. **Wilson, D. L., Hall, M. E., and Stone, G. C.,** Test of some aging hypotheses using two-dimensional protein mapping, *Gerontology,* 24, 426, 1978.
64. **Vaughn, W. J. and Calvin, M.,** Electrophoretic analysis of brain proteins from young adult and aged mice, *Gerontology,* 23, 110, 1977.
65. **Etlinger, J. D. and Goldberg, A. L.,** A soluble ATP-dependent proteolytic system responsible for the degradation of abnormal proteins in reticulocytes, *Proc. Natl. Acad. Sci. USA,* 74, 54, 1977.
66. **Menzies, R. A., Press, G. D., Gold, P. H., Hendley, D. D., and Strehler, B. L.,** On the question of long-lived RNA in mammals, *Cell Tissue Kinet.,* 2, 133, 1969.
67. **Lewis, C. M., 1972,** Protein turnover in relation to Orgel's error theory of aging, *Mech. Ageing Dev.,* 1, 43-47, 1972.
68. **Mende, T. J. and Viamonte, L. M.,** A study of total body turnover in rats of different ages, *Gerontologia,* 11, 208, 1965.
69. **Comolli, R., Ferioli, M. E., and Azzola, S.,** Protein turnover of the lysosomal and mitochondrial fractions of rat liver during aging, *Exp. Gerontol.,* 7, 369, 1972.
70. **Menzies, R. A., Mishra, R. K., and Gold, P. H.,** The turnover of ribosomes and soluble RNA in a variety of tissue of young adult and aged rats, *Mech. Ageing Dev.,* 1, 117, 1972.
71. **Foote, R. S. and Stulberg, M. P.,** Efficiency and fidelity of cell-free protein synthesis by transfer RNA from aged mice, *Mech. Ageing Dev.,* 13, 93, 1980.
72. **Frazer, J. M. and Yang, W.-K.,** Isoaccepting transfer ribonucleic acids in liver and brain of young and old $BC3F_1$ mice, *Arch. Biochem. Biophys.,* 153, 610, 1972.
73. **Kurtz, D. I.,** The effect of ageing on in vitro fidelity of translation in mouse liver, *Biochim. Biophys. Acta,* 407, 479, 1975.
74. **Kurtz, D. I.,** Fidelity of protein synthesis with chicken embryo mitochondrial and cytoplasmic ribosomes, *Biochemistry,* 13, 572, 1974.
75. **Popp, R. A., Bailiff, E. G., Hirsch, G. P., and Conrad, R. A.,** Errors in human hemoglobin as a function of age, *Interdiscip. Top. Gerontol.,* 9, 209, 1976.
76. **Bradshaw, B. S., Popp, R. A., and Hirsch, G. P.,** Errors in protein synthesis detected by misincorporation of cysteine: effect with age and X-rays, *Fed. Proc. Fed. Am. Soc. Exp. Biol.,* 37, 1306, 1978.
77. **Clarke, J. M. and Smith, J. M.,** Increase in the rate of protein synthesis with age in *Drosophila subobscura, Nature (London),* 209, 627, 1966.
78. **Harrison, B. J. and Holliday, R.,** Senescence and the fidelity of protein synthesis in Drosophila, *Nature (London),* 213, 990, 1967.
79. **Dingley, F. and Smith, J. M.,** Absence of a life-shortening effect of amino-acid analogues on adult drosophila, *Exp. Gerontol.,* 4, 145, 1969.
80. **Parker, J., Pollard, J. W., Friensen, J. D., and Stanners,** Stuttering: high-level mistranslation in animal and bacterial cells, *Proc. Natl. Acad. Sci. USA,* 73, 1091, 1978.
81. **Holliday, R. and Tarrant, G. M.,** Altered enzymes in ageing human fibroblasts, *Nature (London),* 238, 26, 1972.
82. **Houben, A. and Remacle, J.,** Lysosomal and mitochondrial heat labile enzymes in ageing human fibroblasts, *Nature (London),* 275, 59, 1978.
83. **Lewis, C. M. and Tarrant, G. M.,** Error theory and ageing in human fibroblasts, *Nature (London),* 239, 316, 1972.
84. **Shakespeare, V. and Buchanan, J. H.,** Increased degradation rates of protein in aging human fibroblasts and in cells treated with an amino acid analog, *Exp. Cell Res.,* 100, 1, 1976.
85. **Linn, S., Kairis, M., and Holliday, R.,** Decreased fidelity of DNApolymerase activity isolated from aging human fibroblasts, *Proc. Natl. Acad. Sci. USA,* 73, 2818, 1976.
86. **Kahn, A., Guillouzo, A., Cottreau, D., Marie, J., Bourel, M., Biovin, P., and Dreyfus, J.-C.,** Accuracy of protein synthesis and in vitro aging, *Gerontology,* 23, 174, 1977.
87. **Battala, N. and Loeb, L. A.,** The infidelity of avian myeloblastosis virus deoxyribonucleic acid polymerase in polynucleotide replication, *J. Biol. Chem.,* 249, 4086, 1974.
88. **Sirover, M. A. and Loeb, L. A.,** Infidelity of DNA synthesis: a general property of RNA tumor viruses, *Biochem. Biophys. Res. Comm.,* 61, 360, 1974.
89. **Wheldon, T. E. and Kirk, J.,** An error cascade mechanism for tumor progression, *J. Theor. Biol.,* 42, 107, 1973.

90. **Qvist, R.**, Transfer RNA and aminoacryl tRNA synthetases in hormone dependent and independent mammary tumors of GR mice. I. Comparative study of the amino acid accepting capacity of the tRNA's in the presence of the homologous and heterologous enzymes, *Cancer Biochem. Biophys.*, 1, 215, 1976.
91. **Fujioka, S. and Gallo, R. C.**, Aminoacyl transfer RNA profiles in human myeloma cells, *Blood,* 38, 246, 1971.
92. **Kerr, S. J.**, Interaction of mammalian tRNA methyltransferases with heterologous and homologous tRNA, *Adv. Enzyme Regulation,* 13, 379, 1975.
93. **Borek, E. and Kerr, S. J.**, Atypical transfer RNA's and their origin in neoplastic cells, *Adv. Can. Res.,* 15, 163, 1975.
94. **Volkers, S. A. S. and Taylor, M. W.**, Chromatographic comparison of the transfer ribonucleic acids of rat livers and morris hepatomas, *Biochemistry,* 10, 488, 1971.
95. **Kahn, A., Cottreau, D., Bernard, J. F., and Boivin, P.**, Post transcriptional modification of glucose-6-phosphate dehydrogenase in human leukemias, *Biomedicine,* 22, 539, 1975.
96. **Kahn, A., Boivin, P., Rubinson, H., Cottreau, D., Marie, J., and Dreyfus, J-C.**, Modification of purified glucose-6-phosphate dehydrogenase and other enzymes by a factor of low molecular weight abundant in some leukemic cells, *Proc. Natl. Acad. Sci. USA,* 73, 77, 1976.
97. **Goldstein, S., Wojtyk, R. I., Harley, C. B., Pollard, J. W., and Stannus, C. P.**, Fidelity of protein synthesis in aging human fibroblasts, in *Aging: Its Chemistry,* Dietz, A., Ed., American Association for Clinical Chemistry, Washington, D.C., 1980, 248.
98. **Ryan, J. M., Duda, G., and Cristofalo, V. J.**, Error accumulation and aging in human diploid cells, *J. Gerontol.,* 29, 616, 1974.
100. **Talmud, P. J. and Lewis, D.**, The mutagenicity of amino acid analogues in *Coprinus lagopus, Genet. Res. Camb.,* 23, 47, 1974.
101. **Davies, P. J. and Perry, J. M.**, The modification of induced genetic change in yeast by an amino acid analog, *Molec. Gen. Genet.,* 162, 183, 1978.
102. **Wulf, J. H. and Cutler, R. G.**, Altered protein hypothesis of mammalian aging processes. I. Thermal stability of glucose-6-phosphate dehydrogenase in C57BL/6J mouse tissue, *Exp. Gerontol.,* 10, 101, 1975.
103. **Goren, P., Reznick, A. Z., Reiss, U., and Gershon, D.**, Isoelectric properties of nematode aldolase and rat liver superoxide dismutase from young and old animals, *FEBS Lett.,* 84, 83, 1977.
104. **Barton, R. W. and Yang, W-K.**, Low molecular weight DNA polymerase: decreased activity in spleens of old BALB/c mice, *Mech. Ageing Dev.,* 4, 123, 1975.
105. **Holliday, R. and Stevens, A.**, The effect of an amino acid analog, *p*-fluorophenylalanine on longevity of mice, *Gerontology,* 24, 417, 1978.
106. **Beauchene, R. E., Roder, L. M., and Barrows, Jr., C. H.**, The effect of age and of ethionine feeding on the ribonucleic acid and protein synthesis of rats, *J. Gerontol.,* 22, 318, 1967.
107. **Fulder, S. J. and Holliday, R.**, A rapid rise in cell varients during the senescence of populations of human fibroblasts, *Cell,* 6, 67, 1975.
108. **Holland, J. J., Kohne, D., and Doyle, M. V.**, Analysis of virus replication in ageing human fibroblast cultures, *Nature (London),* 245, 316, 1973.
109. **Pendergrass, W. R., Martin, G. M., and Bornstein, P.**, Evidence contrary to the protein error hypothesis for *in vitro* senescence, *J. Cell. Physiol.,* 87, 3, 1976.
110. **Bozcuk, A. N.**, Testing the protein error hypothesis of ageing in Drosophila, *Exp. Gerontol.,* 11, 103, 1976.
111. **Randerath, E., Chia, L. L. S. Y., Morris, H. P., and Randerrath, K.**, Transfer RNA base composition studies in Morris Hepatomas and rat liver, *Can. Res.,* 34, 643, 1974.
112. **Ekstrom, R., Liu, D. S. H., and Richardson, A.**, Changes in brain protein synthesis during the life span of male Fisher rats, *Gerontology,* 26, 121, 1980.

Chapter 6

# AN OVERVIEW OF CELL CULTURE AS A MODEL SYSTEM FOR THE STUDY OF AGING

**Vincent J. Cristofalo and Denise G. Ragona**

## TABLE OF CONTENTS

## I. INTRODUCTION

The phenomenon of aging has intrigued humankind since antiquity. However, the dramatic increase over the last half century in the number of people aged 65 years or older[1] has amplified and intensified interest in the biological, clinical, and social aspects of this universal process. For the most part, biological and clinical research in gerontology has focused both on describing the aging process and delineating the mechanisms that control this time-dependent, deteriorative event. Several levels of biological organization, from whole organisms to isolated cells, have been used in this work.

Investigations with whole organisms have included studies on humans and on animal model systems ranging from rodents to nonhuman primates. Though humans are the ultimate primary focus of aging research, they are relatively poor subjects for the scientific study of aging. Their very longevity (mean life span, 71 years; maximum life span, 115 years)[2] makes the study of an individual from birth to death (longitudinal study) a difficult undertaking. The use of cross-sectional studies has circumvented the life span problem to some extent, but the genetic heterogeneity and the constantly changing environment of humans makes tightly controlled experimentation difficult.

The development of animal model systems for the study of aging has minimized many of the problems inherent to the use of human subjects. Animal species exhibit many of the same aging characteristics as humans and so can serve as working models for human aging. Generally, animal life spans are shorter, their genetics better understood, and their environment more easily controlled. In addition, the range of experiments that can be performed with animals is considerably larger than that for humans.

The development of in vitro models for the study of aging has expanded the possibilities of gerontological research since it allows workers to ask questions and to perform technical manipulations not easily done with whole organisms. These in vitro systems include organ and tissue explants and isolated cell cultures. The prolonged maintenance of organ and tissue explants has been described[3,4] but has seen little use in aging studies. It remains, however, a potentially useful tool for observing the effects of age on the structure and function of specific tissue-organ systems, free from the complications inherent in studies of an integrated organism.

## II. HISTORICAL BACKGROUND

The human diploid, fibroblast-like cell cultures are among the most widely used cellular models for the study of aging. The use of cells in culture as a model for aging is a relatively recent approach, stemming from the concept that isolated cells, once freed from the constraints and controls of a complex organism, would be able to live forever.[5,6] The apparent inability of the first cell culture workers to maintain cells in vitro for indefinite periods of time was assumed to be due to methodological deficiencies, and the expectation was that technological advancements would overcome this failure. An apparent milestone was reached when Carrel and Ebeling,[5-8] in experiments begun at the start of this century, reported that fibroblast-like cells from chick embryo heart tissue could be cultured indefinitely and were essentially immortal. This work had a profound influence on gerontological research for many years, as it was interpreted to be conclusive evidence that cellular aging was not an intrinsic property but rather a supracellular phenomenon. Additional experimental support for the unlimited proliferative capacity of animal cells in vitro came from laboratories in which "L" cells, derived from mouse mesenchymal tissue[9] and HeLa cells, derived from a human cervical tumor[10] were used.

In 1961, Hayflick and Moorhead reported, in what has since become a classic paper,

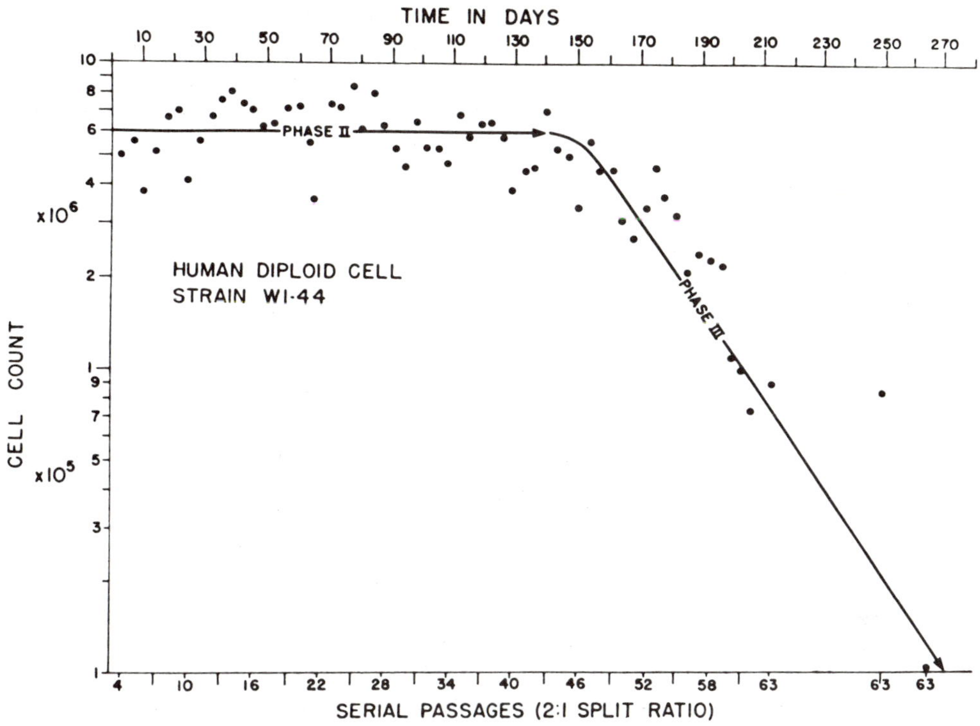


FIGURE 1. Cell counts determined at each passage of human diploid cell strain WI-44. The initial plateau during Phase II, with no apparent loss of biological function as measured by constant doubling time, is followed by Phase III, where doubling time increases exponentially. (From Hayflick, L., *Exp. Cell Res.*, 37, 614, 1965. With permission.)

that normal human fibroblast-like cells from fetal, neonatal, and adult tissues could proliferate in culture for only finite periods of time, i.e., they underwent a limited number of population doublings and then senesced or became incapable of further division and died.[11] Figure 1 illustrates typical data obtained by Hayflick and Moorhead for the life history of human fetal lung cells in culture. After establishment in culture (Phase I), there is a period during which cell proliferation is rapid and relatively constant (Phase II). This is followed by a period of declining proliferative capacity during which the cells undergo many physiologic changes until eventually the culture is lost (phased out or Phase III). The average number of population doublings achieved before senescence was found to be about 50 (range 35 to 63) for cells derived from fetal lung and about 20 (range 14 to 29) for cells from adult lung. In the last 18 years the observations of Hayflick and Moorhead have been confirmed in other human cells and also in cell cultures from other species.[12,13]

In 1957, Swim and Parker[14] presented evidence that the variation in life span of fibroblast-like cell cultures was a function of the tissue of origin and not due to such technical difficulties as inadequate nutrition, pH variation, toxic metabolic products, microcontamination, or depletion of some essential metabolite. Hayflick and Moorhead[11] expanded on this theme and showed that cellular degeneration with time was not related, at least in any simple way, to environmetal factors. They mixed young and old cell populations that were distinguishable by karyotypic markers (Barr bodies) and were derived from different sexes and grew them together. The time required for each component to disappear from the mixture compared to unmixed controls was noted. The old cells in the mixture stopped growing at the same population doubling level (PDL) as did old control cells and young cells in the mixture grew vigorously and stopped dividing only after reaching the same number of PDLs. These results showed that the limited life span of human diploid cells in culture was an intrinsic event that expressed aging at the cellular level and that, therefore, these cells would be a potentially useful model system for the study of the mechanisms of senescence.[11,15]

The conflict between the data showing limited life span[11] and those showing immortality of certain cell types was resolved when it was noted that the cell types previously reported to be "immortal" were almost always (except for Carrel's chick cultures) abnormal in one or more important properties: chromosome morphology and/or number; virus content; or tumorgenicity.[11] The apparent immortality of Carrel's cultures was later suggested by Hayflick[16] to stem from the inadvertent introduction of fresh, viable fibroblasts which would have contaminated the chick embryo extract used in the growth medium.

## III. RELEVANCE TO AGING IN VIVO

The suggestion that tissue culture might reflect aging changes has its roots in earlier studies. Carrel and Ebeling[17] demonstrated that the age-associated changes that occur in plasma can inhibit cell growth in vitro. Also, the time required for the initiation of cell migration from explanted tissue fragments has been shown to increase with age.[18-20] However, it has not been possible to demonstrate a direct relationship between aging in vitro and aging in and of the whole organism, primarily because so little is known about the basic process of senescence. An additional difficulty is that death is the endpoint often used in evaluating aging. While an old organism contains old cells, it is clear that organisms do not die because they "run out" of cells. Death is a stochastic event and the time and cause are subject to great variability. Though we cannot use cell cultures to ask direct questions about why people die, we can use them as model systems to learn about the cellular aspects of the process of senescence. For example, we can learn about the general characteristics of aging cells and whether or not differentiation occurs in these cells. We can examine whether aging is correlated with the accumulation of errors. We can study the mechanisms underlying the failures in proliferative capacity as well as other functional changes that accompany decrements in proliferative ability. Cell cultures can also be used to investigate the cellular effects of environmental agents known to be associated with aging in vivo such as radiation,[21] oxygen,[22] pollutants,[23] and carcinogens.[24] Finally, we can employ normal cells in culture to study the factors controlling the initiation and progression of cell proliferation and mitotic potential as these are related to the two principal age-associated diseases, cancer and atherosclerosis.[25] In essence, we can use cells in culture to investigate mechanisms and to test theories of aging.

### A. The Latent Period

The latent period is defined as the time required for cells to migrate out from an explanted tissue which has been placed in an appropriate culture medium. Several independent laboratories, using chick or rat tissue, have demonstrated that the latent period increases with increasing donor age not only during the active growth period of the donor but even into its old age.[26-29] Waters and Walford[30] and Soukupovâ and Hnêvkovský[31] extended this observation to human tissues. Waters and Walford[30] showed that the latent period was directly proportional to the age of the donor (Table 1), i.e., the time required for the initiation of fibroblast, but not epithelial, outgrowth increased as donor age increased. However, considerable variability was noted.

### B. Limited Life Span In Vivo

The observation that the proliferative activity of normal cells generally declines in vivo gives further support for a relationship between aging *in situ* and aging in vitro. LeBlond[32] showed that for some populations in vivo, the rate of cell division gradually

**Table 1**
**SKIN CELLS FROM DONORS OF DIFFERENT AGES**

| | | Degree and Type of Outgrowth[b] | | | | |
|---|---|---|---|---|---|---|
| Skin donor[a] | Age | Biopsy number | 3+ Epithelial | 1+ Fibroblast | 2+ Fibroblast | 3+ Fibroblast |
| A | Neonate | 1 | 8 | 3 1/2 | 5 | 6 |
| | | 2 | 5 | 2 1/2 | 3 | 3 1/2 |
| B | Neonate | 3 | 6 | 5 | — | 8 |
| | | 4 | 8 | 6 | — | — |
| C | Neonate | 5 | 5 | 4 | 5 | — |
| | | 6 | 5 | 3 1/2 | 6 | — |
| D | Neonate | 7 | — | 5 | 13 | — |
| | | 8 | 6 | 5 | 8 | — |
| E | Neonate | 9 | 8 | 2 1/2 | 3 1/2 | 4 1/2 |
| CH[c] | 26 yrs. | 10 | 8 | 5 1/2 | — | 7 |
| | | 11 | 5 1/2 | 4 | 5 1/2 | 7 |
| HWA | 26 yrs. | 12 | 3 | 4 1/2 | 7 1/2 | 9 |
| HWB | 27 yrs. | 13 | 3 1/2 | 5 1/2 | 6 | 6 1/2 |
| EZ[c] | 29 yrs. | 14 | — | 4 1/2 | 5 1/2 | 7 |
| | | 15 | — | 3 | 4 | 7 |
| BL[d] | 31 yrs. | 16 | 2 1/2 | 6 1/2 | — | 12 |
| RW | 44 yrs. | 17 | 3 | 7 | 9 | 9 1/2 |
| | | 18 | 3 | 8 1/2 | 10 1/2 | 11 1/2 |
| PLP | 57 yrs. | 19 | 3 1/2 | 6 1/2 | 8 1/2 | 10 |
| LZ | 57 yrs. | 21 | 3 | 6 | 9 | 10 |
| | | 22 | 3 | 11 | 18 | 19 1/2 |
| SM | 62 yrs. | 23 | 2 | 3 1/2 | 4 | 5 1/2 |
| | | 24 | 3 | 3 1/2 | 4 | 5 |
| | | 25 | 3 1/2 | 6 | 8 1/2 | 9 |
| | | 26 | 9 | 9 | 10 1/2 | 12 1/2 |
| DW[e] | 63 yrs. | 27 | 2 1/2 | 7 1/2 | — | 10 1/2 |
| | | 28 | 3 1/2 | 4 | 5 1/2 | 7 |
| ES[e] | 69 yrs. | 29 | 4 | 19 | — | — |
| CMD[e] | 74 yrs. | 30 | 6 | 7 1/2 | 13 | 14 |
| | | 31 | 4 | 8 | 9 | 12 |
| MS | 77 yrs. | 32 | 4 | 7 1/2 | 10 | 10 1/2 |
| | | 33 | 11 | 8 | 9 | 10 |
| PLD[e] | 77 yrs. | 34 | 4 | 6 | — | 7 1/2 |
| | | 35 | 4 | 6 | — | 7 1/2 |
| MJH[e] | 80 yrs. | 36 | 4 | — | 6 | 7 |
| | | 37 | >30 | — | 7 | 9 |
| RS[e] | 80 yrs. | 38 | 4 | 12 | 13 | 13 1/2 |
| | | 39 | 4 | 6 | 7 1/2 | 8 |

[a] More than one biopsy, designated by number, was taken from most donors.
[b] 1+ means 1 to 6 cells growing out from explant; 2+ means 7-25 cells growing out of explant; 3+ means greater than 25 cells growing out from explant.
[c] Female.
[d] Chinese.
[e] Taking medication.

From Waters, H. and Walford, R. L., *J. Gerontol.*, 25, 381, 1970. With permission.

but continually declined after an initial peak. Similar observations have been reported in detailed studies of mouse tissues.[33-36] Lesher and Sacher[33] showed that the generation time of mouse duodenal crypt cells is nearly 50% longer in old, as compared to young animals. In 1971, Buetow[37] tabulated and reviewed the literature on age-associated changes in cellular proliferation rates in vivo; in general, there was a decline in mitotic activity in a wide variety of human and rodent tissues.

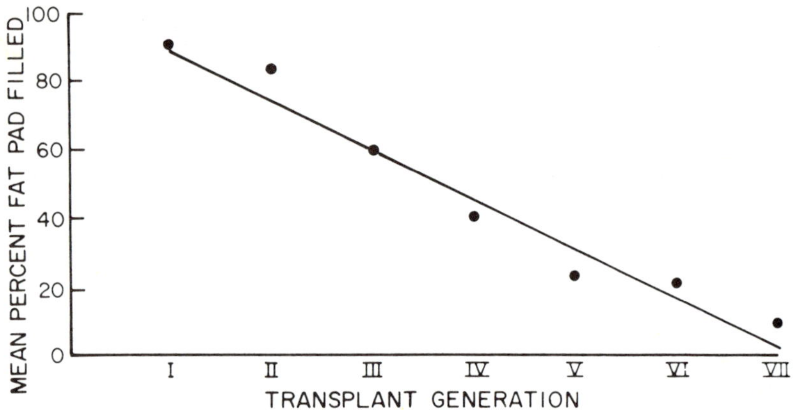


FIGURE 2. Decline in growth rate of mammary tissue during serial propagation. This plot summarized results of eight transplant lines, and each point represents 80 to 100 transplants. The regression is approximately linear, and the slope indicates a 15% loss of growth potential at each passage. Line fitted by method of least squares. (From Finch, C. E. and Hayflick, L., *Handbook of the Biology of Aging,* Van Nostrand Reinhold, New York, 1976. With permission.)

Similar conclusions have been reached using age chimeras and a serial transplantation technique in which normal, somatic tissue is transplanted into new, young inbred hosts each time the current recipient approaches old age. Data from several independent laboratories in which skin,[38,39] hemopoietic cells,[40-44] and mammary tissue[24,45,46] have been used suggest that, in general, normal somatic cells serially transplanted to isogeneic hosts appear to show a decline in proliferative capacity and cannot survive indefinitely, although the survival time of some transplants has been greater than that of the host average life span.

Krohn[38,39] transplanted mouse skin *ad seriatum* and found a decline in the vitality of the transplant. Daniel and co-workers,[24,46] using a procedure first developed by DeOme et al.,[45] transplanted mouse mammary glands into gland-free mammary fat pads of young, isogeneic female mice. These workers demonstrated that, though there was variation in the maximum time mammary tissue could be propagated, in no instance could indefinite growth be achieved; a decline in proliferative capacity was observed with repeated transplantations (Figure 2). Williamson and Askonas[43] studied the life span of a clone of antibody-producing cells upon serial passage to syngeneic mice and reported that, after a period of high antibody production, an exponential decline began in the fifth transplant generation (Figure 3). This decline was due to a reduction in the total number of antibody-producing cells and not to diminished productivity per cell.

Harrison[47] has studied the ability of cells to repopulate the bone marrow and allow survival of genetically anemic mice. He found that cells from older normal animals were equally able to cure the anemia of the deficient animals as those from young animals. He interprets this as indicating that cell proliferation does not fail in a way that significantly compromises the survival of the animal. This does not mean that proliferating cells do not senesce, but simply that their senescence does not cause the death of the organism.

Although serial transplantation experiments are subject to technical difficulties, including the visualization and identification of transplanted cells, the monitoring of isogenicity, and the objective quantification of aging,[48] the overall thrust of the data generated by this approach suggests that cell aging is an intrinsic, cellular phenomenon and not an artifact of in vitro techniques.

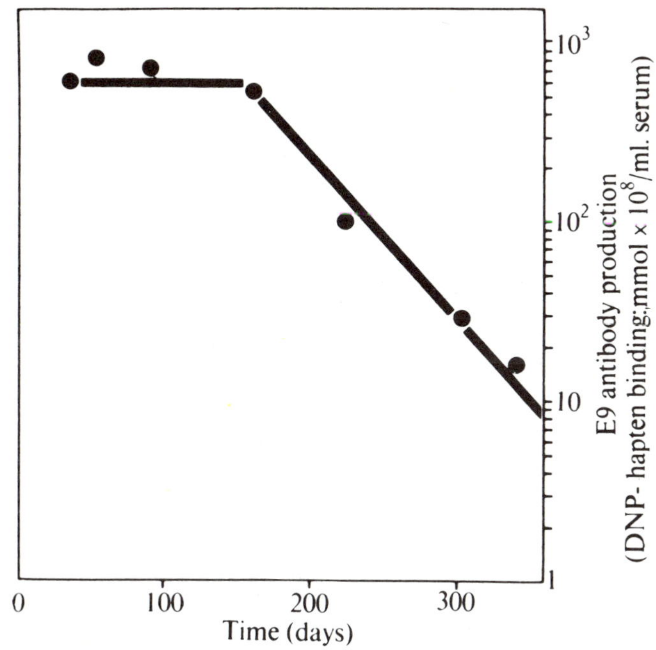


FIGURE 3. Maximum production of E9 antibody in each transplant generation plotted as a function of the age of the clone. Each point represents the time at which the highest producer in each generation was killed for transplantation of clone E9. (From Williamson, A. R. and Askonas, B. A., *Nature (London)*, 238, 337, 1972. With permission.)

## C. Correlation Between Donor Age and Life Span

The most frequently cited evidence for a relationship between aging in vitro and aging *in situ* is the observation that the life span of cells in culture is inversely proportional to the age of the donor for cells derived from human skin, lung, and liver tissue.[49-52] Martin and co-workers,[49] in their study of human skin fibroblast-like cells, reported a regression of −0.20 (± 0.05) cell doublings per year for ages embyronic to 90 years, i.e., the older the donor the less time the cells lived in culture (Figure 4). Because their study failed to show significant regression in the critical age range of 20 to 100 years,[53] Martin et al.[51] undertook an additional study with a larger number (N = 104) of individuals in this age range. A similar regression (−0.18 ± 0.5 cell doublings per year) was obtained, although the correlation coefficient was only 0.33. Despite the variance, which was attributed to methodological difficulties, the regression was highly significant ($P < 0.001$). Schneider and Mitsui[52] corrected some of the difficulties and reported a statistically significant decrease in the rate of fibroblast outgrowth, in vitro life span, replication rate, and cell number at confluency for cultures derived from old (63 to 92 years) vs. young (21 to 36 years) donors.

Smith et al.[54] compared the clone size distribution of cultures derived from subjects of various ages and found that cultures of fetal origin gave rise to the highest percentage of rapidly growing colonies whereas cultures from old adults yielded the lowest percentage. Rheinwald and Green,[55] using a clonal cell culture system, reported a decreased replicative ability for epidermal cells from old compared to young individuals.

The division potential of cultured human arterial smooth-muscle cells[56] and of mouse aortic and adventitial cells[57] also have been demonstrated to decline with age.

Goldstein,[58] Martin et al.,[49] and others[59,60] have studied cells from individuals with

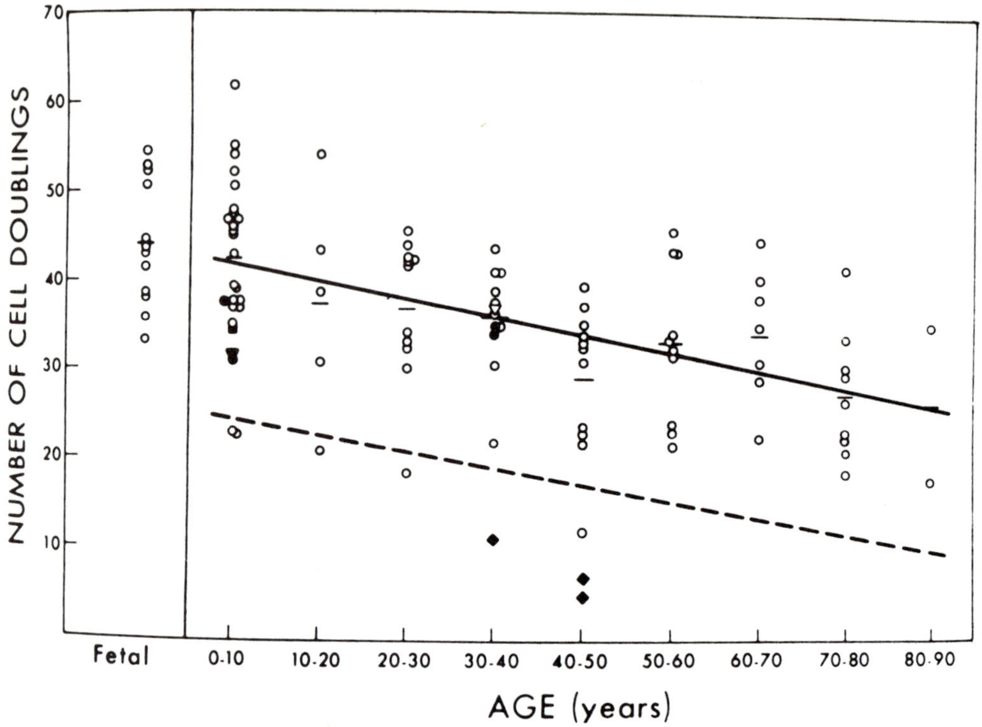


FIGURE 4. The cumulative number of cell doublings achieved by human skin fibroblast cultures plotted as a function of the age of the donor. The calculated linear regression line (solid line) for the control group is drawn between the first and ninth decades and has a regression coefficient of −0.20 ± 0.05 standard deviation cell doublings per year with correlation coefficient of −0.50. The dashed line is the lower 95% confidence limit for the regression line. (From Martin, G. M., Sprague, C. A., and Epstein, C. J., *Lab. Invest.*, 23, 86, 1970. With permission.)

progeria (Hutchinson-Gilford syndrome) and Werner's syndrome; both are diseases of accelerated aging. Victims of progeria begin to show growth deceleration, graying and loss of hair, atherosclerosis, calcification of blood vessels, and osteoporosis as early as 9 years of age.[61] People with Werner's syndrome show similar symptoms, but not until the third or fourth decade of life.[61] The goal, in part, was to determine whether cells from these patients had a reduced proliferative capacity in vitro compared to age-matched controls. It was found that fibroblasts from subjects with these disorders did have a shorter life span in culture than fibroblasts from normal persons of the same age; only 2 to 10 doublings occurred in comparison to the normal 20 to 40 doublings.[49,58] Other investigators have reported a decrease in mitotic activity, DNA synthesis, and cloning efficiency for cells from these patients.[59,60] Although the use of the cells from subjects afflicted with these syndromes has been criticized on the grounds that the diseases represent more of a caricature than a phenocopy of aging,[62] the fibroblast populations derived from these subjects undergo significantly fewer doublings than their age-matched controls. In 1969, Goldstein et al.[63] reported that cells derived from diabetic individuals have a reduced ability to grow and survive in culture, as manifested by a reduced plating efficiency. More recently, Goldstein[64] has presented evidence that a statistically significant regression is not evidenced from his data if diabetic and prediabetic subjects are considered separately. Other genetic disorders that correlate with early onset senescence are the various trisomies, including Down's syndrome.[62]

One approach to correlating cells from young and old donors or from patients with diseases of accelerated aging is to use cultures from closely related animal species that differ markedly in life span. This was pioneered by Sacher and Hart[65] who used two outbred species of mice, *Mus musculus* and *Peromyscus leucopus.* They are similar in DNA content per cell, body size, metabolic rate, body temperature, and brain and organ size, yet *Peromyscus* has an average life span 2.4 times that of *Mus.* Sacher and Hart[65] found that fibroblast cell cultures from the longer-lived *Peromyscus* have 2.5 times the proliferative capacity of fibroblasts from *Mus.*

### D. Life Span Variation in Different Species

Despite the well-documented findings discussed above, a number of criticisms can be leveled at the use of cell culture as a primary model system for the study of aging.

If the loss of proliferative potential with time in vitro is truly a manifestation of aging at the cellular level and relevant to aging in vivo, then this loss should be characteristic of cultures derived from all vertebrate species. As pointed out by Martin,[62] exceptions would lend support to the idea that the limited replicative life span of normal somatic cells is an artifact of technological inadequacies.

Many studies have carefully documented that the spontaneous degeneration of cells with time in culture is characteristic of fibroblast-like cells from human,[11,15] avian,[12,66] reptilian,[67] marsupial,[13] bovine,[68] and rabbit[69] cell cultures. Normal nonfibroblastic cells which have been reported to show a finite life span in culture include human skin,[55] muscle,[70] and kidney cells,[71] and bovine endothelial cells.[72,73]

However, a number of reports involving various rodent cell cultures[74-77] and human hematopoietic cell cultures[78,79] suggest that these cells can maintain their proliferative capacity for what appear to be indefinite periods of time.

One explanation that has been offered for the apparent immortality of these cell lines is that they are not truly normal diploid cells.[62,80] While exhaustive karyological studies have not been performed on all of these cell lines, most of those that have been examined with the newest chromosome banding techniques fail the test of euploidy.[81-83] One exception is human lymphoid tissue in which at least some of the cell lines are euploid;[84] however, they have been shown to contain Epstein-Barr virus and appear to cause tumor growth when injected into suitable hosts[85] and so fail a different test of normalcy.

An apparent exception to the idea that normal cells display a finite life span is the promuscle cell line derived from the early tail regenerate of the lizard (*Anolis carolinensis*).[86] These cells have been continuously cultured for over 300 generations. They appear to have a normal karyotype and fail to cause neoplastic growth when inoculated into irradiated hosts. Similarly, Hadorn[87] has reported that *Drosophila* imaginal disc tissue cultured in vivo in the adult fly abdomen can proliferate indefinitely. Mezger-Freed[88] has discussed the culture of haploid vertebrate cells, which may be normal.

## IV. SOME CHARACTERISTICS OF CELL CULTURE AGING

### A. Population Dynamics of Aging Cell Cultures

Another area of interest concerns the interpretation of data describing the decline of proliferative capacity in aging cell cultures. The fundamental question has been whether this decrease results from a uniform decline in all the cells of the culture or if it reflects culture heterogeneity stemming from an increased fraction of cells that are unable to divide.

Experimental evidence to date appears to favor the latter alternative. Merz and Ross[89] have shown that for very low density populations, the percentage of cells that undergo division within a fixed time period decreases as a function of the number of subcultivations. This decline in the division was not a reflection of a general decrease

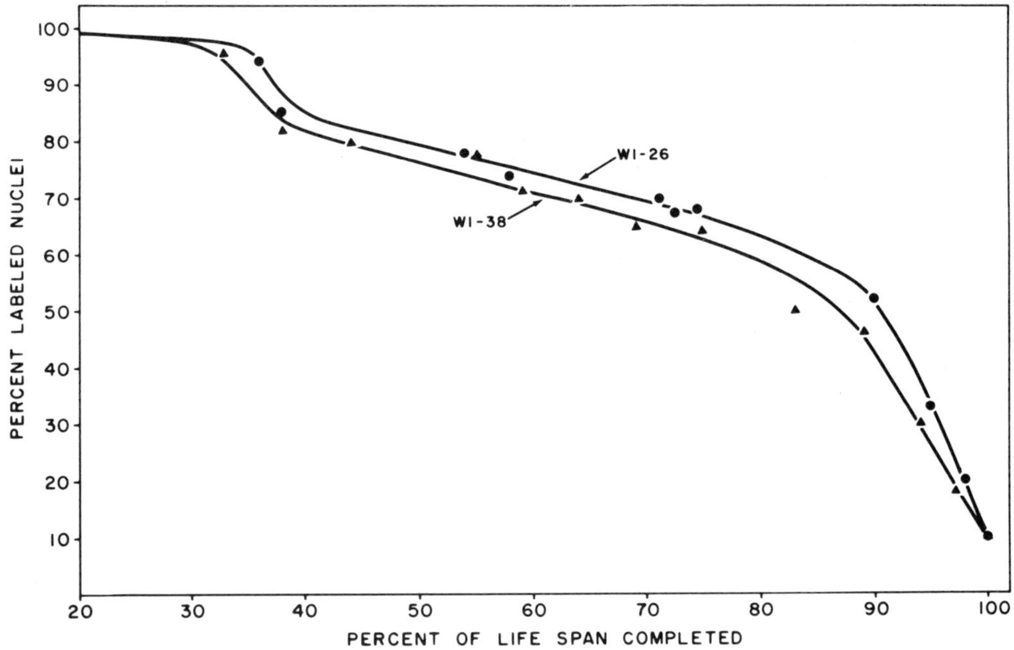


FIGURE 5. Percentage of cells incorporating [$^3$H] thymidine and thus rapidly traversing the cell cycle during the life span of two human diploid cell populations.

in the proliferation rate of all the cells since the population continued to increase exponentially but, rather, was a reflection of an increase in "nondividers". Macieira-Coelho and co-workers[90,91] reported an increased heterogeneity in the length of the division cycle in late passage cells due principally to an increased $G_2$ period and to the fact that the fraction of cells involved in DNA synthesis decreased as a function of culture age. Additional data supporting this interpretation have come from Cristofalo and Sharf,[92] who showed that, for the human diploid cell lines WI-38 and WI-26, the fraction of the population that incorporates $^3$H-thymidine into DNA decreaes exponentially (Figure 5). This fraction is directly proportional to the proliferative capacity of the population. A time-related decline in the proportion of labeled cells also has been reported for adult skin fibroblasts.[93] Subsequent studies by several groups[94-96] have shown that most of the nondividing cells in aging WI-38 populations have a 2C DNA content, an indication that these cells are arrested in the $G_1$ phase of the cell cycle. An increase in unlabeled cells with a 4C DNA content also has been reported. Yanishevsky and Carrano[97] have suggested that these cells are $G_1$ tetraploids.

Increased heterogeneity in the size distribution of late passage cells has been reported by Simons,[98] Macieira-Coelho and Ponten,[91] Cristofalo and Kritchevsky,[99] and Greenberg et al.[102] Wolosewick and Porter[100] also noted this phenomenon in young passage WI-38 cells. In general, cell size increases with age and is associated with a loss of division potential and a decrease in uptake of $^3$H-thymidine.[96,101]

The doubling potential of several hundred clones derived from lung fibroblast-like cell cultures was examined,[89,103,104] and in all cases, there was wide variation in clone size and doubling potential; however, the highest doubling potential of any clone was never higher than the doubling potential of the mass population. Martin, et al.[105] have observed the growth kinetics of clones of human diploid skin cultures and reported extensive heterogeneity in the cultures.

Additional information on the heterogeneity of diploid cell cultures comes from the work of Absher et al.[106] who used microcinematography to follow the interdivision time of clones from populations of various ages. These workers found a gradual lengthening of average interdivision time with successive generation in all geneologies studied, regardless of passage level. However, on the average, cells from old populations had longer interdivision times than cells from young populations.

Thus, the evidence strongly suggests that the loss of proliferative capacity seen in diploid cell populations with time is a well regulated phenomenon derived not from a uniform decrease in reproductive ability but, rather, from a progressive selection process within the population. Individual cells asynchronously proceed through a series of proliferative states ranging from rapidly proliferating to more and more slowly proliferating until finally reaching what appears to be a state of total arrest of DNA synthesis.

### B. Metabolic Time Vs. Replications as Determinants of Life Span

A third major question is whether the onset of decline in proliferative capacity depends on the number of division events that a cell has undergone or on the amount of time a cell has been in culture. In 1967, Hay and Strehler[12] reported that chick cells subcultivated at high population densities underwent significantly fewer doublings than those at low densities. This suggested to them that cells have a limited metabolic potential rather than a limited division potential. These workers attempted to verify this hypothesis experimentally by using an agar-overlay technique which kept the chick cell monolayer attached to the glass surface but unable to divide.[107] After various time periods in this arrested state, the agar was removed from the culture, substrains were established, and subcultivation resumed. Their results showed a progressive loss of proliferative capacity that was directly related to the length of time the culture was maintained under agar. Thus, total life span appeared to be a function of the total time in culture rather than of population doublings. Culture death occurred at the same calendar time for all substrains.

Additional evidence for this conclusion has come from the work of McHale et al.[108] Using the diploid cell line WI-38, they reduced the serum content of the growth medium from 10% to 0.1% (v/v) and were able to maintain the cells for 5 weeks in a viable, stationary state. Upon subcultivation, the serum-deprived cells underwent fewer population doublings than the continuously subcultivated controls (Table 2). Again, culture degeneration occurred at approximately the same calendar time, irrespective of the number of cell doublings. The results of Hay et al.[107] and of McHale et al.[108] have been criticized on the basis that the experimental manipulations themselves (agar overlay, serum deprivation) may inhibit cell division.[109]

Evidence in support of the idea that the number of division events is the determining factor for the onset of senescence also has been reported.[110-112] Daniel and Young[110] studied the proliferation of mouse mammary epithelium during serial transplantation (Section III.B) and showed that transplanted lines in which cells were allowed to proliferate continuously, senesced before sister lines in which cell division was partially restricted. They concluded that senescence was dependent on the number of cell divisions rather than on the passage of time. A similar conclusion was reached by Dell'Orco et al.[111] who maintained fetal and adult fibroblast-like cells in a nondividing state for various periods of time (21 to 177 days) by reducing the serum content of the growth medium to 0.5%. When the serum was replaced and subcultivation resumed, it was observed that the continuously dividing control cultures and those cultures maintained on low serum for 177 days phased out at approximately the same population doubling level (Table 3). So, while the total number of division events was the same, one group of cultures had lived 287 days and the other only 72 days, indicating that life span is related more to the number of divisions than to time in culture. Parallel results also have been reported by Goldstein and Singal.[112] More recent experiments

Table 2
RELATIONSHIP OF CULTURE DOUBLINGS AND TIME TO THE ONSET OF PHASE III IN WI-39 CELLS

| | Group | Onset of Phase III[a] | | |
|---|---|---|---|---|
| | | Passage level (Total doublings) | Subsequent culture doublings after passage 38 | Subsequent time (days) after passage 38[b] |
| A | Controls continuously subcultivated[c] | 44 | 5 | 35 |
| B | 3-Week stationary phase at passage 38[d] | 41 | 2 | 33 |
| C | 5-Week stationary phase at passage 38[d] | 39 | 0 | 35 |

[a] Cultures did not reach confluency and exhibited degenerative morphological changes.
[b] Actually, the day of final subcultivation. All sets within a group were subcultivated at the same time.
[c] Cultures were split 2:1 every 5 to 6 days.
[d] After this time, cultures were split 2:1 every 5 to 6 days. Groups A, B, and C were replicates from a single pooled source. Four sets of cultures in each group were passed independently. All sets within a group were subcultivated at the same time and reached Phase III at the same passage level.

From McHale, J. S., Mouton, M. L., and McHale, J. T., *Exp. Gerontol.*, 6, 89, 1971. With permission.

from our lab (Cristofalo et al., unpublished), using conditions similar to those of Dell'Orco et al.,[111] have shown that in young cells phase-out is determined primarily by culture doublings. However for older populations, events during the maintenance period shortened life span somewhat. Chronological time, then, appears to be significantly less important than division events.

### C. Possible Mechanism of Cell Aging

One of the most controversial questions in gerontological research today concerns the mechanism(s) that limits the proliferative potential of diploid cells in culture. There are currently two schools of thought regarding this problem; one proposes that aging is the result of a genetic program and is a deterministic process, the other suggests that aging is the result of random events and is a stochastic phenomenon. These groups, however, need not be mutually exclusive.

Deterministic hypotheses are grounded in two basic observations: each species has its own characteristic mean and maximum life span, and individual members of a given species display parallel patterns of aging changes. An example of the deterministic school of thought is the terminal differentiation theory which suggests that the decline in proliferative potential of cells in vitro is the result of a sequential process leading to a postreplicative, terminally differentiated cell.[104,105,109,113] Martin et al.[113] have suggested that the limited replicative life span of cultivated somatic cells be regarded as a two-stage process. In the first stage, growth is shown and is paralleled by a step-wise in vitro differentiation. The second stage involves the "true" senescence of this postreplicative terminally differentiated cell. Martin et al.[113] defines true senescence as deleterious changes in the structure and function of a cell.

Experimental efforts to distinguish the terminal differentiation theory from various stochastic and error theories have centered on cell fusion techniques. Norwood et al.[114]

**Table 3**
**EXTENSION OF IN VITRO CALENDAR TIME OF WI-38 AND WLW CELLS AFTER INCUBATION WITH WLW SERUM MEDIUM**

| Cell strain | Experiment | P[a] | A-time[b] (days) | P at Phase III[c] Arrested | P at Phase III[c] Control | Days in culture[d] Arrested | Days in culture[d] Control |
|---|---|---|---|---|---|---|---|
| WI-38 | 1 | 23 | 21 | 42 | 41 | 96 | 75 |
| | | 27 | 21 | 50 | | 130 | 65 |
| | 2 | 25 | 39 | 50 | 41 | 116 | 49 |
| | | 25 | 66 | 49 | | 133 | 49 |
| | | 27 | 102 | 51 | | 175 | 45 |
| ALW | 1 | 8 | 21 | 16 | 17 | 64 | 37 |
| | | 15 | 21 | 17 | | 36 | 9 |
| | 2 | 8 | 21 | 18 | 19 | 80 | 50 |
| | | 13 | 21 | 18 | | 56 | 31 |
| | 3 | 11 | 21 | 20 | 18 | 79 | 42 |
| | | 11 | 59 | 18 | | 109 | 42 |
| | | 11 | 99 | 16 | | 133 | 42 |

[a] Passage number of cells when exposed to medium containing 0.5% serum.
[b] Days of incubation with medium containing 0.5% serum.
[c] Passage number at entrance into Phase III.
[d] Days in culture from indicated passage number[a] until entrance into Phase III.

From Dell'Orco, R. T., Mertens, J. G., and Kruse, P. F., Jr., *Exp. Cell Res.*, 84, 363, 1974. With permission.

fused young and senescent human skin fibroblasts and found that the young cells failed to reinitiate DNA synthesis in the old cells. Moreover, DNA synthesis in the young cells themselves was repressed. If, however, senescent cells were fused to HeLa cells or to virus-transformed cells, DNA synthesis was reinitiated in the senescent cell.[115] Wright and Hayflick[116] used cytochalasin B to enucleate the cells and fused these cytoplasts with whole cells of various ages. The data they obtained suggested that it was the nucleus that was primarily involved in senescence.

One important fact to be derived from these studies is that senescence can be "reversed" by fusion with transformed cells. Senescence can also be delayed by inclusion of physiologic levels of hydrocortisone in the culture medium.[117] Thus, senescence can be modulated and the modulating agents can be used as probes in attempting to understand the molecular mechanisms regulating senescence.

Perhaps the most widely known of the stochastic theories is the error theory of Orgel.[118,119] This theory suggests that aging results from a random accumulation of errors that occur during the processes of replication, transcription, and translation. Mistakes in "information transfer" eventually involve those products that are themselves part of the transfer machinery such that the error is amplified. Originally, Orgel[118] deduced that the error frequency would increase exponentially and lead ultimately to an error catastrophe and death of the cell. Later he concluded that, due to existing cellular repair mechanisms, such a catastrophe need not occur.[119]

Experimental efforts aimed at testing the error theory have centered on determining the presence of error-containing proteins in young and old cells by using such parameters as changes in heat inactivation kinetics and an increase in cross-reactive, enzymatically inactive molecules. Holliday and Tarrant[120] reported that the proportion of thermolabile glucose-6-phosphate-dehydrogenase (G6PD) increased from 4% to 20% as cultures of MRC-5 cells (human fetal lung fibroblast-like cells) senesced. Goldstein and Moerman[121] have reported age-associated increases in heat-labile G6PD, 6-phosphogluconate dehydrogenase and hypoxanthine-guanine phosphoribosyl transferase from normal skin cultures. However, Pendergrass et al.[122] were unable to demonstrate any thermolabile G6PD using senescent cultures of human male infant skin fibroblasts even though the techniques were adequate to detect the enzyme. Danot and co-workers[123] were unable to detect any differences in the thermostability of the enzyme aldolase in young and senescent mouse fibroblast-like cells. Experimental evidence against the error theory also has been reported by Holland et al.,[124] Tomkins et al.,[125] and Ryan et al.[126] The basis for the experimental differences outlined above is obscure and may be due to various technical difficulties in the procedures. Other stochastic theories of aging include the somatic mutation theory,[127] the free radical theory,[128] and the cross-linking theory.[129]

Burnet[130] has proposed his intrinsic mutagenesis theory in an attempt to link the deterministic and the stochastic theories of aging. He suggests that there may be a deterministic character to the stochastic process of error accumulation in that the mutability of key polymerases may be under genetic control.

## V. SUMMARY AND CONCLUSIONS

One of the major questions about the biology of aging is whether aging is a cellular phenomenon or only a supracellular phenomenon that involves integrative functions among cell and tissue types. For many years it was thought that cells were immortal. However, the benchmark work of Hayflick and Moorhead[11] indicated that cells in culture, under relatively controlled environmental conditions, undergo senescence and ultimately die. This senescence has been shown to be independent of any simple direct effect of medium deficiency, contamination by microorganisms or the elaboration of toxic products by the cells. It is an intrinsic effect which Hayflick and Moorhead[11] interpreted as an expression of cellular aging. The observations that normal cells in culture have a limited replicative life span has been repeated many times over the last 15 to 20 years and is now a well-established fact in biology. The remaining controversy concerns primarily the establishment of criteria by which normal cells can be defined, and the stage in ontogeny at which the cultures are established.

The relevance of cell culture senescence to aging of the organism remains highly controversial. It is unlikely that death is caused by failure in proliferative capacity, but perhaps the changes that accompany alterations in proliferative capacity are significant. Of greater importance is the value of cell cultures as model systems to determine fundamental mechanisms of aging and to test the various hypotheses that have been proposed as the basis for aging.

A wide variety of studies have been carried out on fibroblast-like cultures as they age. Most of these studies have been reviewed elsewhere.[62,80,109] We emphasize here that the aging of cell populations is the result of changes in individual cells. These changes involve transition from a rapidly dividing state, through a series of more slowly dividing states, and finally an arrested state. In making these transitions, the cells seem to recognize the number of previous mitotic events, rather than the passage of chronologic time.

The course of cell senescence is modifiable. Senescence can be delayed by the inclusion of physiologic levels of hydrocortisone in the medium and senescent cells can be reactivated to synthesize DNA by fusion with transformed cells. Cultures treated with hydrocortisone still senesce but senescence occurs after 25 to 50% more doublings. The results of the cell fusion studies are more difficult to interpret since these are only short-term experiments in which one round of DNA synthesis occurs. The principle to be derived from these observations, however, is that the mechanisms of senescence can be changed by manipulation. Thus, these modulating agents become probes for understanding the underlying control system in senescence.

# REFERENCES


1. **Blumenthal, H. T.**, Aging: biologic or pathologic? *Hosp. Prac.*, 13, 127, 1978.
2. **Rockstein, M., Chesky, J. A., and Sussman, M. L.**, Comparative biology and evolution of aging, in *Handbook of the Biology of Aging*, Finch, C. E. and Hayflick, L., Eds., Von Nostrand Reinhold, New York, 1977, chap. 1.
3. **Stoner, G. D., Myers, G., Katoh, Y., Jackson, F., Trump, B. F., Brinkley, B. R., and Harris, C. C.**, Culture of human bronchial epithelial cells, *J. Cell Biol.*, 79, 66a, 1969.
4. **Autrup, H., Barrett, L. A., Jackson, F., Jesudason, M., Stoner, G., Phelps, P., Trump, B., and Harris, C.**, Explant culture of human colon, *Gastroenterology*, 74, 1248, 1977.
5. **Carrel, A.**, On the permanent life of tissues outside of the organism, *J. Exp. Med.*, 15, 516, 1912.
6. **Ebeling, A. H.**, The permanent life of connective tissue outside of the organism, *J. Exp. Med.*, 17, 273, 1913.
7. **Carrel, A.**, Present condition of a strain of connective tissue twenty-eight months old, *J. Exp. Med.*, 20, 1, 1914.
8. **Carrel, A.**, *Man, the Unknown*, Halcyon House, New York, 1935.
9. **Earle, W. R.**, Production of malignancy *in vitro*. IV. The mouse fibroblast cultures and changes seen in the living cells, *J. Natl. Cancer Inst.*, 4, 165, 1943.
10. **Gey, G. O. and Gey, M. K.**, The maintenance of human normal cells and tumor cells in continuous culture. I. Preliminary report: cultivation of mesoblastic tumors and normal tissue and notes on methods of cultivation, *Am. J. Cancer*, 27, 45, 1936.
11. **Hayflick, L. and Moorhead, P. S.**, The serial cultivation of human diploid cell strains, *Exp. Cell Res.*, 25, 585, 1961.
12. **Hay, R. J. and Strehler, B. L.**, The limited growth span of cell strains isolated from the chick embryo, *Exp. Gerontol.*, 2, 123, 1967.
13. **Simons, J. W. I. M.**, A theoretical and experimental approach to the relationship between cell variability and aging *in vitro*, in *Aging in Cell and Tissue Culture*, Holečková, E. and Cristofalo, V. J., Eds., Plenum Press, New York, 1970, 25.
14. **Swim, H. E. and Parker, R. F.**, Culture characteristics of human fibroblasts propagated serially, *Am. J. Hyg.*, 66, 235, 1957.
15. **Hayflick, L.**, The limited *in vitro* lifetime of human diploid cell strains, *Exp. Cell Res.*, 37, 614, 1965.
16. **Hayflick, L.**, Cell senescence and cell differentiation *in vitro*, in *Aging and Development*, Band 4, Bredt, H. and Rohen, J. W., Eds., FK Schattauer Verlag, Stuttgart, 1972, 1.
17. **Carrel, A. and Ebeling, A. H.**, Age and multiplication of fibroblasts, *J. Exp. Med.*, 34, 599, 1921.
18. **Carrel, A. and Burrows, M. T.**, Cultivation of adult tissues and organs outside of the body, *JAMA*, 55, 1379, 1910.
19. **Carrel, A. and Burrows, M. T.**, Cultivation of sarcoma outside of the body, *JAMA*, 55, 1554, 1910.
20. **Carrel, A. and Burrows, M. T.**, On the physiochemical regulation of the growth of tissues, *J. Exp. Med.*, 13, 562, 1911.
21. **Lorenz, E., Jacobson, L. O., Heston, W. E., Shimkin, M., Eschenbrenner, A. B., Deringer, M. K., Doniger, J., and Schweisthal, R.**, Effects of long-continued total body gamma irradiation on mice, guinea pigs and rabbits. III. Effects on life span, weight, blood picture and carcinogenesis and the role of the intensity of radiation, in *Biological Effects of External X and Gamma Irradiation*, National Nuclear Energy Series, McGraw-Hill, New York, 1954, 24.
22. **Rigby, B. J., Mitchell, T. W., and Robinson, M. S.**, Oxygen participation in the *in vivo* and *in vitro* aging of collagen fibres, *Biochem. Biophys. Res. Commun.*, 79, 400, 1977.
23. **Cowdry, E. V. and Suntzeff, V.**, Influence of age on epidermal carcinogenesis induced by methylcholanthrene in mice, *Yale J. Biol. Med.*, 17, 47, 1944.
24. **Daniel, C. W., DeOme, K. B., Young, J. T., Blair, P. B., and Faulkin, L. J.**, The *in vivo* life span of normal and preneoplastic mouse mammary glands: a serial transplantation study, *Proc. Natl. Acad. Sci. USA*, 61, 52, 1968.
25. **Upton, A. C.**, Pathobiology, in *Handbook of the Biology of Aging*, Finch, C. E. and Hayflick, L., Eds., Van Nostrand Reinhold, New York, 1977, chap. 21.
26. **Cohn, A. E. and Murray, H. A.**, Physiological ontogeny. Chicken embryos. IV. The negative acceleration of growth with age as demonstrated by tissue cultures, *J. Exp. Med.*, 42, 275, 1925.
27. **Hoffman, R. S., Goldschmidt, J., and Doljanski, L.**, Comparative studies on the growth capacity of tissues from embryonic and adult chickens, *Growth*, 1, 228, 1937.
28. **Medawar, P. B.**, The growth, growth energy and aging of chicken's heart, *Proc. R. Soc. (London) Ser. B*, 129, 332, 1940.
29. **Soukupová, M. and Holečková, E.**, The latent period of explanted organs of newborn, adult and senile rats, *Exp. Cell Res.*, 33, 361, 1964.

30. **Waters, H. and Walford, R. L.**, Latent period for the outgrowth of human skin explants as a function of age, *J. Gerontol.*, 25, 381, 1970.
31. **Soukupovâ, M. and Hnêvkovský, P.**, The influence of donor age on the behavior of human embryonic tissue *in vitro, Physiol. Bohemoslov.*, 21, 485, 1972.
32. **LeBlond, C. P.**, Classification of cell populations on the basis of their proliferative behavior, National Cancer Institute Monograph No. 14, Congdon, C. C. and Mori-Chavez, P., Eds., 1964, p. 119.
33. **Lesher, S. and Sacher, G. A.**, Effects of age on cell proliferation in mouse duodenal crypts, *Exp. Gerontol.*, 3, 211, 1968.
34. **Thrasher, J. O.**, Age and the cell cycle of the mouse esophageal epithelium, *Exp. Gerontol.*, 6, 19, 1971.
35. **Cameron, I. L.**, Minimum number of cell doublings in an epithelial population during the life span of the mouse, *J. Gerontol.*, 27, 157, 1972.
36. **Cameron, I. L.**, Cell proliferation and renewal in aging mice, *J. Gerontol.*, 27, 162, 1972.
37. **Buetow, D. E.**, Cellular content and cellular proliferation changes in the tissues and organs of the aging mammal, in *Cellular and Molecular Renewal in the Mammalian Body*, Cameron, I. L. and Thrasher, J. O., Eds., Academic Press, New York, 1971, 87.
38. **Krohn, P. L.**, Review lectures on senescence. II. Heterochronic transplantation in the study of aging, *Proc. R. Soc. (London) Ser. B*, 157, 128, 1962.
39. **Krohn, P. L.**, Transplantation and aging, in *Topics of the Biology of Aging*, Krohn, P. L., Ed., John Wiley & Sons, New York, 1966, 125.
40. **Till, J. E. and McCullough, E. A.**, A direct measurement of the radiation sensitivity of normal bone marrow cells, *Radiat. Res.*, 14, 213, 1961.
41. **Siminovitch, L., Till, J. E., and McCullough, E. A.**, Decline in colony-forming ability of marrow cells subjected to serial transplantation into irradiated mice, *J. Cell. Comp. Physiol.*, 64, 23, 1964.
42. **Cudkowicz, G., Upton, A. C., and Shearer, G. M.**, Lymphocyte content and proliferative capacity of serially transplanted mouse bone marrow, *Nature (London)*, 201, 165, 1964.
43. **Williamson, A. R. and Askonas, B. A.**, Senescence of an antibody-forming cell clone, *Nature (London)*, 238, 337, 1972.
44. **Harrison, D. E.**, Normal production of erythrocytes by mouse marrow continuous for 73 months, *Proc. Natl. Acad. Sci. USA*, 70, 3184, 1973.
45. **DeOme, K. B., Faulkin, L. J., Bern, H. A., and Blair, P. B.**, Development of mammary tumors from hyperplastic alveolar nodules transplanted into gland-free mammary fat pads of female C3H mice, *Cancer Res.*, 19, 515, 1959.
46. **Young, L. J. T., Medina, D., DeOme, K. B., and Daniel, C. W.**, The influence of host and tissue age on life span and growth rate of serially transplanted mouse mammary gland, *Exp. Gerontol.*, 6, 49, 1971.
47. **Harrison, D. E.**, Proliferative capacity of erythropoietic stem cell lines and aging: an overview, *Mech. Ageing Dev.*, 9, 409, 1979.
48. **Daniel, C.**, Cell longevity *in vivo*, in *Handbook of the Biology of Aging*, Finch, C. E. and Hayflick, L., Eds., Van Nostrand Reinhold, New York, 1977, 122.
49. **Martin, G. M., Sprague, C. A., and Epstein, C. J.**, Replicative life span of cultivated human cells: effects of donor's age, tissue and genotype, *Lab. Invest.*, 23, 86, 1970.
50. **LeGuilly, Y., Simon, M., Lenoir, P., and Bourel, M.**, Long-term culture of human adult liver cells: morphological changes related to *in vitro* senescence and effect of donor's age on growth potential, *Gerontologia*, 19, 303, 1973.
51. **Martin, G. M., Ogburn, C. E., and Sprague, C. A.**, Effects of age on cell division capacity, in *Aging: A Challenge to Science and Society*, Dannon, D., Shock, N. W., and Marcois, M., Eds., Oxford University Press, 1981, 124.
52. **Schneider, E. L. and Mitsui, Y.**, The relationship between *in vitro* cellular aging and *in vivo* human age, *Proc. Natl. Acad. Sci. USA*, 73, 3584, 1976.
53. **Kohn, R. R.**, Aging and cell division, *Science*, 188, 203, 1975.
54. **Smith, J. R., Pereira-Smith, O. M., and Schneider, E. L.**, Colony size distributions as a measure of *in vivo* and *in vitro* aging, *Proc. Natl. Acad. Sci. USA*, 75, 1353, 1978.
55. **Rheinwald, J. G. and Green, H.**, Serial cultivation of strains of human epidermal keratinocytes: the formation of keratinizing colonies from single cells, *Cell*, 6, 331, 1975.
56. **Bierman, E. L.**, The effect of donor age on the *in vitro* life span of cultured human arterial smooth-muscle cells, *In Vitro*, 14, 955, 1978.
57. **Martin, G. M., Ogburn, C., and Sprague, C.**, Senescence and vascular disease, *Adv. Exp. Biol. Med.*, 61, 163, 1975.
58. **Goldstein, S.**, Lifespan of cultured cells in progeria, *Lancet*, 1, 424, 1969.
59. **Danes, B. S.**, Progeria: a cell culture study on aging, *J. Clin. Invest.*, 50, 2000, 1971.

60. **Menhaus, A. J., deJong, B., and ten Kate, L. P.,** Fibroblast culture in Werner's syndrome, *Hum. Genet.,* 13, 244, 1971.
61. **Reichel, W., Garcia-Bunuel, R., and Delallo, J.,** Progeria and Werner's syndrome as models for the study of normal human aging, *J. Am. Geriatr. Soc.,* 19, 369, 1971.
62. **Martin, G. M.,** Cellular aging: clonal senescence (Part I), *Am. J. Pathol.,* 89, 484, 1977.
63. **Goldstein, S., Littlefield, J. W., and Soeldner, J. S.,** Diabetes mellitus and aging: diminished plating efficiency of cultured human fibroblasts, *Proc. Natl. Acad. Sci. USA,* 64, 155, 1969.
64. **Gleason, R. E. and Goldstein, S.,** Age effect and replicative life span of fibroblasts of diabetic, prediabetic, and normal donors. another look at the data, *Science,* 202, 1217, 1978.
65. **Sacher, G. A. and Hart, R. W.,** Longevity, aging and comparative cellular and molecular biology of the house mouse, *Mus musculus* and the white-footed mouse, *Peromyscus leucopus, Birth Defects: Original Articles Series,* 14, 71, 1971.
66. **Ponten, J.,** The growth capacity of normal and Rous virus-transformed chicken fibroblasts *in vitro, Int. J. Cancer,* 6, 323, 1970.
67. **Goldstein, S.,** Growth of cultured cells from the Galapagos tortoise, *Exp. Cell Res.,* 83, 297, 1974.
68. **Lithner, F. and Ponten, J.,** Bovine fibroblasts in long-term tissue culture: chromosome studies, *Int. J. Cancer,* 1, 579, 1966.
69. **Haff, R. F. and Swim, H. E.,** Serial propagation of three strains of rabbit fibroblasts: their susceptibility to infection with vaccinia virus, *Proc. Soc. Exp. Biol. Med.,* 93, 200, 1956.
70. **Haushka, S. D.,** Cultivation of muscle tissue, in *Growth, Nutrition and Metabolism of Cells in Culture,* Rothblat, G. H. and Cristofalo, V. J., Eds., Academic Press, New York, 1977, 67.
71. **Nichols, W.,** personal communication.
72. **Schwartz, S. M.,** Selection and characterization of bovine aortic endothelial cells, *In Vitro,* 14, 966, 1978.
73. **Mueller, S. N., Rosen, E. M., and Levine, E. M.,** Cellular senescence in a cloned strain of bovine aortic endothelial cells, *Science,* 208, 1980.
74. **Petursson, G., Coughlin, J. G., and Meylan, C.,** Long-term cultivation of diploid rat cells, *Exp. Cell Res.,* 33, 60, 1964.
75. **Krooth, R. S., Shaw, M. W., and Campbell, B. K.,** A persistent strain of diploid fibroblasts, *J. Natl. Cancer Inst.,* 32, 1031, 1964.
76. **Yaffe, D.,** Retention of differentiation potentialities during prolonged cultivation of myogenic cells, *Proc. Natl. Acad. Sci. USA,* 61, 477, 1968.
77. **Valenti, C. and Friedman, E. A.,** Long-term cultivation of diploid rabbit skin cells, *Texas Rep. Biol. Med.,* 26, 363, 1968.
78. **Moore, G. E. and Sandberg, A. A.,** Studies on a human tumor cell line with a diploid karyotype, *Cancer,* 17, 170, 1964.
79. **Moore, G. E. and McLimans, W. F.,** The life span of the cultured normal cell: concepts derived from studies of human lymphoblasts, *J. Theor. Biol.,* 20, 217, 1968.
80. **Hayflick, L.,** Cellular aging, in *Handbook of the Biology of Aging,* Finch, C. E. and Hayflick, L., Eds., Van Nostrand Reinhold, New York, 1977, 159.
81. **Deaven, L. L. and Petersen, D. F.,** The chromosomes of CHO, an aneuploid Chinese hamster cell line: G-band, C-band and autoradiographic analyses, *Chromosoma,* 41, 129, 1973.
82. **Puck, T. T., Waldren, C. A., and Tjio, J. H.,** Some data bearing on the long-term growth on mammalian cells *in vitro,* in *Symposium on Topics in the Biology of Aging,* Krohn, P. L., Ed., Interscience, New York, 1966, 101.
83. **Martin, G. M. and Ogburn, C. E.,** Cell, tissue and organoid cultures of blood vessels, in *Growth Nutrition and Metabolism of Cells in Culture,* Rothblat, G. and Cristofalo, V. J., Eds., Academic Press, New York, 1977, 1.
84. **Povey, S., Gardiner, S. E., Watson, B., Mowbray, S., Harris, H., Arthur, E., Steel, C. M., Blenkinsop, C., and Evans, H. J.,** Genetic studies on human lymphoblastoid lines: isozyme analysis on cell lines from forty-one different individuals and on mutants produced following exposure to a chemical mutagen, *Ann. Hum. Genet.,* 36, 247, 1973.
85. **Deal, D. R., Gerber, P., and Chisari, F. V.,** Heterotransplantation of two human lymphoid cell lines transformed *in vitro* by Epstein-Barr virus, *J. Natl. Cancer Inst.,* 47, 771, 1971.
86. **Simpson, S. B., Jr. and Cox, P. G.,** Studies on lizard myogenesis, in *Research in Muscle Development and the Muscle Spindle,* Banker, B. Q., Przybylski, R. J., Van der Meulen, J. P., and Victor, M., Eds., Exerpta Medica, Amsterdam, 1972, 72.
87. **Hadorn, E.,** Dynamics of determination, in *Major Problems in Developmental Biology,* Locke, M., Ed., 25th Symposium of the Society for Developmental Biology, Academic Press, New York, 1967.
88. **Mezger-Freed, L.,** Haploid vertebrate cell cultures, in *Growth, Nutrition and Metabolism of Cells in Culture,* Rothblat, G. and Cristofalo, V. J., Eds., Academic Press, New York, 1977, 57.
89. **Merz, G. S. and Ross, J. D.,** Viability of human diploid cells as a function of *in vitro* age, *J. Cell. Phys.,* 74, 219, 1973.

90. **Macieira-Coelho, A., Ponten, J., and Phillipson, L.**, The division cycle and RNA synthesis in diploid human cells at different passage levels *in vitro, Exp. Cell. Res.*, 42, 673, 1966.
91. **Macieira-Coelho, A. and Ponten, J.**, Analogy in growth between late passage human embryonic and early passage human adult fibroblasts, *J. Cell Biol.*, 43, 374, 1969.
92. **Cristofalo, V. J. and Sharf, B. B.**, Cellular senescence and DNA synthesis, *Exp. Cell Res.*, 76, 419, 1973.
93. **Vincent, R. A. and Huang, P. C.**, The proportion of cells labeled with tritiated thymidine as a function of population doubling level in cultures of fetal, adult, mutant and tumor origins, *Exp. Cell Res.*, 102, 31, 1976.
94. **Macieira-Coelho, A., Loria, E., and Beruman, L.**, Relationship between cell kinetic changes and metabolic events during cell senescence *in vitro*, in *Cell Impairment in Aging and Development*, Cristofalo, V. J. and Holečková, E., Eds., Plenum Press, New York, 1975, 51.
95. **Yanishevsky, R., Mendelsohn, M. L., Mayall, B. H., and Cristofalo, V. J.**, Proliferative capacity and DNA content of aging human diploid cells in culture: a cytophotometric and autoradiographic analysis, *J. Cell. Phys.*, 84, 165, 1974.
96. **Schneider, E. L. and Fowlkes, B. J.**, Measurement of DNA content and cell volume in senescent human fibroblasts utilizing flow multiparameter single cell analysis, *Exp. Cell Res.*, 98, 298, 1976.
97. **Yanishevsky, R. and Carrano, A. V.**, Prematurely condensed chromosomes of dividing and non-dividing cells in aging human cell cultures, *Exp. Cell Res.*, 90, 169, 1975.
98. **Simons, J. W. I. M.**, The use of frequency distributions of cell diameters to characterize cell populations in tissue culture, *Exp. Cell Res.*, 45, 336, 1967.
99. **Cristofalo, V. J. and Kritchevsky, D.**, Cell size and nucleic acid content in the diploid human cell line WI-38 during aging, *Med. Exp.*, 19, 313, 1969.
100. **Wolosewick, J. and Porter, K.**, Stereo high-voltage electron microscopy of whole cells of the human diploid line, WI-38, *Am. J. Anat.*, 147, 303, 1976.
101. **Bowman, P. D., Meek, R. L., and Daniel, C. W.**, Aging of human fibroblasts *in vitro, Exp. Cell Res.*, 93, 184, 1975.
102. **Greenberg, S. B., Grove, G. L., and Cristofalo, V. J.**, Cell size in aging monolayer cultures, *In Vitro*, 13, 297, 1977.
103. **Smith, J. R. and Hayflick, L.**, Variation in the life span of clones derived from human diploid cell strains, *J. Cell Biol.*, 62, 48, 1974.
104. **Smith, J. R., Pereira-Smith, O. M., and Schneider, E. L.**, Colony size distributions as a measure of *in vivo* and *in vitro* aging, *Proc. Natl. Acad. Sci. USA*, 75, 1353, 1978.
105. **Martin, G., Sprague, C. A., Norwood, T. H., and Pendergrass, W. R.**, Clonal selection, attenuation and differentiation in an *in vitro* model of hyperplasia, *Am. J. Pathol.*, 74, 137, 1974.
106. **Absher, P. M. and Absher, R. G.**, Clonal variation and aging of diploid fibroblasts, *Exp. Cell Res.*, 103, 247, 1976.
107. **Hay, R. J., Menzies, R. A., Morgan, H. P., and Strehler, B. L.**, The division potential of cells in continuous growth as compared to cells subcultivated after maintenance in stationary phase, *Exp. Gerontol.*, 3, 35, 1968.
108. **McHale, J. S., Mouton, M. L., and McHale, J. T.**, Limited culture life span of human diploid cells as a function of metabolic time instead of division potential, *Exp. Gerontol.*, 6, 89, 1971.
109. **Cristofalo, V. J.**, Animal cell cultures as a model system for aging, *Adv. Gerontol. Res.*, 4, 45, 1972.
110. **Daniel, C. W. and Young, L. J. T.**, Influence of cell division on an aging process, *Exp. Cell Res.*, 65, 27, 1971.
111. **Dell'Orco, R. T., Mertens, J. G., and Kruse, P. F., Jr.**, Doubling potential calendar time and donor age of human diploid cells in culture, *Exp. Cell Res.*, 84, 363, 1974.
112. **Goldstein, S. and Singal, D. P.**, Senescence of cultured human fibroblasts: mitotic versus metabolic time, *Exp. Cell Res.*, 88, 359, 1974.
113. **Martin, G. M., Sprague, C. A., Norwood, T. H., Pendergrass, W. R., Bornstein, P., Hoehn, H., and Arend, W. P.**, Do hyperplastoid cell lines differentiate themselves to death? *Adv. Exp. Med. Biol.*, 53, 67, 1975.
114. **Norwood, T. H., Pendergrass, W. R., Sprague, C. A., and Martin, G. M.**, Dominance of the senescent phenotype in heterokaryons between replicating and post-replicating human fibroblast-like cells, *Proc. Natl. Acad. Sci. USA*, 71, 2231, 1974.
115. **Norwood, T. H., Pendergrass, W. R., and Martin, G. M.**, Reinitiation of DNA synthesis in senescent human fibroblasts upon fusion with immortal cells, *J. Cell Biol.*, 64, 551, 1975.
116. **Wright, W. E. and Hayflick, L.**, Nuclear control of cellular aging demonstrated by the hybridization of anucleate and whole cultured normal human fibroblasts, *Exp. Cell Res.*, 96, 113, 1975.
117. **Cristofalo, V. J.**, Metabolic aspects of aging in diploid human cells, in *Aging in Cell and Tissue Culture*, Holečková, E. and Cristofalo, Eds., Plenum Press, New York, 1970, 83.
118. **Orgel, L. E.**, The maintenance of the accuracy of protein synthesis and its relevance to aging, *Proc. Natl. Acad. Sci. USA*, 49, 517, 1963.

119. **Orgel, L. E.**, Aging of clones of mammalian cells, *Nature (London)*, 243, 441, 1973.

120. **Holliday, R. and Tarrant, G. M.**, Altered enzymes in ageing human fibroblasts, *Nature (London)*, 238, 26, 1972.

121. **Goldstein, S. and Moerman, E. J.**, Defective proteins in normal and abnormal human fibroblasts during aging *in vitro*, *Interdisc. Top. Gerontol.*, 10, 24, 1976.

122. **Pendergrass, W. R., Martin, G. M., and Bornstein, P.**, Evidence contrary to the protein error hypothesis for *in vitro* senescence, *J. Cell. Physiol.*, 87, 3, 1975.

123. **Danot, M., Gershon, H., and Gershon, D.**, The lack of altered enzyme molecules in "senescent" mouse embryo fibroblasts in culture, *Mech. Ageing Dev.*, 4, 289, 1975.

124. **Holland, J. J., Kohne, D., and Doyle, M. V.**, Analysis of virus replication in ageing human fibroblast cultures, *Nature (London)*, 245, 316, 1973.

125. **Tomkins, G. C., Stanbridge, E. J., and Hayflick, L.**, Viral probes of aging in the human diploid cell strain WI-38, *Proc. Soc. Exp. Biol. Med.*, 146, 385, 1974.

126. **Ryan, J. M., Duda, G., and Cristofalo, V. J.**, Error accumulation and aging in human diploid cells, *J. Gerontol.*, 29, 616, 1974.

127. **Crowley, C. and Curtis, H. J.**, The development of somatic mutations in mice with age, *Proc. Natl. Acad. Sci. USA*, 49, 626, 1963.

128. **Harman, D.**, Aging: a theory based on free radical and radiation chemistry, *J. Gerontol.*, 11, 298, 1956.

129. **Bjorksten, J.**, Aging, primary mechanism, *Gerontologia*, 8, 179, 1963.

130. **Burnet, F. M.**, Implications of a somatic mutation approach to aging for gerontological research, *Interdisc. Top. Gerontol.*, 11, 30, 1977.

Chapter 7

# EVIDENCE AGAINST CELLULAR AGING THEORIES

Robert R. Kohn

## TABLE OF CONTENTS

## I. INTRODUCTION

Advancing arguments against something does not provide explanations of phenomena, and the critic rarely attains a niche in the history of science. However, in a developing field it is very useful to identify trivial or misleading observations and notions in order for the attention of investigators to be directed to more productive lines of work. Progress in science is often hindered not so much by difficulty of problems as by uncertainty over which problems scientists should attempt to solve. Approaches to research are further complicated by the overwhelming pressures on scientists to generate elegant data at regular intervals. Under such circumstances, most scientists cannot resist the appeal of working on manageable models which may, however, be illegitimate in terms of explaining important phenomena in nature. When faced with the choice of finding definitive answers to trivial questions or tentative answers to the most important and difficult questions, many scientists simply cannot afford the luxury of the latter. A late twentieth century substitute for Occam's Razor might be that when there are several hypotheses available to explain a phenomenon, the investigator should favor the one that enables him to do the kind of experiments he likes to do, and the kind of experiments that are certain to yield publishable data.

Aging processes are usually defined as those normal processes, occurring in all members of a population, that are progressive and irreversible. Such processes are very widespread in nature and at all levels of biological organization. However, when we talk about aging, unless otherwise noted, we are referring to aging processes in human beings, and more specifically, to the debilities and losses of function that progress in very predictable and characteristic ways after growth cessation in all members of a human population, even in the presence of optimal nutrition, environment, activity pattern, and genetic background. And when we consider a *theory* of aging, we are considering processes at the most basic level, at the level of molecules, cells, or tissues, that would appear capable of explaining aging as it is recognized in intact human beings. The phrase *Cellular Aging Theory* denotes the view that primary, intrinsic processes occurring in cells are the basic cause of aging as it is recognized in intact human beings.

There are several rules that are useful in evaluating a theory of aging. The argument was advanced that we are interested in human aging. This being the case, there is little reason to be concerned with data on aging of lower forms of life such as insects, rotifers, or nematodes. The cell populations and tissue organization of these animals differ so markedly from human beings that there is no reason to believe that they and man age by similar mechanisms. On the other hand, it is quite likely that all mammals have important aging processes in common, and that information on aging in one mammalian species will hold for others. Secondly, a process that truly *causes* aging would be a primary intrinsic process wherever it occurs; it should not be secondary to some other biological process. The process should be progressive and irreversible because aging is progressive and irreversible. It should occur in all members of the population because aging occurs in all members of a population. Such a process should be conspicuous after maturity because aging is most conspicuous during the postmature period. And of course, the process must be capable of explaining, at least in part, such characteristic manifestations of human aging as arteriosclerosis, decreased organ perfusion, degenerative joint disease, less compliant lungs, and declining function of every physiological process.[1] These criteria will be used in this essay in the evaluation of cellular aging theories.

There are very many theories of aging that deal with changes in cells. However, these theories fall into three categories that will provide the framework for the discussions to follow: (1) there is dying out of cells, a progressive loss of large amounts of cells with the passage of time, (2) cells that normally divide, lose their capacity to divide with increasing age and become functionally impaired or die out, and (3) cells, while remaining viable, progressively lose some capacity or function.

## II. CELL TYPES

In order to consider the categories of aging theories and to evaluate observations, it is necessary to appreciate the different types of cells that might be affected. Cell populations can be classified in several ways. The classification scheme most relevant to theories of aging describes three different kinds of cell populations:

**Dynamic cell populations** — these populations consist of stem cells that divide continuously or periodically giving rise to specialized cells that divide less frequently. The latter give rise to highly specialized cells that carry out one or a small number of specific functions. They do not have the capacity to divide. These specialized postmitotic cells have life spans that are characteristic for each cell type. As cells die, they are replaced by new cells from stem cell division, so that the entire population is in a more-or-less steady state. Examples are epithelial cells, gland cells of the gastrointestinal tract, spermatozoa and precursors, and the erythrocyte and granulocyte series. The postmitotic cells in these populations clearly age and die. The important question is whether or not anything in these populations changes over the life span of an animal or plays a role in aging of the intact animal.

**Long-lived fixed postmitotic cells** — the full complement of these cells is present at or around the time of birth. The cells do not divide over the life span, although some may have the capacity to divide under very special curcumstances. Examples are neurones, skeletal, and cardiac muscle cells.

**Reverting postmitotic cells** — these are specialized cells that are quiescent, not dividing unless they receive a stimulus. When stimulated, they undergo a series of divisions and then become quiescent again. Examples are fibrocytes, chondrocytes, osteocytes, endothelial cells, lymphocytes, and liver cells.

## III. AGING OF CELL POPULATIONS

To advance a theory of aging based on cellular changes, we must identify changes in cells that are primary and intrinsic, and that occur during the period of animal aging. Many aspects of cell proliferation and function are different during growth and development, as compared to the postmature period. There are many reports in the aging literature in which some comparisons are made between cells from a growing and developing animal and cells from an old animal, and inferences are made about changes during aging. To have a legitimate relationship to aging of an animal, cell changes should certainly occur during the period of aging — that is, they should progress after maturity.

Many reports of differences in cellular processes during aging are difficult to interpret because the processes are homeostatically regulated. Enzyme levels, rates of protein synthesis and degradation, and rates of cell division rise and fall depending on functional demand, diet, activity patterns, and environmental stresses. Aging animals are debilitated, sluggish, and have altered patterns of feeding and sleeping. Whatever the causes of aging, many cellular processes would be secondarily altered in the older animals. In evaluating any cellular change with age, it would be important to determine if the change is reversible, and therefore homeostatically regulated.

Similarly, secondary cellular changes in many organs could occur because of primary changes in some regulatory organ system, such as the cardiovascular or respiratory system.

In considering reported cellular changes with age, where it is implied that such change supports a cellular theory of aging, it is important to keep in mind the possibility that such change might be secondary and reversible.

### A. Loss of Cells

There are several reasons for *a priori* doubts that cell loss plays an important role in the aging syndrome. For one, the reserve of cells in various organs is enormous. Homeostasis can be maintained with part of one kidney, one lung, a fraction of liver, the loss of much stomach and intestine, and with much of the brain destroyed. If cell loss were important in aging, it would have to be very great indeed. Secondly, many tissues are composed of dynamic cell populations that reconstitute themselves, and many tissues have marked powers of regeneration. For significant cell loss to occur in such tissues, there would have to be an age-related loss in the ability of cells to divide. This question will be dealt with in a later section, but for the time being we should recognize that the notion that there is an age-related decrease in the ability of cells to divide is a very tenuous one. Finally, if cell loss were widespread and occurring at random, an old individual would simply be smaller than a younger one. In order to explain debilities, there would have to be selective cell loss at certain sites with subsequent marked imbalances between different cell populations, again a tenuous notion, as will be brought out.

Cell loss has been shown to occur most clearly during growth and development. In the embryo, cell loss occurs during invaginations, separation of tissues, endochondral ossification, and disintegration of such structures as gills and tails and Mullerian and Wolffian duct components. The thymus gland of mice is largest at around 6 weeks of age, and then loses weight very rapidly while the mouse is growing and developing.[2] The number of ova in human ovaries is greatest at around 6 months gestation, and drops off rapidly during subsequent gestation.[3]

After maturity, no clear irreversible losses of cells in dynamic populations have been shown. There is no change in cellularity of mouse intestinal mucosa with age, but the number of proliferating stem cells drops from about 126 per crypt in 100-day-old mice to 89 per crypt in 825-day-old animals.[4] Since total cellularity remains constant in the face of a smaller stem cell population, the life span of postmitotic cells must increase with age. Similarly, the number of cells is constant with age in rat tongue and palate epithelium.[5] In these cell populations, there is a slight decrease in numbers of progenitor cells with age, but those that are present divide more frequently, giving rather stable cell populations.

Some studies have revealed cell loss with age, but not in all individuals. Thus, numbers of human Leydig cells have been reported to decrease with age, except that some very old individuals have as many cells as young people.[6] Unless a change occurs in every individual, it cannot be used to explain debilities of age that occur in every individual. In reviewing a variety of dynamic cell populations during aging of animals, no pattern of decreasing cell numbers become apparent.[7]

Losses of long-lived fixed postmitotic cells with age would be more likely to have serious consequences than would losses of cells from dynamic populations, because the former cannot be replenished from a progenitor cell pool. A study of rat skeletal muscle showed a loss of red fibers between 12 and 24 months of age, but little or no change in numbers of white fibers over that period.[8]

The postmitotic cells that have received the most attention have been neurones. The concept that neurone loss is part of the aging process has found its way into popular journalism and it is now widely believed that large numbers of neurones drop out of everyone's cerebral cortex every day. Counts of neurones in histological sections of various parts of the human cerebral cortex indicated little or no change at some sites with increasing age, but show significant drops over the life span in the superior temporal gyrus and postcentral gyrus.[9] However, the possibility was not excluded in that study that numbers of neurones did not change, but that there was an apparent decrease in the sections studied because of increased numbers of non-neuronal cells. Furthermore, the greatest rate of decrease was early in life, during the growth period. The probability of neurones being lost did not increase with neurone age, as would be the case if loss were due to intrinsic aging processes.

No loss of neurones with age was demonstrated in the rat cerebral cortex.[10] And no change with age has been shown in several human brain stem nuclei.[11] A study of mouse brain showed no neuronal loss when the mice started dying off at a rapid rate, and a significant loss only in a very small number of very old survivors.[12] The number of Purkinje cells has been reported to decrease, on the average, about 25% over the human life span.[13] However, the study revealed an enormous variability in number of cells at each age, with large fractions of the oldest populations having as many Purkinje cells as many young and mature individuals.

Additional contradictory and inconclusive reports could be cited. The world literature on neurone loss with age from 1894 to 1972 has been reviewed.[14] It was concluded that no consistent pattern of neurone loss could be demonstrated.

Thus, while some decrease in cell numbers probably occurs in some tissues of some aging animals and human beings, cell loss cannot be viewed as a generalized and extensive aging process. And the notion that cell loss plays a significant role in the diseases and generalized debilitation that characterize the aging syndrome is not supported by the available data.

### B. Loss of Capacity to Divide

The question of the ability of cells to divide as a function of age is actually part of the question of cell number or loss of cells with age, which was just considered. The main reason for considering cell division as a separate topic is that there is widespread use of models for the study of aging based on the view that failure of cell division is important in aging. The use of such models followed the report that cultures of human diploid fibroblasts died out after about 50 doublings.[15] It became accepted by many individuals who wanted to work in the aging field that similar dying out of stem cells or reverting postmitotic cells occurred in vivo and played a role in overall aging. More critical investigators did not believe so much in the dying out of stem cells in vivo, but tentatively accepted the notion that changes occurring over time in these cultures was somehow similar to changes occurring over time in vivo and that cell cultures could be studied as models for important aging processes. Such models are expedient and manageable, and can be readily used to generate large amounts of data. It is not surprising that they have been so widely used and that their study has resulted in an enormous literature.

It should be noted that fibroblasts are reverting postmitotic cells. They are quiescent in an adult animal. When stimulated by tissue injury or stress, they undergo a series of divisions, synthesize extracellular macromolecules, and become quiescent again. A culture in which cells double every week is a highly artifactual system because of selection of cell lines, environment, or both. Fifty doublings would yield about 1000 liters of cells. Such uncontrolled growth never occurs in nature. It is not difficult to suggest causes for the dying out of such cultures, and to question the view that any phenomenon observed in aging cultures is similar to an important aging process in an aging animal.

A useful approach to the question of the legitimacy of culture models is to determine if there is any loss of ability of cells to divide or any defect in reverting postmitotic cells during aging of an animal. The regeneration of liver following partial hepatectomy occurs at similar rates in mature and old rats.[16] Similarly, the proliferative response of bone marrow cells to acute blood loss is not impaired in old rats.[17] As noted earlier, the numbers of cells present and the ability to generate cells in intestinal, palate, and tongue epithelia are not significantly diminished in old animals.[4,5] On the other hand, spermatogonial stem cells, a population of stem cells not necessary for life, appeared to show some decrease in number after maturity.[18] With reference to a limit to potential doublings, thought to be around 50 from human cell culture investigations, chronic labeling studies indicated a lifetime number of doublings, on the average, of around 565 in mouse tongue epithelium.[7] As noted above, a review of findings on dynamic and reverting postmitotic cell populations indicated some increases and some decreases with age; no pattern of decline was revealed.[7]

The ability of cells from old animals to divide and function has been shown most dramatically in transplantation experiments. Results of transplanting bone marrow and spleen cells from young and old mice into irradiated recipients indicated that tissues from the old donors could generate immunocompetent cells as effectively as could the cell population from the younger animals.[19] Similarly, genetically anemic mice could be cured by bone marrow transplants from very old donors.[20]

Even more impressive results have been obtained from serial transplantation experiments. In such studies, an easily identified tissue is transplanted to an animal. When that animal gets old, the same tissue is removed and transplanted to another recipient. This is repeated when the second recipient gets old, and so on, until the tissue can no longer be identified. Serially transplanted marrow showed normal proliferation and function for at least 84 months in mice, almost three times the life span of the original donors.[20] Comparable studies undertaken with prostate gland[21] and skin[22] indicate that the cells comprising these organs can proliferate and function much longer than the life span of the original donor. Even when serially transplanted tissues eventually disappear, there is little reason to believe the loss is due to cellular aging. It is more likely caused by the periodic manipulations involved in transplantation and by healing and inflammatory responses of the hosts.

Returning to the human diploid fibroblast model, if capacity to divide in vitro is related to aging, the number of potential doublings should decrease with donor age. In other words, during aging, individuals should be using up the limited number of cell doublings that they started with. In the first extensive study dealing with this question, skin biopsies were obtained from a large number of human beings, and the number of cell doublings on culture in vitro was determined, up to the point where the cells disappeared.[23] There was a suggestion of a decrease in total doublings between birth and maturity, but no difference was apparent between 20 and 90 years of age. There was marked variability at each age. In the 40 to 50-year-old age group, for example, the number of doublings ranged from about 12 to 40. In a similar study by other workers, there was also marked variability at each age, with cultures from some of the oldest individuals showing the greatest number of doublings in vitro.[24] Another study concluded that potential doublings did not decrease with age of donor in the absence of diabetes or predisposition to diabetes,[25] but on re-examination of the data,[26] it was decided that there was a decrease with age that was statistically significant. However, many old individuals yielded cultures that gave as many doublings as did the cultures from young individuals, and there was very marked variability at each age. For example, the number of doublings at 20 years of age appeared from inspection of the graph to be around 42-76, and in the 70 to 80-year-old group to be around 28-65. In yet another study of doublings in vitro of fibroblasts obtained from human beings of different ages, it was concluded that there was a statistically significant decline with age, but the number of doublings of the young group (21 to 36 years of age) varied between 21 and 71, and that the old group (63 to 92 years of age) between 2 and 57.[27] Doubling time in that study was found to be 20.8 ± 0.8 (mean ± std. error of the mean) hours for the young group and 24.3 ± 0.9 for the old. Another determination of doubling rate for cultures from three individuals 20 to 30 years old and from five individuals around 60 years old revealed about 0.9 doubling per day for the young group and about 0.7 for the old.[28]

From all of these studies it would appear that some cultures from some old individuals have decreased numbers of doublings. It would be worth knowing why this is so. Have certain cell lines been selected at some sites in aging individuals? Is a given number of doublings a true marker for that individual, or would repeat biopsies, or biopsies of different sites give different doublings for a given individual? It is certainly clear that the using up of potential doublings is not generalized or inevitable in members of an aging population. It is also of interest that maximum number of doublings in vitro of cells from different species does not correlate with life span.[29]

There has been a great deal of work done on the question of cell division and the maintenance or loss of dynamic cell populations during aging. The findings have been reviewed elsewhere.[30,31] The representative reports cited here fail to support a cellular theory of aging. That is, they do not support the view that the *inevitable* generalized deterioration that characterizes aging is *caused* by an *inevitable* intrinsic loss of the capacity of cells to divide.

### C. Defects in Structure and Function

Several theories of aging are based on the view that while there may be no significant loss of cells, there is a widespread alteration of cell function, or accumulation of cellular defects that play important roles in overall aging of an animal. The most common experimental approach to this question has been to measure, in organs of animals of different ages, levels of enzymes or other proteins, amounts of some cellular component such as hormone receptors, rates of synthesis and turnover, or some aspect of translation or transcription. A majority of these studies cannot be interpreted adequately because of flaws in concept and design. During growth of an animal, most cellular processes operate at greater rates than when growth ceases. Rats and mice grow until at least 7 months of age, and mice do not attain physiological maturity in terms of maximal function until around 7 months of age.[32] However, there is an enormous number of reports in the aging literature in which 3- and 18-month old rats or mice are compared. It cannot be known if any age differences observed occur during growth or during aging. Any differences reported might not take place after 1 year of age.

A major conceptual problem with most studies of cell function is caused by the functions under study being labile, or homeostatically regulated. They are reversible or go up or down depending on diet, activity pattern, presence or absence of stress, and so on. Old animals are debilitated and diseased, and they eat less and sleep more than younger animals. It would not be surprising if, for example, one sampled liver of young and old animals for enzyme levels and found a difference. It has been implied in many reports of such studies that an altered level of something represents a primary, intrinsic, basing aging process.

By now, probably most enzymes and other intracellular components and organelles have been measured in a variety of tissues of animals of different ages. Findings have been summarized.[1,30] The overall conclusion would be that there is no general pattern; some substances go down with age, some go up, and some show no change. And where changes with age have been observed, it is not known if they are primary and irreversible.

A more useful approach has been to stimulate cells to produce something, hopefully at a maximum rate, and look for age differences in capacity to function. When enzyme levels in several rat tissues were depleted by nutritional deficiency, and rates of synthesis were determined on return to adequate diets, no significant age-related differences in rates of synthesis were apparent.[33] Tissues of rats of different ages have been induced to synthesize enzymes at maximum rates; synthesis of tyrosine aminotransferase in response to steroids, of glucokinase in response to glucose, and of NADH: cytochrome c reductase in response to phenobarbitol were ultimately at the same level in animals of different ages.[34,35] However, in some cases there was a lag period between administration of the inducer and synthesis of the enzyme that was clearly age-dependent. It is possible that in older animals there are lower steady-state levels of organelles and molecules required for the synthesis of inducible enzymes, and that simply more time is required initially to generate these components. Resting levels of testosterone are decreased with age in the rat. However, stimulation with human chorionic gonadotropin results in similar testosterone secretion by Leydig cells in old and young animals.[36]

The turnover rates of mitochondria[37] and of ribosomes[38] of a variety of organs were found not to differ significantly between adult and old rats. Thus, the complex reactions required for the synthesis and degradation of these organelles do not appear to be affected by age.

A popular cellular aging theory proposes that errors accumulate in the synthesis of proteins. A study comparing immature to old mice found that aldolase activity per immunoreactive unit of enzyme decreased with age in liver but not in muscle.[39,40] In other words, it decreased in an organ where the significance is doubtful, namely in liver which can generate new cells when required, but did not show a change in muscle, which does not regenerate and in which a change would be permanent and significant. Other studies with human salivary gland alpha amylase[41] and rat insulin[42] have not demonstrated any loss of activity per unit protein with age. Any molecules that might be found altered with age could have undergone denaturation, partial degradation, or aggregation with other molecules, and not have resulted only from errors in synthesis.

Some alterations in cellular ultrastructure with age have been reported; these have been reviewed.[1] The most striking change is the accumulation of the pigmented material, lipofuscin. Lipofuscin accumulates in many tissues, but most notably in fixed postmitotic cells such as cardiac muscle and neurones.[43,44] It is an insoluble, granular material that appears to consist of oxidatively polymerized unsaturated lipid plus variable amounts of other lipids, proteins, and enzymes. It is not known if lipofuscin accumulation is harmful to cells.

The enormous number of studies of cell function in animals of different ages has failed to demonstrate any generalized or marked decrease that is known to be intrinsic to the cells, that is irreversible, that coincides with overall aging of the animal, and that is capable of explaining any important aspect of the aging syndrome.

## IV. CONCLUSIONS

### A. Future of Cellular Aging

The reports cited here were selected to demonstrate certain lines of work in the relationships between cell properties and aging, and to show there is no proved extensive cell loss or irreversible change in cellular function that coincides with aging or that could explain major aspects of the aging syndrome. That is, evidence against cellular aging theories has been presented. Such evidence does not, of course, prove the nonexistence of important aging processes in cells, and it is certainly possible that such processes eventually will be discovered. Enough information is available, however, to indicate the types of studies that are likely to be useful and those that are probably not worth doing.

If questions are being asked about human aging, it would certainly be desirable to study human material. If this is not feasible, other mammals would probably be appropriate in many cases. There is little justification for the use of invertebrate or cell culture models in the study of mammalian aging. The part of the life span studied should extend from growth cessation out to old age. It is particularly important that one not draw conclusions from a comparison of young animals to old animals.

There is no evidence that new cells in organs of old animals differ from new cells in younger animals. Thus, there is no reason to study cells in organs that can generate new cells readily if one is looking for primary, intrinsic changes with age. Liver, epithelia, and bone marrow would be poor choices; it would make more sense to study skeletal and cardiac muscle and neurones.

There is little to be gained by the continual measurement, under resting conditions, of labile cell components such as enzymes, hormone receptors, or factors involved in protein synthesis. If one postulates a loss in capacity to synthesize such factors, they should be induced or caused to be synthesized at maximal rates. Studies should be undertaken of stable cell components such as macromolecules, membrane components, and intracellular aggregates such as lipofuscin in long-lived fixed postmitotic cells such as cardiac muscle and neurones. Also, searches for altered or defective molecules in such cells may be productive.

The most useful studies suggested here are difficult, and unlikely to yield elegant data in a hurry. However, many of the expedient models used in past studies have enabled investigators to generate clear and reproducible data that are of little value in understanding mechanisms of aging.

### B. What Causes Aging?

The manifestations of age in terms of debility, disease, and organ function are very striking, and certainly must be caused by something. One who lists all the factors that have not been shown to be responsible is obliged to present some more likely possibilities. As noted above, some cellular changes may be discovered to be important causes of aging. However, certain other tissue components have been shown to change very conspicuously during aging.

Extracellular macromolecules such as collagen and elastin comprise 40% or more of the total body protein, have many important functions, are relatively inert metabolically, and are highly polymerized; high polymers such as paint, rubber, and plastics become stiff and brittle with age. Collagen and elastin also become stiff and brittle with age. Changes in these substances with age, and possible consequences have been reviewed,[1] and it it has been argued that studies of extracellular macromolecules should have a high priority in research on aging.

## V. SUMMARY

A theory of aging, unless otherwise defined, would propose that certain normal, universal processes at the molecular, cellular, or tissue level cause the aging syndrome in all members of a human population in spite of the optimization of all genetic and environmental factors.

There is no significant generalized cell loss during aging that is capable of explaining the characteristic debilities and generalized physiological decline. No primary, intrinsic loss of capacity of stem cells to divide has been shown to occur during aging. No irreversible loss of function with age has been shown in dynamic cell populations. No primary, irreversible loss of capacity to synthesize enzymes with age has been demonstrated. Thus, available data do not support a cellular aging theory.

Important primary cellular aging processes may eventually be identified. These would most likely take place in stable components of long-lived fixed postmitotic cells such as muscle and neurones. Such processes, to play roles in aging, must progress after growth cessation and must be irreversible, rather than homeostatically controlled. Models such as invertebrate animals and cell cultures are of doubtful value.

Studies of the aging of extracellular macromolecules would be useful.

## REFERENCES


1. **Kohn, R. R.,** *Principles of Mammalian Aging,* 2nd ed., Prentice-Hall, Englewood Cliffs, N.J., 1978.
2. **Hirokawa, K. and Makinodan, T.,** Thymic involution: effect on T cell differentiation, *J. Immunol.,* 114, 1659, 1975.
3. **Baker, T. G.,** Gametogenesis, *Acta Endocrinol.,* 71 (suppl. 166), 18, 1972.
4. **Lesher, S.,** Chronic irradiation and ageing in mice and rats, in *Radiation and Ageing,* Lindop, P. J. and Sacher, G. A., Eds., Taylor & Francis Ltd., London, 1966, 183.
5. **Sharav, Y. and Massler, M.,** Age changes in oral epithelia. Progenitor population, synthesis index and tissue turnover, *Exp. Cell Res.,* 47, 132, 1967.
6. **Kaler, L. W. and Neaves, W. B.,** Attrition of the human Leydig cell population with advancing age, *Anat. Rec.,* 192, 513, 1978.
7. **Cameron, I. L.,** Cell proliferation and renewal in aging mice, *J. Gerontol.,* 27, 162, 1972.
8. **Tauchi, H., Yoshioka, T., and Kobayashi, H.,** Age change of skeletal muscles of rats, *Gerontologia,* 17, 219, 1971.
9. **Brody, H.,** Organization of the cerebral cortex. III. A study of aging in the human cerebral cortex, *J. Comp. Neurol.,* 102, 511, 1955.
10. **Brizzee, K. R., Sherwood, N., and Timiras, P. S.,** A comparison of cell populations at various depth levels in cerebral cortex of young adult and aged Long-Evans rats, *J. Gerontol.,* 23, 289, 1968.
11. **Vijayashankar, N. and Brody, H.,** Aging in the human brain stem: a study of the nucleus of the trochlear nerve, *Acta Anat.,* 99, 169, 1977.
12. **Johnson, H. A. and Erner, S.,** Neuron survival in the aging mouse, *Exp. Gerontol.,* 7, 111, 1972.
13. **Hall, T. C., Miller, A. K. H., and Corsellis, J. A. N.,** Variations in the human Purkinje cell population according to age and sex, *Neuropathol., Appl. Neurobiol.,* 1, 267, 1975.
14. **Hanley, T.,** 'Neuronal fall-out' in the ageing brain: a critical review of the quantitative data, *Age and Ageing,* 3, 133, 1974.
15. **Hayflick, L.,** The limited *in vitro* lifetime of human diploid cell strains, *Exp. Cell Res.,* 37, 614, 1965.
16. **Bucher, N. L. and Glinos, A. D.,** The effect of age on regeneration of rat liver, *Cancer Res.,* 10, 324, 1950.
17. **Grant, W. C. and LeGrande, M. C.,** The influence of age on erythropoiesis in the rat, *J. Gerontol.,* 19, 505, 1964.
18. **Suzuki, N. and Withers, H. R.,** Exponential decrease during aging and random lifetime of mouse spermatogonial stem cells, *Science,* 202, 1214, 1978.
19. **Harrison, D. E. and Doubleday, J. W.,** Normal function of immunologic stem cells from aged mice, *J. Immunol.,* 114, 1314, 1975.
20. **Harrison, D. E.,** Normal function of transplanted marrow cell lines from aged mice, *J. Gerontol.,* 30, 279, 1975.
21. **Franks, L. M.,** Cellular aspects of aging, *Exp. Gerontol.,* 5, 281, 1970.
22. **Krohn, P. L.,** Heterochronic transplantation in the study of ageing, *Proc. R. Soc. [Biol.],* 157, 128, 1962.
23. **Martin, G. M., Sprague, C. A., and Epstein, C. J.,** Replicative life-span of cultivated human cells, *Lab. Invest.,* 23, 86, 1970.
24. **Goldstein, S., Littlefield, J. W., and Soeldner, J. S.,** Diabetes mellitus and aging: Diminished plating efficiency of cultured human fibroblasts, *Proc. Natl. Acad. Sci. USA,* 64, 155, 1969.
25. **Goldstein, S., Moerman, E. J., Soeldner, J. S., Gleason, R. E., and Barnett, D. M.,** Chronologic and physiologic age affect replicative life-span of fibroblasts from diabetic, prediabetic, and normal donors, *Science,* 199, 781, 1978.

26. **Gleason, R. E. and Goldstein, S.,** Age affect and replicative life-span of fibroblasts of diabetic, prediabetic, and normal donors: another look at the data, *Science,* 202, 1217, 1978.
27. **Schneider, E. L. and Mitsui, Y.,** The relationship between *in vitro* cellular aging and *in vivo* human age, *Proc. Natl. Acad. Sci. USA,* 73, 3584, 1976.
28. **Rowe, D. W., Starman, B. J., Fujimoto, W. Y., and Williams, R. H.,** Abnormalities in proliferation and protein synthesis in skin fibroblast cultures from patients with diabetes mellitus, *Diabetes,* 26, 284, 1977.
29. **Stanley, J. F., Pye, D., and MacGregor, A.,** Comparison of doubling numbers attained by cultured animal cells with the life span of species, *Nature (London),* 255, 158, 1975.
30. **Finch, C. E. and Hayflick, L., Eds.,** *Handbook of the Biology of Aging,* Van Nostrand Reinhold, New York, 1977.
31. **Martin, G. M.,** Cellular aging — clonal senescence, *Am. J. Pathol.,* 89, 484, 1977.
32. **Hensley, J. C., McWilliams, P. C., and Oakley, G. E.,** Physiological capacitance: a study in physiological age determination, *J. Gerontol.,* 19, 317, 1964.
33. **Barrows, C. H., Jr. and Roeder, L. M.,** Effect of age on protein synthesis in rats, *J. Gerontol.,* 16, 321, 1961.
34. **Adelman, R. C.,** Age-dependent effects in enzyme induction — a biochemical expression of aging, *Exp. Gerontol.,* 6, 75, 1971.
35. **Adelman, R. C. and Freeman, C.,** Age-dependent regulation of glucokinase and tyrosine aminotransferase activities of rat liver *in vivo* by adrenal, pancreatic and pituitary hormones, *Endocrinology,* 90, 1551, 1972.
36. **Harman, S. M., Danner, R. L., and Roth, G. S.,** Testosterone secretion in the rat in response to chorionic gonadotrophin: alterations with age, *Endocrinology,* 102, 540, 1978.
37. **Menzies, R. A. and Gold, P. H.,** The turnover of mitochondria in a variety of tissues of young adult and aged rats, *J. Biol. Chem.,* 246, 2425, 1971.
38. **Menzies, R. A., Mishra, R. K., and Gold, P. H.,** The turnover of ribosomes and soluble RNA in a variety of tissues of young adult and aged rats, *Mech. Ageing Dev.,* 1, 117, 1972.
39. **Gershon, H. and Gershon, D.,** Inactive enzyme molecules in aging mice: liver aldolase, *Proc. Natl. Acad. Sci. USA,* 70, 909, 1973.
40. **Gershon, H. and Gershon, D.,** Altered enzyme molecules in senescent organisms; mouse muscle aldolase, *Mech. Ageing Dev.,* 2, 33, 1973.
41. **Helfman, P. M. and Price, P. A.,** Human parotid $\alpha$-amylase — a test of the error theory of aging, *Exp. Gerontol.,* 9, 209, 1974.
42. **Adelman, R. C.,** Impaired hormonal regulation of enzyme activity during aging, *Fed. Proc. Fed. Am. Soc. Exp. Biol.,* 34, 179, 1975.
43. **Strehler, B. L.,** On the histochemistry and ultrastructure of age pigment, *Adv. Gerontol. Res.,* 1, 343, 1964.
44. **Munnell, J. F. and Getty, R.,** Rate of accumulation of cardiac lipofuscin in the aging canine, *J. Gerontol.,* 23, 154, 1968.

Chapter 8

# AUTOIMMUNITY AND AGING

**Susan R. S. Gottesman and Roy L. Walford**

## TABLE OF CONTENTS

## I. INTRODUCTION

The immune system functions in maintaining the homeostasis of the body against external and internal disturbances. With age an imbalance in homeostasis and an increase in autoimmunity occurs in mammals.

Three processes and their interrelationships will be stressed in this review: first, the normal development and maturation of the immune system particularly as it controls for autoreactive clones; second, the decline with aging in the system's response to exogenous challenges; and third, the development of autoimmunity in both short-lived autoimmune susceptible mouse strains and humans, and in normal elderly members of the species. Emphasis will be placed on the functioning of the thymus-derived cells of the immune system since they serve important regulatory roles. Autoimmune aspects of the diseases of aging have been extensively reviewed elsewhere.[1,2] Autoimmunity plays a role in many of the diseases seen in the elderly and it is therefore important to study autoimmune diseases from a gerontological view. Deregulation of self/nonself discrimination might also be a primary mechanism in the pathogenesis of the basic aging process.[1]

## II. THE IMMUNE SYSTEM

The early theory that the B cell is responsible for humoral immunity while the T cell functions in cell mediated responses is no longer tenable. A complex network of interrelationships exists which has not yet been fully defined. Because of this, assays of the immune system may yield results whose underlying mechanisms are still unclear.

### A. Ontogeny

The yolk sac, and then the fetal liver are the first sites of development of hemopoietic stem cells.[3] Towards the end of gestation the bone marrow and spleen assume this function. The stem cell pool contains precursors for hemopoietic and lymphoid cell lines.[4]

Mature B cells are predominantly spleen-seeking and stationary whereas many T cells are long-lived, recirculating, and node-seeking.[5] T cells mature in the thymus; B cells in the bursa of Fabricius in chickens.[6] An analogous structure in mice and humans has not been found, and B cell maturation is probably distributed among various lymphoid tissues. Maturation of B and T cells is followed by sequential appearance of cell surface markers.

### B. Lymphoid Subpopulations and Surface Markers

#### *1. B Cells*

Surface immunoglobulin is the most distinctive feature of B cells and is often used as a tool to separate them from a mixed population.[7] Later in differentiation many B cells display surface Fc and complement receptors and Ia surface antigens.[7] The neonatal animal acquires first the ability to respond to T independent antigens and then T dependent antigens.[8] Ease of tolerance induction changes in a parallel manner.[8]

The surface markers are not exclusively on B cells, and not on all B cells. Rosette formation with erythrocytes coated with antibody and complement (EAC), followed by density gradient centrifugation and lysis of red cells, isolates cells bearing complement receptors.[7] Antibody coated erythrocytes (EA) are used in a similar manner to detect Fc receptor bearing cells. Fluorescent antibodies are used to enumerate Fc receptor and surface Ig bearing cells. Assays detecting Ig bearing cells may sometimes react with Fc receptors as well. Although the two populations overlap, Fc receptors are also present on some T cells.[9]

#### *2. Thymus-Derived Cells*

In mice the thymus appears midway in gestation and becomes infiltrated with lymphocytes by 12 to 14 days.[10] Immature incompetent T cells occupy the cortex, express thymus leukemia (TL) surface antigen, and are cortisone and radiation sensitive.[11,12] The mature cells of the medulla are TL-,Thy-1 +, relatively cortisone and radiation resistant, and capable of immunological activity.[11] The Thy-1 marker is also found on peripheral T cells and nonlymphoid tissue such as brain and skin.[13] Antisera to Thy-1 plus complement is used to eliminate T cells from a mixed population, and fluorescent labeled anti-Thy-1 is used to enumerate them.

Thymic epithelial cells produce thymic hormones, which influence T cell differentiation.[14] The hormones are assayed in vitro by incubation with immature T cells, resulting in the appearance of surface markers but not functional capacity.[15] To demonstrate hormonal activity in vivo thymic tissue is transplanted in diffusion chambers or thymic extract is injected into thymectomized or genetically athymic (nude) hosts.[16] Contamination of preparations with endotoxin or ubiquitin, which effect the immune system, complicate these experiments.[16] It is unclear where and how these hormone products exert their influence normally.

T cells, not fully competent when exported from the thymus,[17] differentiate peripherally into specific helper, cytotoxic, suppressor, or memory cells. These are distinguishable by different Lyt surface markers[18,19] (Table 1). In adult mouse spleens, the Thy-1 + cells are 50% Lyt-123 +, 33% Lyt-1 +, and 6 to 8% Lyt-23 +. Lyt-123 + cells are the first peripheral Thy-1 + cells to appear in ontogeny and decline rapidly after adult thymectomy. Lyt-1 + and Lyt-23 + cells appear later and are resistent to the early effects of adult thymectomy.[18]

**Table 1**
**TWO SYSTEMS OF CLASSIFICATION OF T CELL SUBPOPULATIONS**

| Symbol | Functions | Location | Life span | Thy-1 expression | Ly[a] phenotype | Ia | FcR[b] | ALS |
|---|---|---|---|---|---|---|---|---|
| $T_1$ | Amplifier<br><br>Suppressor | Lymph<br>Thymus | Short | High | Ly123 | + | ? | resist |
| $T_2$ | Helper<br>Cytotoxic<br>Suppressor | Lymph nodes<br>Spleen | Long | Low | Ly1<br>Ly23 | + | + | suscept. |
| Ly123 | Precursor<br>Amplifier<br>Suppressor | Thymus<br>Spleen | Short | Higher | | | | |
| Ly1 | Helper-B<br>Helper-CTL<br>MLC responder | Periphery | Long | Low | | | −<br>+<br>+/−[c] | |
| Ly23 | Cytotoxic<br>Suppressor | Periphery | Long | Low | | I-J | | |

[a] Assignment of Ly phenotypes to $T_1/T_2$ groups is approximate. There is not an absolute identity of the subpoplulations.
[b] Expression of surface receptor for Fc.
[c] The Fc receptor is expressed on only a subgroup of the MLC responder cells.

Negative selection experiments have shown helper cells to be Lyt-1 + and cells cytotoxic for allogeneic targets to be Lyt-23 + .[20] Lyt-1 + cells also amplify Lyt-23 + cell function.[21] Lyt-1 + cells respond to I region determinants and Lyt-23 + cells to K/D determinants of the major histocompatibility complex of the mouse[21] (H-2) (Figure 1) (Section II.C). Suppressor cells are Lyt-23 + and, in some cases, Lyt-123 + .[22,23]

The immune associated (Ia) antigens, products of the I region of the mouse H-2 system, are serologically detectable on B cells[24] with lower concentrations found on macrophages, sperm, epidermal cells,[25] and a T cell subpopulation.[26] Products of different subregions of I are expressed on cells with different functions. T cell subpopulations are therefore identified by expression of different Lyt antigens and I subregion products in addition to differential sensitivity to irradiation and drug treatment.[5]

A sequence of glass wool followed by nylon wool columns can be used to enrich for different mouse cells.[27] Macrophages and dead cells stick to glass wool, B cells adhere to nylon wool, and T cells pass through both. Purity is usually checked with antibody to surface markers.

$T_1$-$T_2$ is an older classification system of T subpopulations. $T_1$ cells are defined as being short-lived (based on life span after adult thymectomy), resistant to antilymphocyte serum (ALS), rich in Thy-1 antigen, and relatively abundant in the spleen.[28] $T_2$ are long-lived, sensitive to ALS, poor in Thy-1, and abundant in lymph nodes and peripheral blood.[28] Some Lyt-123 + cells correspond to $T_1$ while the $T_2$ population contains cells which are Lyt-1 + and Lyt-23 + (Table 1)[5]; however, these assignments are not clear-cut.

Human T cells can be separated from other mononuclear cells by forming rosettes with sheep erythrocytes (E rosettes).[29] Subpopulations are in the process of being defined by means of specific antisera.[30]

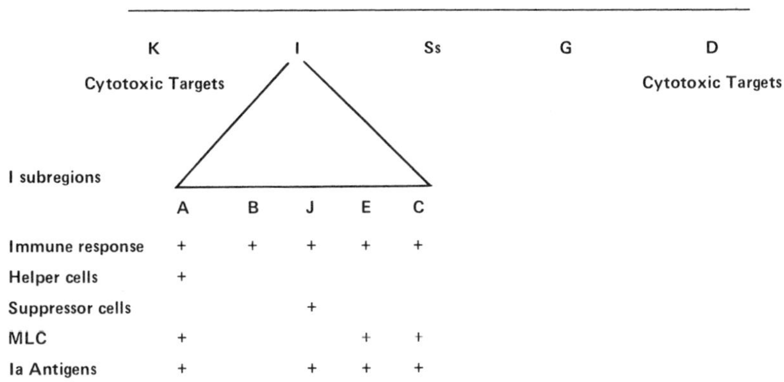


FIGURE 1. Map of mouse major histocompatibility complex (H-2) and the immune functions controlled for by each region.

### *3. Macrophages*

Phagocytic cells found in primitive invertebrates represent the beginnings of the development of immune defenses.[31] In higher vertebrates, macrophages retain their function as scavengers but are also required for antibody formation in vitro.[32] They were first believed to function in presenting the antigen by lining up determinants on their surfaces and forming a sort of bridge between helper T and antibody producing B cells.[32] A requirement for histocompatibility among the three interacting cells demonstrated a degree of specificity in the macrophage (Section II.D). Macrophage subpopulations may also be activated to perform nonspecific cytotoxic and suppressive functions.

Macrophages are characterized by their adherence properties, surface markers, phagocytic properties, and sensitivity to carregeenan. They stick firmly to plastic surfaces and G10 or glass wool columns,[27] and express Ia antigens and Fc receptors.[25] Uptake of iron filings and separation by magnets, or uptake of latex beads followed by density separation is used to enrich for them. Carregeenan is a chemical toxic to macrophages and is often used in in vivo studies.[33]

## C. The Main Histocompatibility Complex

The main histocompatibility complex (MHC) codes for surface glycoproteins which govern rejection of grafts from genetically nonidentical donors.[5] MHCs have been described in a large number of species (HLA in humans, H-2 in mice). It is the most highly polymorphic system known in mammals. Minor histocompatibility gene systems have also been defined, particularly in mice.

A current map of the mouse H-2 gene is shown in Figure 1. The K and D region determine strong transplantation antigens. The cell mediated cytotoxicity reaction in vitro and graft and tumor rejection in vivo are used to measure response to these determinants (Section II.E).[34] Response (antibody production) to certain antigens is genetically controlled by the I region of H-2.[35] The I region is divided into subregions which govern helper (A and C) or suppressor (J) functions. It is involved in genetic control not only of the level of antibody response but also of many aspects of cell-cell interactions, possibly by means of soluble factors.[36] It codes for structures stimulating mixed lymphocyte culture (MLC) and graft-vs.-host (GVH) reactions (Section II.E) and for the serologically defined Ia antigens[37] (Section II.B). The Ss and G regions govern levels of complement components and other serum proteins.

Associations have been uncovered between the MHC and disease susceptibility, including malignancies, autoimmune and inflammatory diseases.[2] In humans, the association with autoimmune diseases is particularly strong. In mice, several genes controlling resistance to oncogenic viruses (i.e., Gross leukemia virus) are linked to H-2.[38]

Susceptibility to spontaneous late-life occurring cancers is strongly linked to the H-2 system in mice.[39] Strains have been specifically bred for spontaneous autoimmune disease, and some controlling genes are closely linked to H-2.[40] The H-2 system may also influence the rate of decline of immune response capacity and maximum life span.[39] Studies are in progress to demonstrate a link between specific HLA antigens and human life span.

## D. Assays of Humoral Immunity

### *1. In Vitro Assays*

#### *a. Plaque-Forming Cell (PFC) Assay*

Humoral immune function may be measured in terms of antibody production in the PFC assay after in vivo or in vitro sensitization.[41] In in vitro stimulation, responding cells (i.e. splenocytes) are incubated with antigen for several days. The sensitizing antigen is usually then used to coat the surface of sheep erythrocytes (SRBC) — the indicator cell. A lawn of modified SRBC is placed in agarose in small dishes and dilutions of responder cells and then complement are added.[41] The antibody produced will diffuse out and, with the complement, form an area of lysis or clear plaque around each responder cell. Plaques of individual cells can be counted, reflecting the concentration of responder cells.[41]

Sensitization and T dependent antibody production are dependent on B cells, T cells, and macrophages.[32] T independent antigens, i.e., DNP-Ficoll and SIII, do not require T helper cell function but, in the case of SIII, are regulated by T suppressor cells.[42]

#### *b. Mitogen Induced Antibody Production*

*E. coli* lipopolysaccharide (LPS), a B cell mitogen, directly stimulates antibody production by B cells.[43] This polyclonal activation by LPS does not directly correlate with its properties as mitogen.

### *2. In Vivo Methods*

#### *a. Cell Transfer Technique*

In transfer experiments cell suspensions are injected into syngeneic irradiated (sometimes thymectomized) recipients.[44] Irradiation knocks out the recipient's own lymphoid system so that the activity of sensitized transferred lymphoid cells can be assessed independently. Spleen cells or bone marrow (with thymocytes if thymectomized hosts) are transferred and antigen is given with the cells, or at a specified time later. Stem cells (colony-forming units — CFU) colonizing the spleen are quantified from the number of splenic nodules, each being the product of a single stem cell.[45]

The response depends upon the trafficking and colonizing ability of the donor cells, and is also influenced by the host environment. The assay must be conducted before recovery of the recipient's own cells. The rate of recovery is partially defined by the treatment the host received before cell transfer. Advantages of the cell transfer technique include separate manipulation of the cellular and environmental conditions (i.e., with respect to age of each component) and of the different cell types.

Through limiting dilutions of the different cell types and variations on the assays, one can arrive at estimates for:[46] immunocompetent units (I.U.) per tissue (I.U. is the minimum number of cells required for response); immunologic burst size (IBS) (number of effectors generated per I.U.); antigen doses required for response; and affinity of the antibody.

#### *b. Serum Antibody Levels*

The PFC assay measures the number of antibody forming cells, whereas serum antibody levels reflect the actual amount of circulating antibody. Titers are determined by hemagglutination or hemolysin assays and concentrations of antibody or antigen are varied until a maximum response is obtained.[47] The assays are subject to variations based on antibody affinity and other conditions. Antigen-antibody complexes may form and dissociate. The radioimmunoassay (RIA) on a solid support is less affected by antibody affinity or formation of complexes.[47]

### F. Assays of Cellular Immune Function

#### *1. In Vitro Assays*

#### *a. Mixed Lymphocyte Cultures*

In the MLC assay two incompatible lymphoid populations are co-cultured, the stimulator population having been inactivated with irradiation or mitomycin C. Degree of response by the responder cells is based upon the strength of the histocompatibility differences between the two populations.[48] The response is usually quantitated by measuring uptake of tritiated thymidine. The MLC measures T proliferative response and allows the differentiation of other T cells into cytotoxic effector cells directed against K/D region determinants.[48] The proliferating cell is part of the $T_2$ subpopulation, expresses Lyt-1 antigen,[19] and responds preferentially to I region differences.[49] It is defined as a helper cell which stimulates the generation of cytotoxic T cells,[50] B cell antibody responses and possibly suppressor cells.[5] There may be different helper populations, as the existence of the Fc receptor on only a portion of helper T cells suggests.[51]

#### *b. Cell Mediated Lympholysis (CML)*

The cytotoxic T cell (CTL), which can be generated in vitro in the MLC or in vivo by injection of incompatible cells, is commonly assayed by a chromium release assay.[48] $Cr^{51}$-labeled tumor cell targets or mitogen stimulated lymphoblasts of the same MHC type as the sensitizing cell population are co-cultured with the sensitized responder cells for several hours. The amount of chromium released reflects the amount of lysis.

The CTL is generally a Lyt-23+ $T_2$ cell[19] and responds preferentially to K/D differences.[52] However, I region disparate, K/D identical cells can stimulate cytotoxic effectors specific for I region differences[53] and vice versa.[34] In addition, amplifier and suppressor cells function in CML assays.[54,55] Thymocytes, which do not themselves respond in the MLC, can synergize with lymph node and spleen cells.[54] The amplifiers reside in the $T_1$ subpopulations and are probably Lyt-123+.

Suppressor cells are generated during the course of most immune responses;[56] many (i.e., those maintaining induced tolerance in vivo) are $T_2$, Lyt-23+, I-J+ cells.[57] In addition, a group of Lyt-123+ nonspecific suppressor cells exists.[23] The suppressor cell detected depends on the assay and the conditions used to generate it.[58]

The MLC is dependent on T cells and macrophages,[59] its magnitude being determined by the antigenic differences (I region the most effective) and the relative proportions of amplifier, helper, and suppressor T cells.[5] Although the CTLs generated in the MLC are helped by the proliferating T cells, the efficiency of the CTLs is not proportional to the magnitude of proliferation in the MLC.[34] The magnitude of each response can be varied independently.

#### *c. Mitogen Assays*

The mitogen LPS stimulates B cells, concanavalin A (Con A) and phytohemagglutinin (PHA) stimulate T cells, and pokeweed mitogen (PWM) stimulates subpopulations of both [60,61] to proliferate.

Con A may preferentially stimulate the more immature $T_1$ population whereas PHA stimulates both $T_1$ and $T_2$ (Lyt-1+, Lyt-23+, and Lyt-123+).[62] The stimulatory ratio PHA/Con A may reflect the overall maturity of the population. How these mitogen assays relate to the cells responding in the more functional assays (i.e., MLC, antibody help, GVH) is still a matter of speculation.[58,63] In addition to stimulating proliferation and nonspecific helper function, varying the mitogen assay conditions can result in the generation of nonspecific suppressor and cytotoxic cells.[64] Con A induces suppressor cells in mouse and human cell populations.

*2. In Vivo Assays*

***a. Graft Vs. Host Reaction***

In vivo assays are not clearly defined in terms of the cell types operating. GVH is considered the in vivo correlate of the MLC. Lymphoid cells are injected into an incompatible, immunologically inert host; for example, parental cells into an $F_1$ hybrid animal.[65] Spleen or regional lymph node weight measured some days later is taken as an indication of the GVH reactivity.[65] Synergy between donor T subpopulations, similar to that seen in the MLC, has been found in the GVH reaction.[66] Splenomegaly is due to the proliferation of both donor and host lymphocytes, and the accumulation of host cells.[67] Injection of large numbers of immunocompetent cells into a neonatal or immunosuppressed host may lead to runting disease and death.[65] Chronic GVH disease has been proposed as a model of accelerated aging.[1] It shows many features characteristic of age and autoimmune disease.

***b. Delayed Type Hypersensitivity (DTH)***

DTH is manifest as a local cell infiltrate in response to antigen application.[68] Induction of DTH is considered similar to the blastogenesis seen in the MLC assay.[69] The sensitizing moiety may actually be a complex of antigen and self-components.[70] The reaction is due to the release of large quantities of lymphokines, resulting in the attraction of a variety of cells to the site.[70]

***c. Graft Rejection***

Allogeneic graft rejection is due to CTLs whose activity is against K/D differences.[71] Skin graft rejection can, however, occur across I region differences. Skin grafts or a combination of skin grafts and tumor cell injection may be used as in vivo sensitization prior to in vitro cytotoxic assays. With weak histocompatibility differences, several sensitizations are necessary before cytotoxicity can be detected in vitro.[53]

Allogeneic tumor challenge is similar in principle to the allogeneic MLC-CML; however, syngeneic tumor challenge may be more physiologically significant. The animal's competence is measured in terms of the tumor dose required for lethality. Cytotoxic cells in these cases are not just T cells but may be armed or angry macrophages, natural killer cells, or antibody dependent cytotoxic cells (ADCC).[72] Often the cytotoxic cell type detected in in vitro culture depends on the culture conditions.

Slight differences in the conditions used in assays of humoral and cellular immune function lead to great variations in results.[73] Often no clear answers are obtained when attempts are made to identify the subpopulations responding. The system appears to function as a whole — with its parts intertwined (subpopulations) and dependent on each other. Immunoregulatory circuits may exist among T subpopulations.[74] The introduction of antigen disturbs the system and homeostasis is restored by signals generated from within the immune system itself. It is therefore almost impossible to separate the components responding. One is seeing the end results — the reestablishment of homeostasis.

## III. DIFFERENTIATION AND EDUCATION OF T CELLS AND CONTROL OF AUTOIMMUNITY

The education of T cells and the elimination or control of autoreactive clones are interrelated and begin early in the development of the mouse, principally in the thymus. In the thymus, most of the cells are immature[11,12] but a small population of immunocompetent T cells resides in the medulla. It was once hypothesized that immature cortical cells migrate into and mature in the medulla, and are then exported. Evidence indicates, however, that the immunocompetent cells are permanent residents, never exported.[75]

Another striking feature of the thymic residence is the large amount of intrathymic death of cells. Thymocytes proliferate profusely but comparatively small numbers are exported, the majority dying within the organ.[12]

Important questions about the immune system concern the mechanisms behind (1) the elimination of autoreactive cells, (2) the diversity of the response of the cellular immune system, and (3) the presence of an inordinately large number of alloreactive cells. A high frequency of T cells in the total population of an individual are reactive against cells different from that individual at the MHC (alloreactive).

Burnet[76] hypothesized that extensive intrathymic proliferation provided for the generation of diversity, while intrathymic death was due to elimination of autoreactive cells. Jerne[77] refined this concept by proposing that T cell reactivity was first directed only against the MHC specificities of the species. In the thymus, alloreactive T cells would be left alone, while autoreactive cells would be stimulated to proliferate by the self-H-2 antigens of the thymus. As proliferation continued, mutations would accumulate and these would be selected for until little or no reactivity against self remained.

Observations on peripheral control of autoimmunity have concerned tolerance induction. Tolerance induced during the neonatal period is specific and long-lasting.[78] During this period autoreactive clones are supposedly being eliminated or turned off. The introduction of a foreign alloantigen at this time results in its being treated as a self-antigen.

Tolerance in the adult is more difficult to achieve and more easily terminated. Low dose tolerance is a property of T cells alone, whereas in high dose paralysis both T and B cells are turned off.[79] Suppressor T cells have been detected after tolerance induction in both neonates and adults.[78] Their presence threw open the question of clonal deletion vs. active suppression in controlling autoimmunity.

Zinkernagel and Doherty[80,81] showed that T cell killing of virus infected cells required simultaneous recognition of virus and K or D region antigens on the target cells. This requirement held for cytotoxicity to minor histocompatibility antigens[82] and to hapten modified targets.[83] I region compatibility is required for effective interactions between T cells, macrophages, and B cells in antibody production.[84] It is not yet clear whether the requirement for histocompatibility (H-2 restriction) is inborn or learned, or whether it may be altered. In the chimeric mouse model, a thymectomized, lethally irradiated host is restored with thymus and bone marrow grafts. The specificity of the effector cells generated reflects the education of the cells,[82] however, there are questions concerning the physiological validity of this model.[85] In the unmanipulated animal infected with virus, viral antigens are seen in the context of its own histocompatibility antigens and therefore a certain degree of autorecognition and autoreactivity must be part of the immune system. Autoreactivity has also been detected in the humoral immune system (anti-antibodies).

One possibility adduced to explain the appearance of H-2 restriction was that intense alloreactivity masked response to the viral or other antigens introduced, but evidence showed that mere tolerance to histocompatibility antigens does not uncover viral reactivity.[86] A second possibility was that specifity for histocompatibility antigens was determined at the time of priming, according to the context in which the antigen was first seen.[86] Evidence exists that T cell education and restriction of response begins at least as early as the thymic residence. Restriction or preference may occur in the thymus.[87] Prothymocytes may already be partially restricted[86] and further restriction and fine tuning probably occurs in the periphery after thymic education.[85]

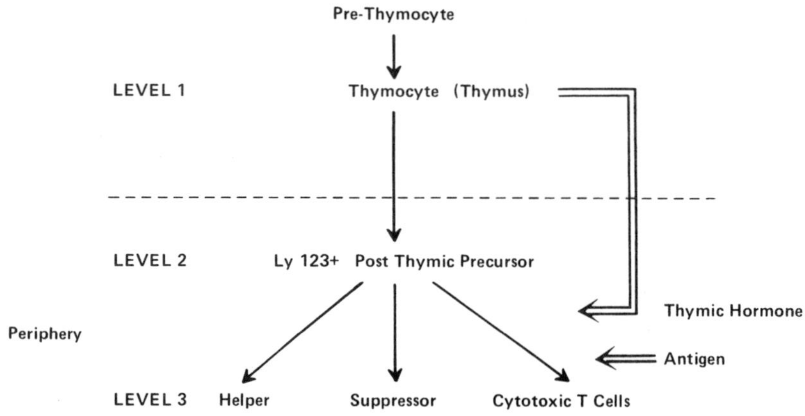


FIGURE 2. Flow chart of the trafficking and maturation pattern of T cells in the mouse. Double arrows indicate influences on T cell maturation.

Figure 2 depicts the traffic pattern of the T cell. Educational processing may parallel this pattern with successive maturation stages, rather than just the thymus, representing another level in T cell education. Fine tuning and sieving out of unwanted reactivity may occur at each stage. In the thymus, deleterious autoreactive cells may be eliminated, inactivated, or in some way controlled. Remaining reactive cells may be educated to react to modified self-antigens present in the thymus ("modified self-antigens" is not used here to distinguish between the modified self or dual recognition hypotheses, but rather to denote antigens recognized in the context of self determinants). The cells exported from the thymus would thus be depleted of the specifically autoreactive cells but not yet be fully competent.[17] In the periphery, a fine tuning process may occur with respect to recognition and a final maturation process will take place, resulting in immunocompetent cells. The first may be influenced by determinants on peripheral epithelial structures in lymphoid organs. The latter may be partially controlled by thymic hormones and antigenic stimulation.[17] Mature T cells then develop (level 3) which express helper, suppressor, and cytotoxic functions. Each level is subjected to regulatory mechanisms. In level 3 suppressor T cells regulate helper and cytotoxic cells (and possibly B cells directly). With further investigation more immunoregulatory circuits and feedback loops have been discovered.[74] These probably exist at each stage (Figure 2). On one hand, they make the system more difficult to study. On the other hand, they allow for reactivity against foreign substances, reactivity against foreign substances that alter membrane determinants, and reactivity against other systems of the body to help maintain homeostasis.

In the above model neonatal tolerance probably fits into level 2. In the neonate, level 3 is not fully developed. At level 2, cross-reactive autoimmune cells are being subjected to further control and the introduction of a large dose of antigen at this stage might well result in paralysis of the system, perhaps with the development of suppressor T cells.

Each maturational stage has its own population of autoreactive T cells, which are subjected to control at that level. It can be predicted that the autoreactive cells existing at the later levels should represent a more cross-reactive population, since the specific deleterious cells would have been eliminated. This model may be used to account for the decline in normal immune response capacity with aging and the concomitant increase in autoimmunity.

# IV. AGING OF THE IMMUNE SYSTEM

## A. Technical Approaches

The most reliable way of approaching aging research is to generate first a life span analysis, then a full maturation curve of the response being studied. Subjects used as the aged population should be in the senescent phase of life while the young controls should be at or slightly beyond the peak of the response.[88] These data are often missing from published experiments, and are noticeably absent from the research on the short-lived autoimmune strains (Section V). This may lead to erroneous interpretations: i.e., when a 15-month-old mouse (with a 32-month life span) is used as "aged" and a 6 to 8-week-old mouse used as the control (most responses peak at about 6 months).[89] Genetic influences play an important role in maturation patterns[89] and generalizing results from one strain to another may not be valid. A conspicuous feature of aging is the tremendous increase in variability, so that pooling cells from several animals may mask changes in the individuals.[46]

## B. Gross Quantitative Changes

### *1. Thymus*

Thymic involution begins at puberty and progresses with advancing age.[90,91] Since many of the immune functions which decline with age are dependent on T cells,[91] it has been suggested that the thymus contains an internal clock for aging of the immune system.[92] However, as thymic function is associated with the hypothalamus-pituitary circuit, the location of such an aging clock might also be in the nervous system. The thymus may influence aging of the immune system but since it appears late in phylogeny its involution cannot be regarded as a general primary cause of aging.

Because a large time gap exists between thymic involution and immune decline, the involuting thymus has been studied to determine what functional capacities it retains. Involution is primarily due to atrophy of the cortical region[90] containing the immature thymocytes. The epithelial cells, presumptive producers of thymus hormones,[14] retain their integrity until a much later age and may be responsible for continued thymus function.

Hirokawa and Makinodan[93] gave young bone marrow and 1 day to 33-month-old thymus grafts to young, thymectomized, irradiated mice, and followed the emergence and functioning of host T cells. With increasing donor age, the grafted thymic tissue lost its capacity to regenerate T cell functions in the following order: restoration of T cell dependent areas of lymph nodes (only newborn grafts would do this); spleen reactivity to PHA and Con A; splenic Thy-1 + cell numbers and splenic T dependent humoral response (SRBC as antigen); and splenic MLC function. Involuted 33-month-old grafts retained some but not total restorative capacity. Partial restoration was observed if a longer time was allowed after grafting. The maximum time waited was 12 weeks.

Stutman et al.[94] exposed neonatally thymectomized mice to thymic grafts for limited periods of time and tested for retention of T cell function. Functional decline in restored animals was more severe than natural decline in intact animals of the same age, therefore it appeared that thymic function was required for a longer time period. T dependent functions did not all decline at the same rate; splenic PHA response being retained longest.

Some functional capacity of the thymus appears to be necessary until fairly late in life.[95] Different subpopulations and therefore, different functions of peripheral T cells display a differential dependency on thymic influence[18] (Section II.B). A pattern reflective of this dependency may emerge in the aging animal whose thymic functions are diminishing. In short-lived autoimmune strains, thymic function declines very early and may follow a different pattern.[96]

In humans, thymic hormonal function, as assayed in vitro, is detectable through age 40,[97] perhaps 60.[98] Sensitivity of assays differ but all detect "hormone" activity well after thymic involution has begun. Epithelial cell remnants in the involuted thymus may still be capable of producing hormone,[99] accounting for the restorative activity seen in 33-month-old thymic grafts in mice.[93] The factors may act on a post-thymic precursor population in the periphery (Section II.B).[100] This population is not self-replicating, hence transplantation of old grafts must take place within a few months after thymectomy to be effective.

Thymic function may therefore be divided into two parts, each declining at a different rate. The thymus provides the site for maturation and education of pre-T stem cells from the bone marrow and may be where T cells learn to distinguish between self and nonself[87] (Section III). Morphologic changes are compatible with the idea that this function declines early, which would have important consequences on the ability of T cells in older animals to distinguish between self and nonself. The production of thymic hormones acting locally and systemically to push the final maturation of T cells may decline much later. Therefore, transplantation experiments must be analyzed with respect to the age of the thymus grafts, the age of the recipients, and the possible relationships between the graft's and host's pre- and post-thymic precursor populations.

*2. Cellular Changes*

The peripheral lymphocyte count in humans and rodents does not change with age, but proportions of subpopulations may be altered. T cells have been reported to decrease or show no detectable change.[89,101-103] In mice, the proportion of Thy-1 + cells in the spleen and peripheral blood is used to represent total T cells.[104] In humans, most assays measure peripheral blood E rosette formation.[105] However, not all human T cells form E rosettes[29,105] and not all mouse T cells express the same quantity of Thy-1.[28,106] Some reports show a decrease in the amount of Thy-1 per cell in old mice.[104,106] Additionally, most studies showing a decline in T cells have noted a concomitant rise in null cells[104,106] (i.e., cells with no distinguishing surface antigens). This may actually be an increase in T cells with surface antigen representation below the level of detection of the assay[106] (Section II.B). Long-lived $T_2$ cells are relatively poor in Thy-1 antigen expression[28] and an increase in the proportion of $T_2$ to $T_1$ cells might account for the above results,[106] although evidence from functional assays does not support this possibility (Section IV.F).[107] Quantitation of Ly subpopulations has not been done with mice older than 1 year of age.[108] In humans, subpopulations of T cells forming E rosettes under specified conditions have been reported to decline; however these have not yet been correlated with functional changes.[109]

B cells are quantified as surface Ig + cells using fluorescent label,[110] and generally show maintenance of constant levels with age. Haaijman et al.[111] quantified cells with cytoplasmic Ig and found a shift from splenic to bone marrow predominance with age. Woda et al.[112] have detected decreased representation of surface markers and diminished capping kinetics for old vs. young rat B cells.

A longitudinal study in humans[103] covering a 10-year period detected no changes in the total lymphoid population, percentage of rosetting T cells, or Ig + B cells.

In summary, there may be small changes in proportions of T subpopulations with age, but the alterations in functional capacity are too great to be accounted for solely on the basis of these subtle changes in cell numbers.

*3. Serum Immunoglobulin*

After adult levels of immunoglobulin are reached in mice there is not much further age-associated change.[113] In humans, serum IgA and IgG may increase while IgM levels remain constant. The overall level of serum immunoglobulins probably does not change with age,[103] although the incidence of autoantibodies increases.[1] Dramatic changes in antibody response are not reflected in total serum immunoglobulin levels.

### C. Stem Cell Competence

The Hayflick phenomenon[114] refers to the fact that normal diploid fibroblasts in culture have a finite life span with a limited doubling capacity, which reflects the age of the donor. Can analogous phenomena of "programed senescence" be found in the stem cell population? Although the bone marrow stem cell concentration decreases with age, the total cellularity increases so that the size of the stem cell pool is unaltered.[115]

The ability of serially transplanted bone marrow cells to repopulate the hemopoietic and lymphopoietic components of lethally irradiated mice declined after five transfers, and was eventually exhausted.[116] However, their ability was intact well past the normal life span of the original donor. Interpretation of such experiments can be difficult. Where donor and recipients are genetically identical, it may not be possible to distinguish donor cell progeny from recovered host cells.[117] Final exhaustion of the stem cells may have been due to stress of repeated transplantation,[116] decreasing ability to home to the spleen (the organ assayed for CFUs),[118] artificial selection of cells transferred resulting in a shift in progeny cells (erythrocytes vs. granulocytes vs. megakaryocytes),[119] or a Hayflick-like phenomenon.[114] The first possibility was considered the most likely. Evidence does exist, however, of altered kinetics of spleen colony formation using old donors[120] and a decreased ability for old spleens to host donated CFUs. The ability to produce red blood cells in genetically anemic mice began to fail after the same number of transfers of young or old bone marrow.[121]

In another set of experiments, bone marrow or spleen was transferred to young irradiated recipients and their ability to restore the SRBC antibody response measured. Makinodan's group[122,123] found that, when assayed a short time after transfer, splenocytes from old mice were less capable than cells from young mice at restoring immune functions. The recipients' capacities recovered after a longer waiting period but the contribution of host vs. donor cells was not distinguished. Using histocompatible but chromosomally distinguishable (T6 marker) donors and recipients, Harrison et al.[124] waited at least 6 months before testing for SRBC antibody response and PHA mitogen response. Donor cell progeny made up the responding population and, given enough time, young and old bone marrow and spleen cells demonstrated equal stem cell capacity.

The experiments cited above differed in the amount of time between cell transfer and testing. Harrison maintains that shortly after grafting responses are due to already differentiated, competent donor cells.[124] These are defective in the old environment and sufficient time must pass to ensure that stem cell function is what is being measured. On the other hand, host cells are known to recover after irradiation.[86] Although the responding cell may be of donor origin (chromosome markers), a recovered host population may amplify these responses. Additionally, all the experiments cited were done at one cell dose with no information presented about the number of CFUs transferred or dose-response relationship.[125] Such assays may be too many steps removed to measure stem cell capacity accurately, and are more informative in determining immunological response ability and burst size of old cells.

There may be subtle changes in the stem cells of old animals but the decline of the immune system and aging of the organism is not attributable to exhaustion of this population.[126]

### D. Humoral Immune System

#### *1. Nonspecific B Cell Responses*

In general B cell responses independent of T cell help do not decline with age as dramatically as T cell responses. Analyses of LPS induced B cell proliferation in mice demonstrated a decreased response late in life.[127,128] The response to PPD showed only a slight decline in some strains[89] while that to PWM (B cells and cortisone-resistant T cells), showed a greater decline.[129] Age-associated changes to B and T cell mitogens appear to be influenced by both H-2 and non-H-2 genes.[89] Certain strains of mice maintain constant levels of response to some mitogens until at least 28 months of age. The response to B cell mitogens in other rodent species decreases with age.[129,130] No alteration in the kinetics or optimal mitogen dose has been found for young vs. old animals.[130,131] Changes in the requirements of stimulation conditions therefore cannot account for the age-associated differences.

Conflicting evidence exists about age-associated changes in polyclonal activation of antibody synthesis by B cell mitogens, one group reporting a significant decrease after 11 months[132] and another[128] only after 30 months of age. The latter results paralleled findings by the same investigators[128] and others[89] on LPS mitogen response. LPS may also be used to stimulate autoantibody production (Section V.D).

*2. T Dependent Antibody Response*

Primary T dependent antibody production shows a marked decline with age both in vivo and in vitro[133] and differs in magnitude and kinetics from the decline in B cell mitogen responses.[127]

Antibody responses to SRBC of spleen cells from donors of various ages were measured in serum[133] and spleen[134] 1 to 2 weeks after cell transfer to irradiated recipients. Deficiencies both in old cells and old host environment were shown, with the cellular component being responsible for most of the decline. Old cells in a young environment may recover further responsiveness after a long time interval.[122,124] Young cells responded better in a young environment than in old hosts,[122] and old cells in old recipients fared the worst.[123] Evidence suggests that the defect in the old environment may be due to a systemic noncellular factor.[135] The minimum dose required for optimal response to SRBC by old mice is increased in vivo but not in vitro.[136] The in vivo deficit must therefore be due to alterations in the old environment rather than in the responding cells. Changes in macrophage function may underlie this "environmental" failure. Makinodan and Albright have shown that in vivo injection of 2-mercaptoethanol can restore impaired primary antibody response of most old mouse strains, particularly when suboptimal antigen (SRBC) doses are used.[137] Similar effects were noted in in vitro studies.[138]

The age-associated decline in cellular response could be due to a decrease in the number of antigen sensitive precursor units (IU) and/or number of antibody producing cells formed by each IU, or IBS. The limiting dilution assay has been used to investigate the number of IU and the dose-response assay to determine the IBS.[46] Price and Makinodan[139] found that both declined with age, the decrease in IBS being more severe. The decreased IBS is more likely due to defective cellular interactions than to changes intrinsic to B cells.[126]

The decline in antibody production with age reflects a loss of IgG and high avidity plaque forming cells (PFC).[140] This may be a preferential loss[140] or, since high avidity PFCs are in the minority normally, a nondiscriminatory decrease might result in the appearance of high avidity PFCs being preferentially lost.[141]

Analyses of the cell type responsible for the above decline show macrophage function to be basically intact (Section IV.E). Circumstantial evidence indicates a severe helper T cell defect,[142] and use of T and B cells from different aged donors has supported this hypothesis.[143,144] There is evidence also for a decline in B cell function but no quantitative figures for T and B cells' individual contributions have been arrived at.

Mixtures of old and young cells, challenged following transfer, have given antibody responses that are less than additive in most experiments,[140,145] suggesting the presence of suppressor T cells. Cases not showing a decrease in the mixtures indicate that variable mechanisms may be operating in aging animals to lower their response.[145]

In the primary response therefore, evidence suggests that: there are fewer responding units; responding units are less capable of continuing or expanding the response; and the products formed are more restricted. Defects of helper T, suppressor T and responding B cells may all be contributory.

The secondary response was first assayed by priming the animals at a young age and challenging at different ages. The response decreased with age, but in these experiments not only was the age at challenge varied, but the interval between priming and challenge also changed. Experiments keeping the time interval constant gave conflicting results. Some showed a normal[46,146] while others showed a decreased secondary response.[143] In human studies the elderly are more competent to respond to secondary challenge than to be primed to a new antigen.[103] It is clear that the secondary response is not as severely affected as primary antibody formation.

### E. Macrophage Function

Morphologically, germinal center formation and antigen localization in the follicles is poor in old mice.[147] However, in vitro analysis has demonstrated macrophages to be somewhat more, not less, active with age. In vitro phagocytosis of opsonized SRBC,[46] lysosomal enzyme activity,[148] and in vitro and in vivo ability to initiate primary and secondary antibody responses[149] have all been reported normal using old macrophages. An increase has been found in old animals in blood clearance time for injected colloidal carbon[150,151] but this might be due to decreased opsonizing ability of old sera.[152]

Increased macrophage activity seen in vitro might alter the immune response in the aged. Overly efficient digestion of antigen might change the antigen dose requirements in vivo.[139] However, these being the same in vitro for young and old cells mitigates against such an interpretation.[136]

Most aging studies on macrophages were conducted before the discovery of Ir gene representation thereon so the situation should perhaps be reevaluated.

### F. Cell Mediated Immunity

#### *1. Nonspecific T Cell Responses*

The proliferative response to PHA is decreased in aged mice[129,153] and humans.[109,154,155] This is not due to changes in optimum culture conditions,[156,157] numbers of membrane receptor sites per cell, or their binding affinity.[157,158] The maturation pattern of PHA response is genetically controlled.[89]

The response to Con A decreases with age in mice and rats[107,130] but not as much as that to PHA. This may indicate a preferential loss of $T_2$ over $T_1$ cells.[62,107] Directly opposite results have been seen on sensitivities of these populations to adult thymectomy[28] and with Thy-1 expression.[106]

Once an old T cell responds (IU), will it undergo as many repeat proliferative cycles (IBS) as a young cell? Using autoradiographic pulse labeling of Con A responding mouse spleen cells, Abraham, Tal, and Gershon[159] found that once old cells respond, they do so with the same capacity as cells from young animals. Studying response of human PBLs to PHA, Weksler's group[154] concluded that old cells are less capable of undergoing repeat divisions. Pulsing PHA-exposed human lymphocytes with a fluorescent label, Tice et al.[160] found that the minimum cell cycle length remained constant but that more old cells showed longer cell cycle times. Studies of cyclic nucleotide patterns in lymphocytes following PHA stimulation suggested that old cells contain intrinsic qualitative defects perhaps contributing to the diminished response.[161]

In summary, evidence clearly reveals a decrease in T cell mitogen response in both rodents and humans, but the mechanism has not been resolved.

## 2. T Cell Mediated Immune Responses

### a. Mixed Lymphocyte Culture

Several groups have demonstrated a decrease with age in the allogeneic MLC response in mice,[162,163] including the response to non-H-2 antigens.[163] One report[164] of normal MLC but decreased T mitogen response used "old" mice 60 to 80 weeks, and controls 8 to 12 weeks of age. These ages are not optimal for such a comparison[88] but the studies do suggest that the T mitogen response may decline earlier than the MLC.

The ability of syngeneic lymph node or spleen cells of different ages to synergize with young thymocytes appears to decline with age.[165,166] The ability of thymocytes to amplify the response did not vary with age[165] although the mature thymocyte population declined in number.[54] It is thus uncertain which of several interacting T cell subpopulations is defective and responsible for the diminished MLC with age. It is also uncertain in this assay as in the above mentioned assays whether, once an old cell responds, it does so with the same capacity as cells from young animals.[163]

### b. Cell Mediated Lympholysis

In vitro CML to H-2 alloantigens declines 4 to 6-fold with age following either in vivo or in vitro stimulation.[167-170] Dose-response curves from old are parallel to those from young animals, and cytotoxic cells from young and old mice seem equally effective in killing capacity.[167,169] Using limiting dilution transfer experiments, Goodman and Makinodan[168] found that the decrease was partly due to the number of immunocompetent precursor units (IU), and partly to diminished proliferative and transforming capacity (IBS), paralleling prior results on antibody response[139] and T mitogen response.[154] The differences observed in CML function between different aged mice may be accentuated by varying the culture conditions.[171] The CML may not decline in all lymphoid compartments at the same rate.[169] Both the MLC and CML have also been reported to decline with age in humans.[109]

### c. Graft Vs. Host Reaction

Three studies[172-174] on GVH reactivity employed the same assay method and two,[172,173] the same mouse strains. Kishimoto et al.[172] found a significant decline with age in lymph nodes and spleen cells while Stutman[173] reported that only the spleen shows a significant but slight decrease. Actually, both these studies yielded almost identical results with the differences being in the interpretations. Stutman[173] compared a long-lived strain with autoimmune susceptible strains of the same chronological age. In the latter mice, the GVH reactivity was greatly depressed and by comparison cellular immunity remained relatively intact with age in the long-lived strains. All studies[172-174] have shown a twofold decrease with age in splenic GVH reactivity, a less dramatic fall off than seen in other T dependent responses although mice up to 30 months old have been examined.[173] The substantial host contribution to splenomegaly in GVH might mask a severe defect in the aged donor population.

### d. Graft Rejection

In old mice, resistance to allogeneic tumor challenge is severely decreased.[168,169,175] The decline seen in vivo (dose rejected) is far more extreme than that seen when in vivo sensitized lymphocytes are assayed in vitro in chromium release assays.[168] Cells from old mice may have some enhancing effect on tumor cell growth in vivo, which would not be detected in vitro.[175] Mean survival time of skin allografts seems not to change significantly in old mice.[173]

Stimulation of cytotoxic lymphocyte (CTL) generation by virus infection decreases with age.[176,177] This is beneficial when the pathology of the disease is caused by the host's reaction to the virus (i.e., lymphocyte choriomeningitis virus).[176] With viruses and bacteria causing direct damage, old mice are more susceptible to chronic, ordinarily subclinical infections.[177] Parallel observations have been made on humans.[178,179]

### G. Suppressor Cell Function

Measuring the antibody response of BALB/c to SIII, a T helper independent antigen, Smith[180] found that the response remained constant from 5 to 100 weeks of age, but the ability to achieve low dose paralysis and ALS enhancement decreased. This was taken as suggestive evidence of an actual decline in suppressor cells, although an age-related increase in amplifier cells was not ruled out. Callard[131] reported that 23-month-old CBA/H mice responded less well than 3 to 6 month olds to SIII antigen, and not because of suppressor T cells since anti-Thy-1 plus complement treatment was without effect. Similar results were obtained with the T helper independent antigen PVP and (C3H × C57Bl)$F_1$ mice aged 7, 24, and 30 months.[144]

Using T dependent antigens and mixing experiments, three groups of investigators have detected an increase in suppressor cells with age. Makinodan et al.[145] assayed BC3F1 mice for SRBC response; Goidl et al.[140] used BALB/c and DNP-BGG as antigen; and Segre et al.[181] also used BC3F1 but with DNP-KLH antigen. Makinodan[145] proposed an increase in suppression as the major but not the sole change in aged cells. Goidl[140] concluded that increased, nonspecific suppressor cells decreased the level of response, while defective helper T cells lowered the affinity of the product formed. Segre et al.[181] found that suppression was due to a T cell and concluded that, with age, T suppressor function first increases, followed by a decrease in T help, and finally by an abrogation of B cell functioning. There was an increase in some strains with age of non-T, nonspecific suppressor cell induced by cyclophosphamide administration,[182] and possibly involved the reestablishment of self tolerance.

Although Krogsrud and Perkins[143] raised objections to the validity of results from mixing experiments due to the combined presence of T cells from young and old mice, their cell transfer experiments led them to conclusions similar to the above. They did not distinguish among decreased frequency of T helper cells, decreased efficiency of T helper cells to collaborate, and increased numbers of T suppressor cells, but hypothesized that all three were operating.

In a review of suppressor cells in aging, Gershon and Metzler[183] point out that the level of response of one subpopulation may depend on the level of another with which it interacts (Section II.E). Results therefore may vary with the assay system. Difficulties arise in separating suppression from help since they probably both change in concert.

Cantor et al.[108] reported that in BALB/c mouse spleens the Lyt-123+ population decreases steadily from 2 weeks to 12 months, Lyt-1+ cells increase from 2 weeks to 6 months, declining slightly at 12 months, and Lyt-23+ cells peak between 6 and 12 months. They suggested that Lyt-123+ cells are responsible for feedback suppression (in the SRBC antibody response) and these decline with age.

It seems therefore that with age there is a decrease in suppressor cells affecting T independent antibody response and an increase in those affecting T dependent responses in the humoral immune system. These results are very different from the majority of those obtained using autoimmune susceptible mice, considered by other criteria to be models of accelerated aging.

Suppressor cells involved in cell mediated immunity have not yet received much attention in gerontologic research. An early study by Gerbase-DeLima et al.[165] reported that splenic suppressor cells may increase in some but not all mouse strains as assayed by their ability to suppress the MLC of young lymph node cells. Bach[171] suggested that an increase in suppressor cells may be demonstrated in a proportion of the aging population under certain culture conditions in the CML. Inhibition of proliferative responses by Con A activated suppressor cells was somewhat decreased in elderly humans although considerable individual variability was encountered[184,185] and problems of allogeneic combinations were not dealt with.

Susceptibility to tumors,[175,186] delayed hypersensitivity,[187] and contact sensitivity[188] have been used to assay suppressor cells. Spleen cells from old donors enhanced tumor growth when given with the challenge to young mice.[175] A spontaneous decrease in suppressor cell function with age was suggested by the ability of cyclophosphamide to enhance the DTH response in young but not old mice.[187] However, the mice tested ranged from 5 weeks to 8 months old and the DTH response was increasing during that age interval. The lack of enhancement in the "old" animals might easily have been due to their reaching the peak of the response! A report of increased suppression for contact sensitivity[188] involved mice 1 month and 5½ months old, and the results extrapolated to indicate that an increase in splenic suppressor cells may be responsible for "the decline in the ability to develop contact hypersensitivity in aging". These very recent reports reemphasize the fact that much "aging" research in immunology is still being conducted without the use of old subjects.[88]

## V. AUTOIMMUNITY

### A. General Theories of Autoimmunity

Although the immune system of the elderly is depressed many autoimmune parameters increase in incidence with age, a dichotomy difficult to reconcile with early concepts about autoimmunity. Autoimmunity was first regarded as hyperreactivity of the immune system.[189] Now the hyperreactivity is known to lie in one component allowed to run awry by defective regulatory mechanisms.[190] The development of autoimmunity secondarily in inherited immunodeficiency states[191] and the occurrence of autoimmunity, immunodeficiency, and cancer in an interrelated fashion[192] are consistent with the idea that the autoimmunity of aging is a consequence of the partial immunodeficiency of aging.[189] The immunodeficiency and autoimmunity of aging may simply reinforce one another.

Burnet[76] and Jerne[77] had hypothesized that cells reactive for "self" were destroyed in the embryo (clonal selection). Somatic mutation occurring in the thymus, particularly in the elderly, might then result in the reappearance of autoreactive clones.[193] However, this mechanism seemed too restricted to explain the high incidence of autoimmune phenomena and the various ways these may be triggered.[196] A modifying hypothesis held that autoreactive clones were not eliminated in the neonate but were suppressed in the thymus and their emergence followed a decrease in suppressive mechanisms.[78] Good and Yunis[190] suggested that autoimmunity might be due to stimulation with foreign antigens cross-reacting with self-antigens (i.e., viral components), with disease being more a result of "forbidden antigens" than forbidden clones.

Reactivity to self antigens is now recognized as a normal part of the immune response.[80] Lymphocytes react to many foreign substances in the context of their own antigens, (Section III) allowing effective interactions with other cells of the immune system and with the antigen. Jerne's network theory[195] provided for autoreactivity in the humoral system with the proposition that antibody levels are controlled by anti-antibodies which react with idiotypic determinants on the original antibody (Section III). This theory can be extended to cellular immunity by hypothesizing idiotypic and anti-idiotypic receptors on lymphocytes.

Alterations during aging in regulatory mechanisms controlling autoreactive cells allow for their increase and detection.[195] Cross-reactive antigens could stimulate already present, autoreactive cells. Thus a decrease in regulation in old age[190] would allow autoimmunity without first necessitating an event as dramatic as somatic mutation, which could however also contribute to autoreactivity.

Talal considered the development of autoimmune disease as a three stage process:[196] first, the physiological mechanism of autorecognition wherein the immune system regulates more than just immunocytes. The finding of anti-receptor antibodies in organ-specific autoimmune diseases suggests that lymphocytes may regulate muscle, nerve, and endocrine systems as well as the immune system. Stage two is characterized by autoimmunity without associated disease. It results from a disturbance in the immune system, perhaps from drugs or a viral infection, is self-limiting, and disappears upon re-establishment of homeostasis. The last stage is overt autoimmune disease; the extension of the disturbance to disease on the basis of genetic abnormalities or tolerance to cross-reactive antigens.

Two age-specific peak incidences of autoimmunity occur in humans in early adult life and in the elderly.[1] Elderly persons showing autoantibodies in their sera, although disease-free, may manifest decreased survival.[197] In addition, many diseases characteristic of the aged have autoimmune aspects which contribute to their pathology. The autoimmune diseases of young adults seem to reflect a "defective" or abnormal adult subpopulation, whereas those of the elderly represent a natural consequence of the aging process. Murine models exist for both groups. An important question is whether the short-lived, autoimmune susceptible strains of mice actually undergo accelerated aging and so can serve as models of the aging process.

### B. Short-lived, Autoimmune Susceptible Murine Models

#### *1. New Zealand Mice (NZ)*

##### ***a. Definitions of Disease***

NZB and (NZB × NZW)$F_1$ hybrids (B/W) develop systemic diffuse autoimmune disease, both usually dying of immune complex deposits in the kidneys (glomerulonephritis). NZB mice develop autoimmune hemolytic anemia, characterized by early appearance of autoantibodies to erythrocytes and thymocytes (3 months).[198] Coomb's positive anemia develops at about 5 months.[199,200] The incidence of antinuclear antibodies (ANA) is low and glomerulonephritis appears late.[201] ANA includes antibodies to RNA and single and double-stranded DNA. It is not clear which is most significant in terms of disease. The autoimmune disease of B/W mice closely resembles systemic lupus erythematosus in humans, with a high incidence of L.E.-like cells, ANA, and glomerulonephritis appearing by 5 months of age.[202] Antibodies to red cells and T cells are less conspicuous than in NZBs. The disease in B/W females is more severe and leads to earlier fatality than in males.[202]

Viral, genetic, and immunological factors contribute to the cause and course of disease in NZB and B/W mice,[189] with modification by hormonal influences.[198,202,203]

C-type leukemia virus particles are easily demonstrated, particularly in NZB mice.[189,204] Gp 70 envelop glycoprotein increases in concentration early (1 month)[205] in both NZB and B/W mice, and both develop antibodies against it.[205] These viral antigen-antibody complexes form part of the deposits in the kidneys.[206] Viral DNA might be integrated into the cell genome and inherited by all offspring. Virus activation may lead to modification of cell surface antigens and the development of autoimmunity as the system reacts against the virus.[189,190] The expression of gp 70 does not correlate with disease activity but detectable levels of gp 70-anti-gp 70 immune complexes precede evidence of renal disease.[205] These viruses are also associated with a high incidence of lymphomas among older NZB or B/W mice.[207] The relationship between viral infection, autoimmunity, and lymphomas is not simple. Autoimmunity cannot be transferred by cell-free filtrates[208,209] whereas lymphomas probably can.[210]

The murine disease is ultimately determined at the gene level. A disease incidence of 100% exists in colonies throughout the world, although environment influences the rate of progression. Whether the genes act by stimulating cross-reactive antigens, by determining viral sensitivity, or by programing for a decline in a vital component of the immune system (tolerance homeostasis, for example) is unknown.

In NZB the incidence of antibody to thymocytes and single-stranded DNA seems to be under the control of two separate genes with two more genes controlling the quantitative response.[211]

Genetic contributions in B/W mice derive from both parents (NZWs do not themselves show autoimmunity yet their genetic contributions modify the nature of the disease).[212] Backcross analysis suggests NZW contributes two, while NZB donates one gene to the disease.[40] Lupus nephritis, characteristic of B/W disease but not found in either parent, probably depends on one gene from each parent.[213] The gene from the NZB parent is loosely linked to H-2D with a crossover frequency of 32.6%.[213] One of two genes derived from NZW is closely linked to H-2 and the other to immunoglobulin structural genes determining the variable region.[40] The genes appear to modify specific aspects of the disease. Integrated viral genomes cannot be eliminated as being one of the genetic factors.

Other so-called autoimmune susceptible strains show similar diseases.[205] MRL/l mice develop a syndrome characterized by massive nonmalignant lymphoproliferation, high concentrations of gp 70 and gp 70 immune complexes, immune complex glomerulonephritis, ANA, and hypergammaglobulinemia.[205,214] The lymphoproliferation is determined by an autosomal recessive mutant gene.[214] These animals show a 50% mortality at 6 months.[205] BXSB mice develop glomerulonephritis with a 50% mortality at 6 months in males and 15 months in females.[205,215] They display low titers of anti-DNA antibody but high concentrations of gp 70-anti-gp 70.[205] Other autoantibodies are also present.

Immunological functions in these animals show early abnormalities preceding clinical evidence of disease. However, their early appearance does not necessarily mean they are causative agents.

### *b. Immunological Deficiencies*

#### 1. General Changes

The immune system of NZ mice seems to undergo accelerated maturation and to decline early. Immunologically, young clinically normal NZ mice appear to resemble adult mice of other strains. Antibody response to T dependent antigens (i.e., SRBC)[198] has developed by 1 week of age, while tolerance is difficult to induce and short-lived as early as several weeks.[198] By 5 weeks of age NZ mice can no longer be made tolerant.

Different results have, however, been reported using different antigens and comparing NZ mice to different normal strains.[216] The precise ages used are important factors as the immune reactivity of NZ mice undergoes dramatic changes during their brief life span. Complete maturation curves have not been generated. Description of a response as hyper- or hypo-reactive is usually done with respect to only one normal strain. Since all immune functions show much variation among strains, it might be more valid to compare the immunological curves of NZ mice to NZ mice whose disease has been accelerated (e.g., by neonatal thymectomy) for analysis of immunological consequences of the disease.

The decline in the immune system of NZ mice is rapid after about 8 months. Although early it still follows clinical evidence of disease by several months.[194] PHA response, GVH reactivity, and graft rejection are all severely depressed. Numbers of Thy-1 + cells in the blood and peripheral lymphoid organs apparently decline beginning at 100 to 200 days of age, suggesting bodily depletion of T cells.[101,198,217-220] This decrease is far more severe than reported for aged animals of long-lived strains (Table 2). The long-lived, recirculating, lymph node seeking T cells may preferentially decline.[218,220] The thymus involutes early and thymic hormone becomes undetectable in young adult NZ mice.[221] Thymic epithelial cell cultures show a premature decline in function. These experiments suggest that a thymic epithelial cell defect may be primary to changes in T cell function[222] and that degeneration is a spontaneous preprogramed event.

### Table 2
### CHANGES IN NORMAL AGING IN MAN AND/OR LONG-LIVED MOUSE STRAINS COMPARED WITH AUTOIMMUNE DISEASES AND WITH POTENTIAL EXPERIMENTAL MODELS OF ACCELERATED AGING

| | | Occurring sooner and/or more intensely | | | | |
|---|---|---|---|---|---|---|
| Parameters | Normal aging | SLE | Autoimmune suscept. mice (NZB, NZB/W) | Chronic GVH reaction | Nude mice | Hypopituitary dwarf mice |
| **Immunological parameters** | | | | | | |
| Thymic atrophy involution | + | ? | + | + | + | + |
| Thymic hormone | ↓ | ↓ | ↓ | ? | ↓ | ↓ |
| Splenomegaly in early phase | + | + | + | + | ? | ? |
| Lymphoid hypoplasia late | + | ? | − | ? | ? | + |
| Plasma cell increase | + | ? | + | + | + | ? |
| Peripheral T cells | = | ↓ | ↓ | ? | ↓ | ↓ |
| Humoral immune response | | | | | | |
| Non-sp. B cell (to mitogen) | ↓ | ? | ↑ | ? | = | ? |
| T-indep. antibody response | ↓ | ? | ↑ | ? | ? | ? |
| T-dep. antibody response | ↓ | ? | ↓ | ↓ | ↓ | ↓ |
| Serum immunoglobulins | ↑/↓ | ? | ? | ↑ | ↓ | = |
| Cellular immunity | | | | | | |
| Response to mitogens | ↓ | ↓ | ↓ | ?[b] | ↓ | ? |
| MLC | ↓ | ↓ | ↓ | ?[b] | ↓ | ↓ |

Table 2 (continued)
CHANGES IN NORMAL AGING IN MAN AND/OR LONG-LIVED MOUSE STRAINS COMPARED WITH AUTOIMMUNE DISEASES AND WITH POTENTIAL EXPERIMENTAL MODELS OF ACCELERATED AGING

| Parameters | Normal aging | Occurring sooner and/or more intensely: SLE | Autoimmune suscept. mice (NZB, NZB/W) | Chronic GVH reaction | Nude mice | Hypopituitary dwarf mice |
|---|---|---|---|---|---|---|
| CML | ↓ | ? | ↓ | ?[b] | ↓ | ↓ |
| GVH | ↓ | ? | ↓ | ?[b] | ↓ | ↓ |
| Graft rejection | = | ? | ↓ | ?[b] | ↓ | ↓ |
| ADCC | ↓ | ↓ | ↓ | ? | ? | ? |
| Suppressor | | | | | | |
| Nonspecific Con A induced | ↓ | ↓ | ↓ | ? | ↓ | ? |
| Antigen-specific | ↑ | ? | ↓ | ? | ? | ? |
| Autoantibodies | | | | | | |
| ANA | + | + | + | + | + | ? |
| Thyroid | + | ? | ? | ? | ? | ? |
| Gastric parietal cell | + | ? | ? | ? | ? | ? |
| Brain-reactive | + | + | ? | ? | ? | ? |
| Thymocytotoxicity | + | + | + | + | ? | ? |
| Relation to HLA or H-2 system | + | + | + | + | – | ? |
| cAMP/cGMP ratios in lymphoid cells | ↓ | ↓ | ? | ? | ? | ? |

| | | | | | | |
|---|---|---|---|---|---|---|
| **Disease of physiologic parameters** | | | | | | |
| Immune complex disease (in kidneys) | + | + | + | + | + | ? |
| Amyloidosis | + | + | ? | + | + | ? |
| Hyperparaproteinemia | + | ? | ? | ? | ? | ? |
| Hemolytic anemia | − | + | + | + | ? | ? |
| Vascular disease | + | + | ? | + | ? | ? |
| Atherosclerosis | + | + | − | ? | ? | ? |
| Arteritis | + | + | ? | ? | ? | ? |
| Hypertension | + | + | ? | ? | ? | ? |
| Arthritis | + | + | ? | ? | ? | ? |
| Disordered carbohydrate metabolism (diabetes or abnormal glucose tolerance) | + | ? | ? | ? | ? | ? |
| Dementia | + | + | ? | ? | ? | ? |
| Cataracts | + | ? | ? | ? | ? | ? |
| ↑ lipofuscin pigment | + | ? | ? | ? | ? | ? |
| Loss of weight, and/or "shrivelling up" of body | + | + | − | + | + | + |
| Collagen changes | + | + | ? | + | + | ? |
| Solubility in weak acid | ↓ | ? | ? | ↓ | ? | ? |
| Alterations in chromatin | + | ? | ? | ? | ? | ? |

**Table 2 (continued)**
**CHANGES IN NORMAL AGING IN MAN AND/OR LONG-LIVED MOUSE STRAINS COMPARED WITH AUTOIMMUNE DISEASES AND WITH POTENTIAL EXPERIMENTAL MODELS OF ACCELERATED AGING**

| | | Occurring sooner and/or more intensely | | | | |
|---|---|---|---|---|---|---|
| Parameters | Normal aging | SLE | Autoimmune suscept. mice (NZB, NZB/W) | Chronic GVH reaction | Nude mice | Hypopituitary dwarf mice |
| ↑ susceptibility to cancer | + | + | + | + | − | − |
| Lymphoid | + | + | + | + | − | − |
| Nonlymphoid | + | ? | ? | ? | − | − |
| Osteoporosis | + | + | ? | ? | ? | ? |
| Characteristic skin changes | + | + | ? | + | + | ? |

[a] + = present; − = absent; ? = no reliable information or not yet studied; ↑ = increase; ↓ = decrease; = = no change; ↑/↓ = variable. In many instances, as described in the text, differing results are reported in the literature. We here give only our interpretation of what is a consensus on each point. See text for details.

[b] Cellular immune functions in chronic GVH reaction are normal, diminished or increased depending on the test system, the antigen, and, most importantly, the time of testing with respect to the course of the GVH disease.

### 2. B Cells

B cells, which produce the autoantibodies, have not often been studied independently of T cells in NZ mice, and functional assays have yielded differing results and interpretations. Quantitatively, B cells may remain relatively constant[223] as in normal old animals, or may increase with age until about 40 weeks.[219] Plasma cell proliferation is seen in the peripheral lymphoid organs.[220] Autoimmune strains show a high IgM/IgD ratio of surface immunoglobulin markers which is more characteristic of neonatal animals of normal strains.[224]

Spontaneous total IgM antibody secretion in the spleens and sera of NZB and B/W mice is greater, from 1 day to 10 weeks of age, than spontaneous secretion from C57Bl/6, DBA/2, and NZW mice.[225] The antibodies could not be absorbed by syngeneic thymocytes or erythrocytes, suggesting polyclonal B cell activation. It probably occurs in utero. A similar conclusion was reached by Izni et al.,[226] who assayed spontaneous IgM PFC production to hapten modified sheep red cells (TNP-SRBC) and serum IgM to DNP. They found an increase in NZB, B/W, BXSB, and MRL/1 mice compared with nonautoimmune strains, and hypothesized that the B cell is influenced by a polyclonal activator with activation taking place during the first week of life (not tested before 2 weeks). They did not differentiate between defective T suppression, excessive T help, or B cell hyperreactivity.

Response to T independent phosphorylcholine antigen did not show much change with age in NZB mice from 1 to 62 weeks old[227] whereas response to SIII increased,[228] suggesting a decreased T cell mediated suppression with normal B cell function in aging NZB. Hyperreactivity to SRBC has been detected as early as one week of age, and also attributed to defective T suppressor function.

LPS stimulation is under suppressor T cell influence. LPS stimulation of SRBC PFC, spontaneous PFC formation, and mitogenesis were reported to decrease by 7 to 77 weeks of age in NZB spleens and the defect considered to reside at the B cell level since fewer suppressor cells should lead to an increase.[229] Loss of LPS induced PFC formation has been found by other investigators comparing 3 and 8-month-old NZB mice.[230] However, Ohsugi and Gershwin,[231] measuring LPS induced B colony formation, showed an increase in NZB and asplenic (Dh/ + ) NZB mice compared with four normal strains. These mice were tested from 1 week of age and the responses peaked in the autoimmune strains at 2 months of age.

Measuring LPS and PPD induced anti-TNP SRBC IgM formation in 10-month-old B/W mice, Cohen et al.[232] found the response decreased compared to age-matched normal controls and 5-week-old B/W mice. Removal of Thy-1 + cells did not alter the response. The 10-month-old B/W mice responded normally to B cell mitogens and to a T independent antigen, TNP-Ficoll. The authors hypothesized that the B cells were influenced by a polyclonal B cell activator in vivo which led to commitment of the B cell antibody response.

Naor et al.[233] demonstrated a decrease in PFC TNP-MRBC formation (T independent) after immunization of NZ mice and a severe decline in response to a T dependent antigen, TNP-SRBC. They suggested a deficiency in suppressor cells and probably macrophages.

Investigators finding an increase in B cell reactivity generally began testing their animals early, one day to about two weeks of age.[225,226,231] NZ mice may first show hypersensitivity of B cell function, later a deficiency as the immune system breaks down. Deficiencies in cell mediated immune function, tolerance induction, and thymic hormones may not begin until several weeks of age, causing either a subsequent decrease or increase in B cell function[228,229,233] depending on the T dependence of the function being assayed.

Akizuki et al.[234] transferred autoimmune disease to normal, lethally irradiated, histocompatible recipients using anti-Thy-1 plus complement treated bone marrow cells from B/W mice. This result suggests a primary defect in marrow B cells or stem cells. Tauros et al.[235] mated CBA/N females with male NZB mice and tested their male offspring for B cell function. The CBA/N parent has an X-linked defect in T independent B cell function, while hybrids with NZB mice generally develop autoimmunity. The male F1 hybrid (receiving the CBA/N X gene) resembled the CBA/N parent, whereas the female resembled the NZB parent with respect to expression of autoimmunity.[236] This suggested that genetic defects in NZB and CBA/N mice act on the same B cell subset. By comparing NZB nude mice with normal littermates and BALB/c nudes, Gershwin et al.[237] also detected abnormal B cell activation independent of T cells.

#### 3. Cellular Immune Function

Leventhal and Talal[238] noted a decline in PHA and MLC responses in NZB and in PHA response for B/W animals from 2 to 8 months of age. Rody et al.[239] found that PHA and MLC responses of NZB spleen cells were severely depressed at 18 months and nonexistent at 24 months, compared to 2-month-old NZBs. NZB × A and A (both autoimmune susceptible) showed a similar but less dramatic decline, whereas CBA mice retained most of their function. No differences were detected among 2-month-old NZB, NZB × A, A, or C3H mice; however, the PHA response was depressed as early as 6 months.[240] Mitogen response was maintained better in lymph node than spleen cells.[212] One of the few studies on T cell mediated immunity assaying mice earlier than 2 months and at several ages showed normal PHA and Con A reactivity in NZB spleens from newborns through 6 weeks of age.[241] The Con A response of thymocytes matured earlier than in BALB/c mice but was lower after 3 weeks of age. Only BALB/c was used as normal control so it is difficult to be sure that the NZBs were prematurely responsive.

The syngeneic MLC reaction (T cells proliferate in response to syngeneic non-T cells) is decreased in 4-week-old NZB (the earliest tested) in comparison to several age-matched strains.[242] The lower reactivity of NZB mice is maintained until 10 weeks, then declines further.[242]

GVH reactivity of spleen and lymph node cells is severely depressed in NZB mice by 10 months of age.[173,217,243] However until 5 months of age, which is after clinical signs of autoimmunity, GVH reactivity may be normal compared with other strains. Thymus cells from 10-day-old autoimmune strains were briefly reactive.[212] Splenic reactivity may also develop earlier,[212] however, in normal strains, GVH function continues to increase as this reactivity is declining in autoimmune mice. NZB mice were compared with CBA/H and NZW in this experiment. Another study of the reaction in B/W mice[244] reported that 6-month-old B/W mice simply displayed higher activity than at different ages (peak) and were actually no more responsive than other strains. The response in B/W mice, however, declined earlier.

Skin allograft rejection was impaired in 8-month-old compared to 1-month-old B/W mice.[245,246] The young mice reacted similarly to long-lived strains and their splenocytes could restore the response of older animals.[218] Gershwin et al.[247] showed that 9-month-old B/W mice were killed by tumor grafts at doses normally rejected by younger animals.

In the CML assay, the response of 1-month-old mice was normal and of 9-month-old mice depressed, but 6 month olds showed a heightened reactivity.[247] Testing NZB mice at 1, 3, 8, and 12 months, Fernandes et al.[212] found no hyperreactivity in the CML assay after in vivo sensitization.[212] Only a progressive decline in response was seen, and this was consistently lower than in C57Bl/6 and CBA/H strains from 1 month on. With other sensitizing and target cell types, the response of autoimmune strains remained vigorous until 3 months of age.[212] Four-month-old BXSB mice also showed a decline compared to 2 month olds, while the response by C57Bl/6 mice was increasing.[248] Old (80 weeks) NZB and age-matched DBA/2 mice showed a decrease in CML generation after stimulation in an allogeneic MLC.[249] Conditions required for optimal stimulation were not affected by age.

Most of the above experiments demonstrated normal cellular immunity from about 1 to 5 months of age and severe depression at 8 to 10 months in NZ mice, i.e., after the onset of autoimmunity.[250] Premature maturation cannot be ruled out. The ages tested have been widely scattered and maturation curves of autoimmune and normal strains may cross at the 2-month period when most have been assayed. Changes found during the first several months seem to involve B cells, some in T independent, but mostly in T dependent assay systems. It is possible that alterations in B cell function result from T cell (e.g., suppressor cell) activity, which would imply that early immune changes are due to a very restricted subpopulation of T cells.

Two additional cellular assays, not involving T cell function, have been briefly studied. Natural cytotoxic activity of NZB spleen cells is within the normal range.[251] Antibody-dependent cell mediated cytotoxicity (ADCC) against DNA coated SRBC targets was found to decrease after 4 months of age in B/W mice but not in BALB/c.[252] These results are interesting in light of the hypothesis that ADCC may contribute to tissue damage in autoimmune disease.

#### 4. Suppressor Cells

Much circumstantial evidence suggests that suppressor cells decline early in NZ mice. This would account for immune hyperreactivity and resistance to tolerance induction in young mice, and for autoimmunity later in life by a lack of control of forbidden clones or normally autoreactive cells. A secondary defect in helper T cells might be responsible for immune depression in old NZ mice. While such an interpretation is attractive, most of the data purportedly demonstrating a defective suppressor T cell population does not eliminate the possibility of excessive helper function or of a more basic regulatory problem. Additionally, the evidence for hyperreactivity and resistance to tolerance induction which has formed the basis of the suppressor cell hypothesis can be questioned. We shall first review circumstantial and then direct evidence about suppressor cells in autoimmune susceptible strains of mice.

At 1 week of age NZ mice show heightened response to the T dependent foreign antigens, SRBC or TNP-SRBC, compared to controls.[298,238] This is followed by a severe decline and by 7 months the response is minimal.[228] While hyperreactive in vivo,[253,254] the in vitro response[200,254] of NZB mice to SRBC is reduced at 5 to 6 weeks of age, whereas the response to DNP-Ficoll, a T independent antigen, is normal. The mice also do not exhibit premature responses to pig or chick red cells, so the generality of the too-soon maturation hypothesis may be questioned.[216]

NZB mice respond to SIII at 1 month of age (earliest tested).[228] The response begins increasing at 3 to 4 months, plateaus at 6 months, and is maintained at a high level up to at least 9 to 11 months of age.[228] The increase is not seen in normal strains and has been attributed to a deficiency in suppressor T cells. Young thymocytes can transfer suppression of the response to older NZB mice. Concomitant analysis of the response to SRBC shows a sharp decrease after its peak at 4 to 6 months, supposedly due to a secondary T cell deficiency. Thus the age-specific responses to SIII and SRBC differ in NZB mice.[198,228] Comparing the responses of 6 and 20-week-old NZB and B/W mice to the responses of three normal strains to four antigens (SRBC, KLH, BSA, and HGG), Cerottini et al.[216] found that the relative response among the strains depended on the antigen. They speculated that hyperreactivity may be selective and only include antigens either involved in the autoimmune disease or cross-reactive with such antigens.

Many experiments aimed at decelerating or accelerating disease in autoimmune strains have indirectly tested the hypothesis that suppressor cell abnormalities are involved. Thymectomy at an early age accelerates the disease in B/W males (although not in females who already show rapid and severe development).[255] Thymectomy may eliminate suppressor cells initially present in the male but already missing in the female. Antithymocyte globulin may function similarly to accelerate the disease, even in female B/Ws.[256]

Splenectomy causes first a depression of the IgM antibody response, later an enhancement of IgG response and development of the female disease pattern in B/W males (earlier switch to IgG antibodies and earlier renal disease).[255] These results have been interpreted as being due to elimination of a splenic suppressor population, freeing helper cells to promote the switch to IgG. When a gene producing a natural asplenic condition (Dh/ + ) was introduced onto the NZB background, NZB disease still developed but without high titers of antithymocyte antibody, hypergammaglobulinemia, or lymphocyte infiltrates.[257] The immune functions of such mice showed a greater decline than those of NZBs with intact spleens, however, nonspecific thymocyte suppressor cell activity was retained.[257]

Antithymocyte antibody, prominent in NZB mice, may be selectively reactive against and specifically eliminate suppressor cells thus increasing the severity of the disease.[258] Loss of self-tolerance with emergence of antithymocyte antibodies may precede the decline in suppressor cells,[207] however, these antibodies sometimes do not appear until after a decline in T cell numbers[257] or in thymus function, and after the appearance of antibodies to RNA,[259] and are not found in all autoimmune strains.[260]

Implanting thymi,[190,261] injecting young syngeneic thymocytes[262] or spleen cells,[263] or administration of thymic hormones[264] has postponed or even reversed certain parameters of NZ disease,[190] but with no effect on survival of the mice.[263,264] These treatments were designed to provide additional suppressor T cells. Survival may be prolonged somewhat by induction of tolerance to DNA[265,266] even though total ANA titers can be decreased by other means without affecting survival. Anti-DNA antibodies may be a more significant factor than other ANAs in the progress of the disease.

Difficulties in tolerance induction in 4-week-old NZ mice can be taken as evidence for a supressor T cell defect. However, results of tolerance induction vary with the antigen tested and the normal strain used for comparison.[216] An early cell transfer experiment[225] suggested a possible defect in an NZ bone marrow population. Since high dose tolerance is a function of both T and B cells, it is possible that deficiencies exist in either one or both populations.

Chronic GVH induced by injection of parental NZW cells into B/W mice has been reported to improve survival,[201] although opposite results have been obtained when NZB cells are used as donor.[267] While GVH and autoimmune diseases have many similarities, GVH is also immunosuppressive and in some cases may interfere with the NZ disease.

Low protein diet partially normalizes most of the immunological changes seen in NZB disease,[268] but with a diet high in protein content and low in fat, the life span of these mice was prolonged.[269] In kdkd mutant mice, a short-lived autoimmune susceptible strain, a low caloric diet also had a positive effect on survival.[270]

Drugs affecting the clinical status of autoimmune diseases do influence survival. Cyclophosphamide decreases antibody production, increases tolerance induction, decreases ANA titers and severity of renal disease, and increases the life span of B/W mice.[271-273] It does not affect the concentration of gp 70 but decreases the amount of gp 70-anti-gp 70 complexes.[205] Surviving mice show an increased incidence of tumors, particularly lymphomas.[274] This might reflect a later manifestation of the disease which untreated mice do not live long enough to develop or the reduction of ANA titers allowing oncogenic expression of the viruses carried.

Prostaglandin $E_1$ ($PGE_1$) prolongs survival of female B/W mice without affecting ANA titers[275] but may act on a subclass of B cells which produces ANA of one specificity. Prostaglandin inhibitors enhance production of autoantibodies in vitro even in T cell depleted cultures. With in vivo prostaglandin treatment, cell mediated immune functions are preserved longer[219] and levels of T and B cells are maintained.

Summarizing indirect evidence that a decrease in suppressor cells is instrumental in NZ disease, we may say that: there appears to be an early maturation and hyperreactivity of predominantly B dependent functions; the severity of the autoimmune disease is increased by deletion of T cells early in life; survival is prolonged by administration of drugs, some of which are known to affect T cells. Assays aimed specifically at analyzing suppressor cell function are difficult to interpret since it is uncertain if one is measuring suppressor cells as opposed to helper or other immunoregulatory cells. Transfer experiments of young putative "suppressor cells" may also be explained by a progressively increasing helper T population in the old which is diluted by the injection of young T cells. Additionally, most experiments do not rule out the possibility that B cells may become unresponsive to signals from suppressor T cells.

Krakauer et al.[277] reported a loss of suppressor cells in adult B/W mice. Con A activation of nonspecific T suppressor cells was normal in 4-week-old B/W mice.[277] Their PWM induced IgM response was suppressed by the Con A activated cells. Seventeen-week-old B/W mice produced much less suppressor factor, but were still able to respond to suppressor signals. With NZB mice and LPS stimulation of IgM synthesis, Primi et al.[230] reported opposite results with Con A suppressor cells. Twelve-week and eight-month-old NZBs were capable of generating nonspecific, Con A activated suppressor cells. However, only B cells from 12-week-old animals could respond to the signals. Primi et al.[230] suggested that suppressor cell function is normal in NZB mice and that the defect lies with the B cell.

Roder et al.[278] found an increase with age in B/W mice of a nonphagocytic, radiosensitive, non-T suppressor cell population, which first appeared at 11 weeks of age. These cells suppressed the in vitro anti-SRBC response of 4-week-old B/W spleen cells. The incidence of suppressive activity reached 100% at 35 weeks and was maintained through 20 months of age, paralleling the increase in incidence of antisingle stranded DNA antibodies. The threshold for suppression appeared also to increase with age. This increase in non-T suppressor cell activity might account for the decline in T dependent B cell response seen in these animals after several months of age. Segre et al.[182] noted an increase with age in a nonspecific non-T suppressor cell population induced by cyclophosphamide in normal and NZB mice, and conjectured that these cells function in re-establishing tolerance to self antigens after cyclophosphamide administration and that their increase indicated autoimmune stimulation.

Thymocytes from NZB mice used to suppress the GVH function of 10-week-old NZB spleen cells are effective at 4 weeks, but not at 20 weeks of age.[257] Thymocytes from hereditary asplenic Dh/+ NZB animals, however, are able to suppress at both ages.[257] In another measurement of thymocyte suppressor activity, Dh/+ and +/+ NZB animals develop a similar autoimmune disease and changes in suppressor cell activity may influence conditions secondary to the disease itself.

Klassen et al.[246] suggested that anti-Thy-1 in the proper dose activates T suppressor cells, which then prolong graft rejection. Five-week-old B/W mice required a higher dose of anti-Thy-1 than BALB/c for graft prolongation, whereas anti-Thy-1 had no effect in 17-week-old NZB mice. Suppression could be transferred from 5 or 17-week-old donors to untreated 5-week-old recipients. No suppression was found, however, when 17-week animals were employed as recipients. These results were interpreted as indicating that suppressor cell activity is somewhat decreased in B/W mice but that response to suppression is severely defective in 17-week-old B/W. In an assay of bone marrow derived "pre-T suppressor cells", Dauphinee and Talal[279] similarly concluded that NZB mice were incapable of responding to suppressive signals.

Using an antigen-specific hapten-carrier system, Creighton et al.[280] found no differences in the immune competence of B, helper T, or suppressor T cells in B/W, BXSB, or MRL/1 animals compared with four normal strains. They were tested at a young age and at a later age, before and after clinical signs of disease. The only defect seen was in the older MRL/1 and this was alleviated when the cells were transferred and tested in young hosts. By using several normal strains the investigators were able to determine a normal range for the responses.

Rather than a defect in the usual Lyt-23+ suppressor cell, Cantor et al.[108] suggested that B/W mice have a defect in Lyt-123+ cells. These cells function in feedback suppression and are stimulated by the Lyt-1+ helper T cell. NZB mice up to 1 year of age showed a decrease in Lyt-123+ and an increase in Lyt-1+ and Lyt-23+ cells relative to age-matched BALB/c.

In summary, results of suppressor cell function in NZ mice vary with the ages studied, the manipulations tried, and the assay systems used. Since suppressor cell function is poorly understood in normal strains, it is difficult to say exactly how NZ mice differ from them.

##### 5. Macrophages

Studies on macrophage function in NZ mice are few and results as varied as those dealing with the other components of the immune system.[200,281-283]

### c. Conclusions

It is not possible to be certain from existing studies that immunological changes are a primary rather than secondary effect of disease in autoimmune susceptible strains. However, the changes may still be compared with those seen in normal aging (Table 2). An obvious discrepancy is that evidence is accumulating for an early B cell abnormality (see Raveche and Steinberg for review)[284] whereas most of the changes seen in normal aging involve T cell defects. Immunological maturation in NZ mice is accelerated to certain antigens, with development and subsequent decline occurring faster. NZ mice reportedly show an early maturation, hyperreactivity, and an early and severe decline in response to SRBC. This is hypothesized as being due to a deficiency of suppressor T cells followed by a secondary decline in helper T cells. Normal long-lived strains should follow the same pattern if the NZ mice represent exact models of accelerated aging. Analysis of the Ly types of peripheral T cells of NZ mice do not show curves displayed in time (accelerated maturation) but rather in magnitude.[108] Assays of cell mediated immunity have not shown accelerated maturation in NZ mice, just accelerated decline. Maturation of the SRBC response is more rapid though. The immune decline observed in autoimmune strains is far more severe than that seen in the late age of long-lived mice. While there is depletion of peripheral T cells in autoimmune strains, the same is not observed in long-lived strains.[101] Additionally, in long-lived mice, suppressor cells may be increased rather than decreased in activity (Section IV.G) (Table 2). Autoantibodies may be found in old C57B1/6 mice and in neonatally thymectomized[285] and nude animals without the coexistence of overt autoimmune disease. A summary of features of accelerated aging present or lacking in autoimmune susceptible strains of mice is given in Table 2.

Other factors, of both viral and genetic origin, are doubtlessly involved in determining disease in NZ mice, as well as a defect in the peripheral immune system. As no one factor could be positively correlated with autoimmune disease in the susceptible strains, Datta and Schwartz[286] developed the "leaky gene" hypothesis. They suggested that defects of gene regulation lead to the derepression of multiple unlinked loci that are present in most normal strains. The derepression results in an overproduction of the genes' products, i.e., gp 70 expression, polyclonal B cell activation. Evidence for chromosomal abnormalities in NZB mice lends credence to this hypothesis.

*2. Additional Short-Lived Murine Models*

Nude mice, hypopituitary dwarf mice, and mice undergoing chronic GVH may be considered as potential models of accelerated aging and do show autoimmune manifestations (Table 2). Nonimmune parameters involving the endocrine, neurological, and muscular systems may be indirectly affected by alterations in the immune system.[287]

Nude, hairless mice are born with only a thymic remnant, display neuromuscular and fertility abnormalities, poor growth, and die at an early age of a runting syndrome.[288] They display an increased incidence of ANA and immune complex deposits in the kidneys at an early age as compared to normal littermates,[289] and this is possibly due to a lack of T cell regulation. Similar results are seen in neonatally thymectomized mice. The thymus may in part regulate the aging of other organs.[288]

Hypopituitary dwarf mice show atrophic thymuses, profound, mostly T related, immunological defects, and die at about 5 months of age.[287] They exhibit signs of accelerated aging (Table 2). Growth hormone corrects the deficiency[290] and injection of peripheral T cells extends their life span to more than 1 year.[290] The features of accelerated aging are considered due to thymic deficit secondary to pituitary deficit.

Severe GVH reaction is characterized by thymic atrophy, splenomegaly, and late lymphoid hypoplasia.[291] Wasting due to neonatal thymectomy and GVH reaction reveal similar features although they are more accelerated in the latter. There is an increase in plasma cells, amyloidosis, deposits of amorphous hyaline material, fibroses, diminished collagen solubility, increased lysozyme, anemia, decreased response to foreign antigens, abnormalities in T and B cell collaboration, and increased signs of autoimmunity[1,292] — all changes seen in normal aging (Table 2). Chronic GVH is often accompanied by autoimmune disease. This may be due to the allogeneic effect; the inappropriate and prolonged stimulation by donor T cells (parental) of host B cells ($F_1$ hybrid), resulting in the production of autoantibodies.[292]

*3. Organ-Specific Murine Autoimmune Diseases*

In contrast to the diffuse disease of NZ mice, immunological diseases are known where one organ or system is specifically attacked. In mice, these may occur spontaneously, after manipulation of the immune system, or after deliberate injection of autologous or homologous antigen. Some autologous antigens are more prone than others to stimulate the development of autoimmune disease.

Myasthenia gravis-like disease, thyroiditis, encephalomyelitis, autoimmune orchitis, and amyloidosis may be induced by immunological manipulation. The first may be secondary to development of antireceptor antibodies following injection of isolated acetylcholine receptors and adjuvant.[293] Thyroiditis may occur in mice following neonatal thymectomy,[294] depending on strain susceptibility. Nude mice cannot be made to develop the disease.[395] It is possible that thymectomy must be performed at a crucial period—after peripheralization of helper T cells but before development of suppressor T cell function. Lacking both T cell types, nude mice would be resistant.[295]

Amyloidosis frequently accompanies autoimmune disease, malignancies, chronic infections, and aging. One form of amyloidosis is considered an autoimmune disease based on the components of the amyloid deposit.[296] Other forms can be induced by methods which imply an immunological basis. Senile amyloidosis has not been intensively studied with modern immunochemical methods.

### C. Human Autoimmune Disease

The human population shows a peak of severe autoimmune disease during the third decade of life, generally with higher incidence in females. The immunopathology of these diseases in relation to aging have been discussed elsewhere.[1,2] Autoimmune disorders also frequently accompany hereditary or acquired immunodeficiency and malignancy.[190]

#### *1. Systemic Lupus Erythematosus (SLE)*

Many similarities exist between SLE in humans and the autoimmune disease of B/W mice. With modern treatment, patients with SLE live much longer than previously, long enough to be able to show features of premature or accelerated aging.[297] In fact, SLE, diabetes, and Down's syndrome probably show more signs of being progeroid conditions than any other human maladies.

Multiple cases of SLE are often found in one family and an increased frequency of the disease occurs in first degree relatives of SLE probands.[298,299] Increased concordance has also been found for monozygotic twins.[300] SLE is highly correlated with HLA specificities DRw2 and 3, and severe cases are apt to be HLA-B8 (+). Twin pairs, discordant for disease, have been examined to test whether the "healthy" twin shows immunological abnormalities suggestive of the beginnings of the disease.[301] Analysis of healthy twins, however, does not usually indicate an impaired cellular immune system.[301,302,303]

Mitogen responses, MLCs, and skin tests for delayed hypersensitivity are diminished in SLE. Peripheral T cells tend to decrease[304,305] correlating with disease activity,[306] and lymphopenia is common.[307] Increased null cells reported in SLE may be due to defective maturation of lymphocytes[308] or to blocking factors present in the serum.[309] Thymic hormone preparations given in an attempt to restore T cell number and immunological function in SLE have yielded mixed results,[305] as have similar experiments with NZ mice. For a more extensive review of immune function in SLE see Raveche and Steinberg.[289]

Autoantibodies have been hypothesized to cause tissue damage by an ADCC mechanism in addition to immune complex deposition. ADCC function has been reported as normal[310,311] or decreased,[252,312] rather than increased, in SLE. Differing results may reflect the different target cells (nucleated versus enucleated) employed in the assays.[313]

Nonactivated or Con A activated cells in SLE have been examined for ability to suppress B cell antibody synthesis; including PWM stimulated, antigen stimulated, and spontaneous synthesis. Most results indicate that whereas suppressor cell induction is defective, the ability to respond to suppressive signals remains intact.[314,315] Cell populations from patients with inactive disease have not shown a suppressor cell defect, hence the defect may be reversible.[314] Anti-T autoantibodies in SLE may preferentially act against suppressor T cells.[315,316]

Autoantibodies to DNA, RNA, and lymphocytes are produced in SLE, as in NZ mice.[317] IgM antibodies to RNA have been detected in "normal" relatives of SLE patients while the patients themselves have IgM and IgG antibodies to DNA and RNA. The presence of these antibodies may reflect suseptibility to the disease.[317] IgG antibodies to DNA seem to be associated with a severe clinical course, similar to the situation in NZ mice.[318]

#### *2. Organ-Specific Autoimmune Diseases*

Organ-specific autoimmune diseases may accompany immunodeficiency syndromes or cancers, or may occur independently. Susceptibility is often linked to HLA. Caucasian individuals with HLA-8, W-27, or HLA-7 seem to be at increased risk.[319,320]

A variety of thyroid autoimmune diseases have been described.[321] Antithyroid antibodies are not an uncommon primary or secondary occurrence in humans. Autoimmunity may be implicated also in the pathogenesis of diabetes mellitus and Parkinson's disease, both of which are "diseases of aging."[1]

Myasthenia gravis is a neuromuscular disorder in which the acetylcholine receptors are attacked by autoantibodies.[322] It shows linkage to the MHC.[323] Thymomas and selective IgA deficiencies are found in increased incidence in these patients.[324,325] Thymectomy may sometimes improve survival,[326] but the beneficial effects of thymectomy are not immediate, perhaps signifying that a peripheral T population has to die out. Some abnormalities in cell mediated immunity have been reported.[327,328]

### D. Autoimmunity in Long-Lived Mouse Strains and in Humans

#### *1. Mice*

The long-lived mouse strains offer a number of opportunities for studying autoimmunity and aging, but have received less attention in this regard than short-lived autoimmune susceptible strains. The latter may reflect only one aspect of the autoimmunity-aging relationship.

Autoantibodies occur spontaneously with age in most strains of mice and include antithyroid, antigastric parietal cell, antisperm, and antibrain antibodies.[1] Different strains vary in type of autoantibody, age of appearance, and titers reached.[285] C3H and CBA/H mice develop autoantibodies to lymphoid cells or to enzyme treated red blood cells as they age.[173] The A strain, hybrids of A, and hybrids of NZB develop antibodies to nucleic acids.[240] Neonatal thymectomy accelerates the appearance of ANA even in strains CBA/H and C3H/UmC, which do not ordinarily develop such antibodies.[240] Although thymus transplants, thymic cells, or lymphoid cells can reverse this acceleration in thymectomized mice, these treatments have no effect on correcting the autoimmunity which accompanies normal aging.[190] One of the longest lived strains, C57Bl/6, shows a relatively high incidence of ANA and thymocytotoxic antibody similar to NZB mice,[46,173] but does not manifest the degree of immunopathology characteristic of NZ mice.

Compared to young controls, old (B10C3)$F_1$ mice showed a greatly depressed in vitro response to the trinitrophenyl (TNP) hapten after in vivo TNP-SRBC immunization, but no depression if the immunization was done with TNP-MRBC.[329] Thus the response to nonself declined with age but that to modified self did not.[329] Cross-reactivity to SRBC increased in aged mice after TNP-MRBC, while avidity of TNP antibodies decreased upon TNP-SRBC injection.

When tested against enzyme treated MRBC, in vitro stimulation by the polyclonal activator LPS, of autoantibody-secreting B cells, was increased in 21-month-old C57Bl/6 and (B10C3)$F_1$ but not in BALB/c mice.[330] Cyclophosphamide enhanced the response in young animals, possibly by eliminating suppressor cells and allowing autoreactive cells to manifest, but in old animals cyclophosphamide almost eliminated the response, suggesting the possibility that with age the B cells themselves were affected. There might be different populations of suppressor cells for alloantigens or xenoantigens than for autoantigens.[330]

In a syngeneic GVH assay—quite analogous to an autoimmune situation—Gozes et al.[331] found that spleen cells from 2-year-old C57Bl/6 mice reacted more strongly than cells from young mice. On the other hand, in a semiallogeneic host the old donor cells were less reactive than young cells.

#### *2. Humans*

Autoantibodies are increased in incidence and titer in healthy elderly humans[1,332] and resemble in type those seen in aged long-lived mice. ANA, gastric and thyroid autoantibodies, and rheumatoid factor are most common.[333] They are not necessarily associated with any clinical abnormalities.[334,335] Autoantibodies may be more frequent in women[336] but the great female predominance seen in some of the autoimmune diseases, i.e., SLE, is no longer present.[1] Very late in life the incidence of autoantibodies may decrease[337] suggesting that their presence earlier may correlate with decreased survival. In an unselected population of about 10,000 individuals, a correlation was noted between autoantibodies and subsequent death from vascular disease.[197,338]

In contrast to the above, Pandley et al.[336] maintain that if the human samples are carefully screened and completely healthy, no association is found between antinuclear antibodies and age. Their population was limited to individuals no older than 70 years. If autoantibodies are associated with decreased survival, these "super healthy" persons in their seventh decade might be those destined to live until 90 or 100 years.

Autoantibodies in the normal population may be caused by a variety of circumstances; exposure to a normally sequestered antigen; disturbance caused by a viral infection or inflammatory reaction; decrease in regulatory mechanisms allowing autoreactive cells present to increase or express their potential. The autoantibodies that appear with old age may be directed against the target organs that the immune system normally helps regulate.

Autoantibodies occur with increased frequency in elderly individuals in poor health, but are not necessarily targeted to the organ systems manifesting the clinically apparent decline in vitality.

## VI. CONCLUSIONS

A consensus of similarities and dissimilarities between different autoimmune "models" for accelerated aging and normal aging are given in Table 2. Three separate phenomena require evaluation in considering autoimmunity and aging. The first is that of maturation and education of the immune system (Figure 2) during which xenoreactivity develops while autoreactivity is eliminated. The generation of diversity in the system and the fine tuning and constant self regulation at all levels in development permit immune responses to substances in the context of self antigens, and permit collaboration between different cell types through their surface antigens, yet still control against the development of autoimmune disease.

The second phenomenon, aging of the immune system, is characterized by a severe depression of responses to foreign antigens, with an increase in autoimmune reactivities. One of the most significant features of old age is the increase in variability.

The third consideration is the short-lived autoimmune strains of mice. To what extent do they really represent models of accelerated aging? It may be that they serve as accelerated aging models for a subgroup of the normally aging. Autoimmune parameters during aging might result from a variety of causes, from decontrol at several levels, whereas the disease of NZ mice develops in a consistent pattern. Thus, for old animals which develop autoimmunity due to decontrol at the same level as NZ mice, they probably represent a model for accelerated aging.

Most investigators have not looked very early in development for the defect in NZ mice. Returning to the pattern of development shown in Figure 2, the problem in NZ mice may occur at level 1 or 2, whereas most experiments have evaluated the immune system at level 2 and particularly level 3. Viral and genetic contributions to NZ disease might account for thymic malfunction by expression of the virus or genes in the thymus.

In the chronic GVH (Parental$\rightarrow F_1$) reaction, induction of autoimmune disease probably occurs because of disruption of control at level 3 (Figure 2). This might result from the allogeneic effect, which involves the inappropriate collaboration of parental T and $F_1$ B cells.[292] GVH reaction may therefore be regarded as a model for "accelerated aging" for those old mice who develop autoimmunity as a result of deregulation at level 3. GVH reaction is also associated with immunodeficiency.

Deregulation at any of the three different levels in old mice may result in autoimmunity with more or less cross-reactive aspects. For example, at level 3, challenge by a foreign antigen cross-reactive with self determinants may lead to autoimmune disease. Exposure to self components normally sequestered (i.e., sperm) may also lead to an autoimmune reaction. Hyperimmunization may lead to decontrol at level 2, the cells then maturing into effector cells without stimulating the proper feedback control mechanisms. In level 1 (the thymus), involution may allow cells to leave the thymus with more autoreactivity than normal. It appears as if all facets of the system have a certain degree of autoreactivity normally. Lack of control at any level may result in undesirable or enhanced expression of that autoreactivity, with the appearance of a variable number of manifestations of accelerated aging.

## REFERENCES


1. **Walford, R. L.,** *The Immunologic Theory of Aging,* Munksgaard, Copenhagen, 1969.
2. **Walford, R. L., Weindruch, R., Gottesman, S., and Tam, C. F.,** The immunopathology of aging, in *Annual Review of Gerontology and Geriatrics,* Eisdorfer, C., Starr, B., and Christafalo, V. J., Eds., Springer Pub. Co., New York, 1981.
3. **Stites, D., Caldwell, J., Carr, M., and Fudenberg, H.,** Ontogeny of immunity in humans, *Clin. Immunol. Immunopathol.,* 4, 519, 1975.
4. **Moore, M. and Metcalf, D.,** Ontogeny of the hemopoietic system: yolk sac origin of *in vivo* and *in vitro* colony forming cells in the developing mouse embryo, *Br. J. Haematol.,* 18, 279, 1970.
5. **Snell, G.,** T cells, T cell recognition structures and the major histocompatibility complex, *Immunol. Rev.,* 38, 3, 1978.
6. **Szenberg, A. and Warner, N.,** Dissociation of immunological responsiveness in fowls with a hormonally arrested development of lymphoid tissue, *Nature (London),* 194, 146, 1962.
7. **Hammerling, U., Chin, A., and Abbott, J.,** Ontogeny of murine B-lymphocytes: sequence of B-cells, differentiation from surface-immunoglobulin-negative precursors to plasma cells, *Proc. Natl. Acad. Sci. USA,* 73, 2008, 1976.
8. **Mosier, D., Zitron, I., Mond, J., Ahmed, A., Scher, I., and Paul, W.,** Surface immunoglobulin D as a functional receptor for a subclass of B lymphocytes, *Immunol. Rev.,* 37, 89, 1977.
9. **Stout, R. and Herzenberg, L.,** The Fc receptor on thymus-derived lymphocytes. I. Detecting of a subpopulation of murine T lymphocytes bearing the Fc receptor, *J. Exp. Med.,* 142, 611, 1975.
10. **Owen, J.,** The origin and development of lymphocyte populations, in *Ontogeny of Acquired Immunity,* A Ciba Foundation Symposium, Elsevier, London, 1971, 35.
11. **Leckband, E. and Boyse, E.,** Immunocompetent cells among thymocytes: a minor population, *Science,* 172, 1258, 1971.
12. **Shortman, K. and Jackson, H.,** The differentiation of T lymphocytes. I. The proliferation kinetics and interrelationships of subpopulations of mouse thymus cells, *Cell Immunol.,* 12, 230, 1974.
13. **Scheid, M., Boyse, E., Carswell, E., and Old, L.,** Serologically demonstrable alloantigens of the mouse epidermal cells, *J. Exp. Med.,* 135, 938, 1972.
14. **Kruisbeek, A., Krose, T., and Zijlstra, J.,** Increase in T cell mitogen response in rat thymocytes by thymic epithelial culture supernatants, *Eur. J. Immunol.,* 7, 375, 1977.
15. **Komuro, K. and Boyse, E.,** *In vitro* demonstration of thymic hormone in the mouse by conversion of precursor cells into lymphocytes, *Lancet,* 1, 740, 1972.
16. **Stutman, O. and Good, R.,** Thymus hormones, in *Contemp. Top. Immunobiol.,* 2, 299, 1973.
17. **Stutman, O.,** Relationship to the regulation of lymphocytic differentiation: characterization of a T cell precursor in the mouse spleen, *Transplant. Proc.,* 7, 291, 1975.
18. **Cantor, H. and Boyse, E.,** Functional subclasses of T lymphocytes bearing different Ly antigens. I. Generation of functionally distinct T cell subclasses in a differentiative process independent of antigen, *J. Exp. Med.,* 141, 1376, 1975.
19. **Cantor, H. and Boyse, E.,** Functional subclasses of T lymphocytes bearing different Ly antigens. II. Cooperation between subclasses of Ly+ cells in the generation of killer activity, *J. Exp. Med.,* 141, 1390, 1975.

20. **Kisielow, P., Hirst, J., Shiku, H., Beverly, P., Hoffman, M., Boyse, E., and Oettgen, H.,** Ly antigens as markers for functionally distinct subpopulations of thymus-derived lymphocytes of the mouse, *Nature (London),* 253, 219, 1975.
21. **Peck, A., Alter, B., and Lindahl, K.,** Specificity in T cell mediated lympholysis: identical genetic control of the proliferative and effector phases of allogeneic and xenogeneic reactions, *Transplant. Rev.,* 29, 189, 1976.
22. **Cantor, H., Shen, F., and Boyse, E.,** Separation of helper T cells from suppressor T cells expressing different Ly components. II. Activation by antigen: after immunization, antigen-specific suppressor and helper activities are inherent properties of distinct T cell subclasses, *J. Exp. Med.,* 143, 1391, 1976.
23. **Mosier, D., Mathieson, B., and Campbell, P.,** Ly phenotype and mechanism of mouse neonatal suppressor T cells, *J. Exp. Med.,* 146, 59, 1977.
24. **Benacerraf, B. and McDevitt, H.,** The histocompatibility-linked immune response genes, *Science,* 175, 273, 1972.
25. **Hammerling, G., Mauve, G., Goldberg, E., and McDevitt, H.,** Tissue distribution of Ia antigens: Ia on spermatozoa, macrophages and epidermal cells, *Immunogen.,* 1, 428, 1975.
26. **Niederhuber, J. and Frelinger, J.,** Expression of Ia antigens on T and B cells and their relationship to immune response function, *Transplant. Rev.,* 30, 101, 1976.
27. **Julius, M., Simpson, E., and Herzenberg, L.,** A rapid method for the isolation of functional thymus-derived murine lymphocytes, *Eur. J. Immunol.,* 3, 645, 1973.
28. **Raff, M. and Cantor, H.,** Subpopulations of thymus cells and thymus-derived lymphocytes, *Progr. Immunol.,* 1, 83, 1971.
29. **Taniguchi, N., Miyawaki, T., Moriya, N., Nagaoki, T., Kato, E., and Okuda, N.,** Mitogenic responsiveness and monocyte-lymphocyte interaction of early and late rosette-forming cell populations of human peripheral blood lymphocytes, *J. Immunol.,* 118, 193, 1977.
30. **Ferrara, G., Strelkauskas, A., Longo, A., McDowell, J., Yunis, E., and Schlossman, S.,** Markers of human T cell subsets identified by alloantisera, *J. Immunol.,* 123, 1272, 1979.
31. **Hildemann, W. and Cooper, E.,** Phylogeny of transplantation reactions, *Transplant. Proc.,* 2, 179, 1970.
32. **Shortman, K. and Palmer, J.,** The requirement for macrophages in the *in vitro* immune response, *Cell. Immunol.,* 2, 399, 1971.
33. **Catanzaro, P., Schwartz, H., and Graham, R.,** Spectrum and possible mechanism of carrageenan cytotoxicity, *Am. J. Pathol.,* 64, 387, 1971.
34. **Bach, F.,** Genetics of transplantation: the major histocompatibility complex, *Annu. Rev. Genet.,* 10, 319, 1976.
35. **Benacerraf, B. and Dorf, M.,** The nature and function of specific H-linked response genes and immune suppression genes, in *The Role of Products of the Histocompatibility Gene Complex in Immune Responses,* Katz, D. and Benacerraf, B., Eds., Academic Press, New York, 1976, 225.
36. **Benacerraf, B. and Germain, R.,** The immune response genes of the major histocompatibility complex, *Immunol. Rev.,* 38, 70, 1978.
37. **Shreffler, D. and David, C.,** The H-2 histocompatibility complex and the I immune response region's genetic variation, function, and organization, *Adv. Immunol.,* 20, 125, 1975.
38. **Lilly, F.,** Multigene control of disease susceptibility, in *Genetic Control of Immune Responsiveness,* McDevitt, H. and Landy, M., Eds., Academic Press, New York, 1972, 279.
39. **Smith, G. and Walford, R.,** Influence of the H-2 and H-1 histocompatibility systems upon lifespan and spontaneous cancer incidence in congeneic mice, in *Genetic Effects on Aging, Birth Defects: Original Article Series,* Bergsma, D. and Harrison, D., Eds., March of Dimes, New York, 1978, 281.
40. **Knight, J. and Adams, D.,** Three genes for lupus nephritis in NZB × NZW mice, *J. Exp. Med.,* 147, 1653, 1978.
41. **Mishell, R. and Dutton, R.,** Immunization of dissociated spleen cell cultures from normal mice, *J. Exp. Med.,* 126, 423, 1967.
42. **Baker, P., Barth, R., Stashak, P., and Amsbaugh, D.,** Enhancement of the antibody response to type 3 pneumococcal polysaccharide in mice treated with antilymphocyte serum, *J. Immunol.,* 104, 1313, 1970.
43. **Jones, J. and Kind, P.,** Enhancing effect of bacterial endotoxins on bone marrow cells in the immune response to SRBC, *J. Immunol.,* 108, 1453, 1972.
44. **Makinodan, T., Perkins, E., Shekarchi, I., and Gengozian, N.,** Use of lethally irradiated isologous mice as *in vitro* tissue cultures of antibody-forming cells, in *Mechanisms of Antibody Formation,* Holub, M. and Jaroskova, L., Eds., Publ. House of Czechoslovak Academy Science, Prague, 1960, 182.
45. **Wu, A., Till, J., Siminovitch, L., and McCulloch, E.,** Cytological evidence for a relationship between normal haematopoietic colony-forming cells and cells of the lymphoid system, *J. Exp. Med.,* 127, 455, 1968.

46. **Makinodan, T.**, Immunity and aging, in *Handbook of the Biology of Aging,* Finch, C. and Hayflick, L., Eds., Van Nostrand Reinhold Co., New York, 1977, 379.
47. **Sigal, N. and Klinman, N.**, The B-cell clonotype repertoire, *Adv. Immunol.,* 26, 255, 1978.
48. **Alter, B., Schendel, D., Bach, M., Bach, F., Klein, J., and Stimpfling, J.**, Cell mediated lympholysis: importance of serologically defined H-2 regions, *J. Exp. Med.,* 137, 1303, 1973.
49. **Schendel, D. and Bach, F.**, Genetic control of cell-mediated lympholysis in mouse, *J. Exp. Med.,* 140, 1534, 1974.
50. **Bach, F., Grillot-Courvalin, C., Kuperman, O., Sollinger, H., Hayes, C., Sondel, P., Alter, B., and Bach, M.**, Antigenic requirements for triggering of cytotoxic T lymphocytes, *Immunol. Rev.,* 35, 76, 1977.
51. **Stout, R., Murphy, D., McDevitt, H., and Herzenberg, L.**, The Fc receptor on thymus-derived lymphocytes. IV. Inhibition of binding of antigen-antibody complexes to Fc receptor-positive T cells by anti-Ia sera, *J. Exp. Med.,* 145, 187, 1977.
52. **Bach, F., Bach, M., and Sondel, P.**, Differential function of major histocompatibility complex antigens in T-lymphocyte activation, *Nature (London),* 259, 253, 1976.
53. **Wagner, H., Gotze, D., Ptschelinzew, L., and Rollinghoff, M.**, Induction of cytotoxic T lymphocytes against I region coded determinants. I. *In vitro* evidence for a third histocompatibility locus in the mouse, *J. Exp. Med.,* 142, 1477, 1975.
54. **Gerbase-DeLima, M. and Walford, R.**, Effect of cortisone in delineating thymus cell subsets in advanced age, *Proc. Soc. Exp. Biol. Med.,* 149, 562, 1975.
55. **Rich, S. and Rich, R.**, Regulatory mechanisms in cell-mediated immune responses. I. Regulation of mixed lymphocyte reactions by alloantigen-activated thymus-derived lymphocytes, *J. Exp. Med.,* 140, 1588, 1975.
56. **Rode, H., Uotila, M., and Gordon, J.**, Regulation of the mixed lymphocyte culture by suppressor cells, *Eur. J. Immunol.,* 84, 213, 1978.
57. **Okumura, K., Herzenberg, L., Murphy, D., McDevitt, H., and Herzenberg, L.**, Selective expression of H-2 (I-region) loci controlling determinants on helper and suppressor T lymphocytes, *J. Exp. Med.,* 144, 685, 1976.
58. **Tse, H. and Dutton, R.**, Separation of helper and suppressor T lymphocytes. III. Positive and negative effects of MLR activated T cells, *J. Immunol.,* 120, 1149, 1978.
59. **Bevan, M., Epstein, R., and Cohn, M.**, Effect of 2-mercaptoethanol on murine mixed lymphocyte cultures, *J. Exp. Med.,* 139, 1025, 1974.
60. **Danossy, G. and Greaves, M.**, Lymphocyte activation. II. Discriminating stimulation of lymphocyte subpopulations by phytomitogens and heterologous anti-lymphocyte sera, *Clin. Exp. Immunol.,* 10, 525, 1972.
61. **Andersson, J., Moller, G., and Sjoberg, O.**, Selective induction of DNA synthesis in T and B lymphocytes, *Cell Immunol.,* 4, 381, 1972.
62. **Stobo, J. and Paul, W.**, Functional heterogeneity of murine lymphoid cells. III. Differential responsiveness of T cells to phytohemagglutinin and concanavalin A as a probe for T cell subsets, *J. Immunol.,* 110, 362, 1973.
63. **Watanabe, T., Fathman, C., and Coutinho, A.**, T cells which proliferate in response to Con A included cells which proliferate in the mixed lymphocyte culture, *Eur. J. Immunol.,* 7, 603, 1977.
64. **Jandiniski, J., Cantor, H., Tadakuma, T., Peavy, D., and Pierce, C.**, Separation of helper T cells from suppressor T cells expressing different Ly components. I. Polyclonal activation: suppressor and helper activities are inherent properties of distinct T-cell subclasses, *J. Exp. Med.,* 143, 1382, 1976.
65. **Billingham, R.**, The biology of graft-versus-host reactions, *Harvey Lect.,* 62, 21, 1966.
66. **Tigelaar, R., Gershon, R., and Asofsky, R.**, Graft-versus-host reactivity of mouse thymocytes: effect of *in vitro* treatment with anti-TL serum, *Cell. Immunol.,* 19, 58, 1975.
67. **Nagino, H., Nomoto, K., Kuroiwa, A., Miyazaki, S., Goya, N., and Takeya, K.**, Experimental models for prevention of graft-versus-host reaction in bone marrow transfusion. II. Inability to prevent GVH reaction in an H-2 identical combination, *Int. Arch. Allergy Appl. Immunol.,* 56, 48, 1978.
68. **Huber, B., Devinsky, O., Gershon, R., and Cantor, H.**, Cell mediated immunity: delayed type hypersensitivity and cytotoxic responses are mediated by different T cell subclasses, *J. Exp. Med.,* 143, 1534, 1976.
69. **Phillips, S., Carpenter, C., and Merrill, J.**, Cellular immunity in the mouse. II. Correlation of *in vivo* and *in vitro* phenomenon, *Cell. Immunol.,* 5, 235, 1972.
70. **Crowle, A.**, Delayed hypersensitivity in the mouse, *Adv. Immunol.,* 20, 197, 1975.
71. **Klein, J., Hauptfeld, V., and Hauptfeld, M.**, Involvement of H-2 regions in immune reactions, in *Progress in Immunology II,* Brent, L. and Holborow, J., Eds., Academic Press, New York, 1974, 797.

72. **Herberman, R., Nunn, M., Holden, H., and Lavrin, D.,** Natural cytotoxic reactivity of mouse lymphocyte cells against syngeneic and allogeneic tumors. I. Characterization of effector cells, *Int. J. Cancer,* 16, 230, 1975.
73. **Eardley, D., Kemp, J., Shen, F., Cantor, H., and Gershon, R.,** Immunoregulatory circuits among T cell sets: effect of mode of immunization on determining which Lyl T cell sets will be activated, *J. Immunol.,* 122, 1663, 1979.
74. **Eardley, D., Hugenberger, J., McVay-Boudreau, L., Shen, F., Gershon, R., and Cantor, H.,** Immunoregulatory circuits among T cell sets. I. T helper cells induce other T cell sets to exert feedback inhibition, *J. Exp. Med.,* 1106, 1978.
75. **Elliott, E.,** A persistent lymphoid cell population in the thymus, *Nature (New Biol.),* 242, 150, 1973.
76. **Burnet, F.,** Role of the thymus and related organs in immunity, *Br. Med. J.,* 2, 807, 1962.
77. **Jerne, N.,** The somatic generation of immune recognition, *Eur. J. Immunol.,* 1, 1, 1971.
78. **Streilin, J.,** Neonatal tolerance: towards an immunogenetic definition of self, *Immunol. Rev.,* 46, 125, 1979.
79. **Dresser, D.,** Tolerance induction as a model for cell differentiation, *Br. Med. Bull.,* 32, 147, 1976.
80. **Zinkernagel, R. and Doherty, P.,** Immunological surveillance against altered self components by sensitized T lymphocytes in lymphocytic choriomeningitis, *Nature (London),* 251, 547, 1974.
81. **Zinkernagel, R. and Doherty, P.,** H-2 compatibility requirement for T cell-mediated lysis of target cells infected with lymphocytic choriomeningitis virus. Different cytotoxic T cell specificities are associated with structures coded in H-2 K or H-2 D, *J. Exp. Med.,* 141, 1427, 1975.
82. **Bevan. M.,** In a radiation chimera, host H-2 antigens determine immune responsiveness of donor cytotoxic cells, *Nature (London),* 269, 417, 1977.
83. **Shearer, G., Rehn, T., and Schmitt-Verhulst, A.,** Role of the murine major histocompatibility complex in the specificity of *in vitro* T cell mediated lympholysis against chemically modified autologous lymphocytes, *Transplant. Rev.,* 29, 222, 1976.
84. **Sprent, J.,** Restricted helper function of $F_1$-parent bone marrow chimeras controlled by K-end of H-2 complex, *J. Exp. Med.,* 147, 1838, 1978.
85. **Katz, D., Katz, L., Bogowitz, C., and Skidmore, B.,** Adaptive differentiation of murine lymphocytes. II. The thymic microenvironment does not restrict the cooperative partner cell preference of helper T cells differentiating in $F_1 \rightarrow F_1$ thymic chimeras, *J. Exp. Med.,* 149, 1360, 1979.
86. **Stutman, O.,** Intrathymic and extrathymic T cell maturation, *Immunol. Rev.,* 42, 138, 1978.
87. **Zinkernagel, R., Callahan, G., Klein, J., and Donnert, G.,** Cytotoxic T cells learn specificity for self H-2 during differentiation in the thymus, *Nature (London),* 271, 251, 1978.
88. **Walford, R.,** When is a mouse "old"? *J. Immunol.,* 117, 352, 1976.
89. **Meredith, P. and Walford, R.,** Effect of age on response to T- and B-mitogens in mice congenic at the H-2 locus, *Immunogen.,* 5, 109, 1977.
90. **Hirokawa, K.,** Age-related changes of the thymus-morphological and functional aspects, *Acta. Pathol. Jpn.,* 28, 843, 1978.
91. **Makinodan, T.,** The thymus in aging, *Aging,* 5, 217, 1978.
92. **Burnet, F.,** An immunological approach to aging, *Lancet,* 1, 358, 1970.
93. **Hirokawa, K. and Makinodan, T.,** Thymic involution: effect on T cell differentiation, *J. Immunol.,* 114, 1659, 1975.
94. **Stutman, O., Yunis, E., and Good, R.,** Studies of thymus function. III. Duration of thymic function, *J. Exp. Med.,* 135, 339, 1972.
95. **Stutman, O. and Good, R.,** Duration of thymic function, *Ser. Haematol.,* 7, 505, 1974.
96. **Yunis, E., Fernandes, G., Teague, P., Stutman, O., and Good, R.,** The thymus, autoimmunity, and the involution of the lymphoid system, in *Tolerance, Autoimmunity, and Aging,* Sigel, M. and Good, R., Eds., Charles C Thomas, Springfield, Ill., 1972, 3.
97. **Bach, J., Papiernik, M., Levasseur, P., Dardenne, M., Barois, A., and LeBrigand, H.,** Evidence for a serum factor secreted by the human thymus, *Lancet,* 2, 1056, 1972.
98. **Twomey, J., Goldstein, G., Lewis, V., Bealmear, P., and Good, R.,** Bioassay determination of thymopoietin and thymic hormone levels in human plasma, *Proc. Natl. Acad. Sci. USA,* 74, 2541, 1977.
99. **Bach, M. and Beaurain, G.,** Respective influence of extrinsic and intrinsic factors on the age-related decrease of thymic secretion, *J. Immunol.,* 122, 2505, 1979.
100. **Stutman, O.,** Humoral thymic factors influencing post thymic cells, *Ann. N.Y. Acad. Sci.,* 249, 89, 1975.
101. **Stutman, O.,** Lymphocyte subpopulations in NZB mice: deficit of thymus-dependent lymphocytes, *J. Immunol.,* 109, 602, 1972.
102. **Kay, M. and Makinodan, T.,** Immunobiology of aging: evaluation of current status, *Clin. Immunol. Immunopathol.,* 6, 394, 1976.
103. **Adler, W. and Nagel, J.,** Studies of immune function in a human population, in *Immunological Aspects of Aging,* Segre, D. and Smith, L., Eds., Dekker, New York, 1980.

104. **Olsson, L. and Claesson, M.**, Studies on subpopulations of 0 bearing lymphoid cells, *Nature (New Biol.)*, 244, 50, 1973.
105. **Carosella, E., Mochanko, K., and Braun, M.**, Rosette-forming T cells in human peripheral blood at different ages, *Cell. Immunol.*, 12, 323, 1974.
106. **Brennan, P. and Jaroslow, B.**, Age-associated decline in theta antigen on spleen thymus-derived lymphocytes, *Cell. Immunol.*, 15, 51, 1975.
107. **Meredith, P., Gerbase-DeLima, M., and Walford, R.**, Age-related changes in the PHA:Con A stimulatory ratios of cells from spleens of a long-lived mouse strain, *Exp. Gerontol.*, 10, 247, 1975.
108. **Cantor, H., McVay-Boudreau, L., Hugenberger, J., Naidorf, K., Shen, F., and Gershon, R.**, Immunoregulatory circuits among T-cell sets. II. Physiologic role of feedback inhibition in vivo, *J. Exp. Med.*, 147, 1116, 1978.
109. **Kishimoto, S., Tomino, S., Inomata, K., Kotegawa, S., Saito, T., Kuroki, M., Mitsuya, H., and Hisamitsu, S.**, Age-related changes in the subsets and functions of human T lymphocytes, *J. Immunol.*, 121, 1773, 1978.
110. **Diaz-Jouanen, E., Strickland, R., and Williams, R.**, Studies of human lymphocytes in the newborn and the aged, *Am. J. Med.*, 58, 620, 1975.
111. **Haaijman, J. and Hijmans, W.**, Influence of age on the immunological activity and capacity of CBA mouse, *Mech. Ageing Dev.*, 7, 375, 1978.
112. **Woda, B., Yguerabide, J., and Feldman, J.**, Mobility and density of AgB, "Ia", and Fc receptors on the surface of lymphocytes from young and old rats, *J. Immunol.*, 123, 2161, 1979.
113. **Haaijman, J., Van Den Berg, P., and Brinkhof, J.**, Immunoglobulin class and subclass levels in the serum of CBA mice throughout life, *Immunology*, 32, 923, 1976.
114. **Hayflick, L.**, The limited *in vitro* lifetime of human diploid cell strains, *Exp. Cell. Res.*, 37, 614, 1965.
115. **Chen, A.**, Age related changes in hematopoietic stem cell populations of a long-lived mouse, *J. Cell. Physiol.*, 78, 225, 1971.
116. **Harrison, D., Astle, C., and DeLaittre, J.**, Loss of proliferative capacity in immunohemopoietic stem cells caused by serial transplantation rather than aging, *J. Exp. Med.*, 147, 1526, 1978.
117. **Harrison, D.**, Proliferative capacity of erythropoietic stem cell lines and aging: an overview, *Mech. Ageing Dev.*, 9, 409, 1979.
118. **Davis, M., Upton, A., and Satterfield, L.**, Growth and senescence of the bone marrow stem cell pool in RFM/Un mice, *Proc. Soc. Exp. Biol. Med.*, 137, 1452, 1971.
119. **Trentin, J.**, Determination of bone marrow stem cell differentiation by stromal hemopoietic inductive microenvironments (HIM), *Am. J. Pathol.*, 65, 621, 1971.
120. **Deitchman, J. and Makinodan, T.**, Effect of age on the rate of proliferation of lymphohematopoietic stem cells, *Proc. 10th Int. Congr. Gerontol.*, 2, 12, 1975.
121. **Harrison, D.**, Normal function of transplanted marrow cell lines from aged mice, *J. Gerontol.*, 30, 279, 1975.
122. **Albright, J. and Makinodan, T.**, Growth and senescence of antibody-forming cells, *J. Cell. Physiol.*, 67, 185, 1966.
123. **Price, G. and Makinodan, T.**, Immunologic deficiencies in senescence. II. Characterization of extrinsic deficiencies, *J. Immunol.*, 108, 413, 1972.
124. **Harrison, D., Astle, C., and Doubleday, J.**, Stem cell lines from old immunodeficient donors give normal responses in young recipients, *J. Immunol.*, 118, 1223, 1977.
125. **Popp, D. and Popp, R.**, Hemopoietic stem cell heterogeneity: use of cell cycle-specific drugs to look for age-associated alterations, *Mech. Ageing Dev.*, 9, 441, 1979.
126. **Makinodan, T., Good, R., and Kay, M.**, Cellular basis of immunosenescence, in *Immunology and Aging*, Makinodan, T. and Yunis, E., Eds., Plenum Press, New York, 1977.
127. **Makinodan, T. and Adler, W.**, The effects of aging on the differentiation and proliferation potentials of cells of the immune system, *Fed. Proc. Fed. Am. Soc. Exp. Biol.*, 34, 153, 1975.
128. **Gerbase-DeLima, M., Wilkinson, J., Smith, G., and Walford, R.**, Age-related decline in thymic independent immune function in a long-lived mouse strain, *J. Gerontol.*, 29, 261, 1974.
129. **Mathies, M., Lipps, L., Smith, G., and Walford, R.**, Age-related decline in response to phytohemagglutinin and pokeweed mitogen by spleen cells from hamsters and a long-lived mouse strain, *J. Gerontol.*, 28, 425, 1973.
130. **Kruisbeek, A.**, Age-related changes in Con A and LPS-induced lymphocyte transformation. I. Effect of culture conditions on mitogen response of blood and spleen lymphocytes from young and aged rats, *Mech. Ageing Dev.*, 5, 125, 1976.
131. **Callard, B., Basten, A., and Waters, L.**, Immune function in aged mice. II. B-cell function, *Cell. Immunol.*, 31, 26, 1977.
132. **Andersson, J., Coutinho, A., and Melchers, F.**, Frequencies of mitogen-reactive B cells in the mouse. I. Distribution on different lymphoid organs from different inbred strains of mice at different ages, *J. Ex. Med.*, 145, 1511, 1977.

133. **Makinodan, T. and Peterson, W.,** Growth and senescence of the primary antibody forming potential of the spleen, *J. Immunol.,* 93, 886, 1964.
134. **Kishimoto, S. and Yamamura, Y.,** Immune responses in aged mice: changes of antibody-forming cell precursors and antigen-reacting cells with ageing, *Clin. Exp. Immunol.,* 8, 957, 1971.
135. **Goodman, S., Chen, M., and Makinodan, T.,** An improved primary response from mouse spleen cells cultured *in vivo* in diffusion chambers, *J. Immunol.,* 104, 148, 1972.
136. **Williamson, A. and Askonas, B.,** Senescence of an antibody-forming cell clone, *Nature (London),* 238, 337, 1972.
137. **Makinodan, T. and Albright, J.,** Restoration of impaired immune functions in aging animals. III. Effect of mercaptoethanol in enhancing the reduced primary antibody responsiveness *in vivo, Mech. Ageing Dev.,* 11, 1, 1979.
138. **Nordin, A. and Adler, W.,** The effect of aging on *in vitro* cellular interactions, in *Developmental Immunobiology,* Siskind, G., Litwin, S., and Weksler, M., Eds. Grune & Stratton, New York, 1979, 215.
139. **Price, G. and Makinodan, T.,** Immunologic deficiencies in senescence. I. Characterization of intrinsic deficiencies, *J. Immunol.,* 108, 403, 1972.
140. **Goidl, E., Innes, J., and Weksler, M.,** Immunologic studies of aging. II. Loss of IgG and high avidity plaque-forming cells and increased suppressor cell activity in aging mice, *J. Exp. Med.,* 144, 1037, 1976.
141. **Segre, D. and Segre, M.,** Age-related changes in B and T lymphocytes and decline of humoral immune responsiveness in aged mice, *Mech. Ageing Dev.,* 6, 115, 1977.
142. **Friedman, D. and Globerson, A.,** Immune reactivity during aging. I. T-helper dependent and independent antibody responses to different antigens, *in vivo* and *in vitro, Mech. Ageing Dev.,* 7, 289, 1978.
143. **Krogsrud, R. and Perkins, E.,** Age-related changes in T cell function, *J. Immunol.,* 118, 1607, 1977.
144. **Friedman, D. and Globerson, A.,** Immune reactivity during aging. II. Analysis of the cellular mechanisms involved in the deficient antibody response in old mice, *Mech. Ageing Dev.,* 7, 299, 1978.
145. **Makinodan, T., Albright, J., Good, P., Peter, C., and Heidrick, M.,** Reduced humoral immune activity in long-lived mice: an approach to elucidating its mechanisms, *Immunology,* 31, 903, 1976.
146. **Finger, J. and Hof, F.,** Influence of pertussis vaccine and bacterial endotoxin on blood leukocyte counts and numbers of pre-existing antibody-forming cells in aged mice, *Gerontologia,* 18, 63, 1972.
147. **Chino, F. and Makinodan, T.,** Relationship between immunologic activity and pathology of aged mice, *Fed. Proc. Fed. Am. Soc. Exp. Biol.,* 29, 896, 1968.
148. **Heidrick, M.,** Age-related changes in hydrolase activity of peritoneal macrophages, *Gerontologist,* 12, 28, 1972.
149. **Heidrick, M. and Makinodan, T.,** Presence of impairment of humoral immunity in nonadherent spleen cells of old mice, *J. Immunol.,* 111, 1502, 1973.
150. **Aoki, T., Teller, M., and Robitaille, M.,** Aging and carcinogenesis. II. Effect of age on phagocytic activity of the reticuloendothelial system and on tumor growth, *J. Natl. Canc. Inst.,* 34, 255, 1965.
151. **Cantrell, W. and Elko, E.,** Effect of age on phagocytosis of carbon in the rat, *Exp. Parasitol.,* 34, 337, 1973.
152. **Aoki, T. and Teller, M.,** Aging and cancerigeneis. III. Effect of age on isoantibody formation, *Cancer Res.,* 26, 1648, 1966.
153. **Hori, Y., Perkins, E., and Halsall, M.,** Decline in phytohemagglutinin responsiveness of spleen cells from aging mice, *Proc. Soc. Exp. Biol. Med.,* 144, 48, 1973.
154. **Inkeles, B., Innes, J., Kuntz, M., Kadish, A., and Weksler, M.,** Immunological studies of aging. III. Cytokinetic basis for the impaired response of lymphocytes from aged humans to plant lectins, *J. Exp. Med.,* 145, 1176, 1977.
155. **Weksler, M. and Hutteroth, T.,** Impaired lymphocyte function in aged humans, *J. Clin. Invest.,* 53, 99, 1974.
156. **Hung, C., Perkins, E., and Yang, W.,** Age-related refractoriness of PHA-induced lymphocyte transformation. I. Comparable sensitivity of spleen cells from young and old mice to culture conditions, *Mech. Ageing Dev.,* 4, 29, 1975.
157. **Callard, R. and Basten, A.,** Immune function in aged mice. I. T-cell responsiveness using phytohemagglutinin as a functional probe, *Cell. Immunol.,* 31, 13, 1977.
158. **Hung, C., Perkins, E., and Yang, W.,** Age-related refractoriness of PHA-induced lymphocyte transformation. II. $^{125}$I-PHA binding to spleen cells from young and old mice, *Mech. Ageing Dev.,* 4, 103, 1975.
159. **Abraham, C., Tal, Y., and Gershon, H.,** Reduced *in vitro* response to concanavalin A and lipopolysaccharide in senescent mice: a function of reduced number of responding cells, *Eur. J. Immunol.,* 7, 301, 1977.

160. **Tice, R., Schneider, E., Kram, D., and Thorne, P.,** Cytokinetic analysis of the impaired proliferative response of peripheral lymphocytes from aged humans to phytohemagglutinin, *J. Exp. Med.,* 149, 1029, 1979.
161. **Tam, C. and Walford, R.,** Cyclic nucleotide levels in resting and mitogen-stimulated cell suspensions from young and old mice, *Mech. Ageing Dev.,* 7, 309, 1978.
162. **Konen, T., Smith, G., and Walford, R.,** Decline in mixed lymphocyte reactivity of spleen cells from aged mice of a long-lived strain, *J. Immunol.,* 110, 1216, 1973.
163. **Merhav, S. and Gershon, H.,** The mixed lymphocyte response of senescent mice: sensitivity to alloantigen and cell replication time, *Cell. Immunol.,* 34, 354, 1977.
164. **Walters, C. and Claman, H.,** Age-related changes in cell-mediated immunity in BALB/c mice, *J. Immunol.,* 115, 1438, 1975.
165. **Gerbase-DeLima, M., Meredith, P., and Walford, R.,** Age-related changes, including synergy and suppression, in the mixed lymphocyte reaction in long-lived mice, *Fed. Proc. Fed. Am. Soc. Exp. Biol.,* 34, 159, 1975.
166. **Meredith, P., Tittor, W., Gerbase-DeLima, M., and Walford, R.,** Age-related changes in the cellular immune response of lymph node and thymus cells in long-lived mice, *Cell. Immunol.,* 18, 324, 1975.
167. **Menon, M., Jaroslow, B., and Keosterer, R.,** The decline of cell-mediated immunity in aging mice, *J. Gerontol.,* 29, 449, 1974.
168. **Goodman, S. and Makinodan, T.,** Effect of age on cell-mediated immunity in long-lived mice, *Clin. Exp. Immunol.,* 19, 533, 1975.
169. **Shigemoto, S., Kishimoto, S., and Yamamura, Y.,** Change of cell-mediated cytotoxicity with aging, *J. Immunol.,* 115, 307, 1975.
170. **Bach, M.,** Lymphocyte mediated cytotoxicity. Effects of aging, adult thymectomy, and thymic factor, *J. Immunol.,* 119, 641, 1977.
171. **Bach, M.,** Influence of aging on T-cell subpopulations involved in the *in vitro* generation of allogeneic cytotoxicity, *Clin. Immunol. Immunopathol.,* 13, 220, 1979.
172. **Kishimoto, S., Shigemoto, S., and Yamamura, Y.,** Immune response in aged mice. Change of cell-mediated immunity with aging, *Transplantation,* 15, 455, 1973.
173. **Stutman, O.,** Cell-mediated immunity and aging, *Fed. Proc. Fed. Am. Soc. Exp. Biol.,* 33, 2028, 1974.
174. **Perkins, E. and Cacheiro, L.,** A multi-parameter comparison of immunocompetence and tumor resistance in aged BALB/c mice, *Mech. Ageing Dev.,* 6, 15, 1977.
175. **Gozes, Y. and Trainin, N.,** Enhancement of Lewis lung carcinoma in a syngeneic host by spleen cells of C57B1/6 old mice, *Eur. J. Immunol.,* 7, 159, 1977.
176. **Doherty, P.,** Diminished T cell surveillance function in old mice infected with lymphocyte choriomeningitis virus, *Immunology,* 32, 751, 1977.
177. **Kay, M.,** Long-term subclinical effects of parainfluenza (SENDAI) infection on immune cells of aging mice, *Proc. Soc. Exp. Biol. Med.,* 158, 326, 1978.
178. **Heine, K., Stobbe, H., Klatt, R., Sahi, J., and Herrmann, H.,** Lymphocyte function in the aged, *Heinetica Med. Acta,* 35, 484, 1969.
179. **Girard, J., Paychere, M., Clievas, M., and Fernandes, B.,** Cell-mediated immunity in an ageing population, *Clin. Exp. Immunol.,* 27, 85, 1977.
180. **Smith, A.,** The effects of age on the immune response to Type III pneumococcal polysaccharide (SIII) and bacterial lipopolysaccharide (LPS) in BALB/c, SJL/J, and C3H mice, *J. Immunol.,* 116, 469, 1976.
181. **Segre, D., and Segre, M.,** Humoral immunity in aged mice. II. Increased suppressor T cell activity in immunologically deficient old mice, *J. Immunol.* 116, 735, 1976.
182. **Segre, D., Greeley, E., and Segre, M.,** Cyclophosphamide induction of non-T suppressor cells and their possible role in self tolerance, in *Immunological Aspects of Aging,* Segre, D. and Smith, L., Eds., Dekker, New York, 1980.
183. **Gershon, R. and Metzler, C.,** Suppressor cells in aging, in *Immunology and Aging,* Makinodan, T. and Yunis, E., Eds., Plenum Press, New York, 1977, 103.
184. **Hallgren, H. and Yunis, E.,** Suppressor lymphocytes in young and aged humans, *J. Immunol.,* 118, 2004, 1977.
185. **Kishimoto, S., Tomino, S., Mitsuya, H., and Fujiwara, H.,** Age-related changes in suppressor functions of human T cells, *J. Immunol.,* 123, 1586, 1979.
186. **Spellman, C. and Daynes, R.,** Immunoregulation by ultraviolet light. III. Enhancement of suppressor cell activity in older animals, *Exp. Gerontol.,* 13, 141, 1978.
187. **Mitsuoka, A., Morikawa, S., Baba, M., and Harada, T.,** Cyclophosphamide eliminates suppressor T cells in age-associated central regulation of delayed hypersensitivity in mice, *J. Exp. Med.,* 149, 1018, 1979.

188. **Roupe, G. and Lindholm, L.**, Demonstration of a thymus-derived, splenic suppressor cell responsible for the age-dependent decrease in contact hypersensitivity in the adult mouse, *J. Invest. Dermatol.*, 72, 178, 1979.
189. **Kay, M.**, Autoimmune disease: the consequence of deficient T-cell function? *J. Am. Geriatr. Soc.*, 24, 253, 1976.
190. **Good, R. and Yunis, E.**, Association of autoimmunity, immunodeficiency, and aging in man, rabbits and mice, *Fed. Proc. Fed. Am. Soc. Exp. Biol.*, 33, 2040, 1974.
191. **Petty, R., Palmer, N., Cassidy, J., Tubergen, D., and Sullivan, D.**, The association of autoimmune diseases and anti-IgA antibodies in patients with selective IgA deficiency, *Clin. Exp. Immunol.*, 37, 83, 1979.
192. **Spector, B.**, Immunodeficiency-cancer registry: 1975 update, in *Genetics of Human Cancer*, Mulvihill, J., Miller, R., and Fraumeni, F., Eds., Raven Press, New York, 1977, 339.
193. **Walford, R.**, Antibody diversity, histocompatibility systems, disease states, and ageing, *Lancet*, 2, 1226, 1970.
194. **Talal, N.**, Immunological and viral factors in autoimmune disease, *Med. Clin. North Am.*, 61, 205, 1977.
195. **Weigle, W.**, Cyclical production of antibody as a regulatory mechanism in the immune response, *Adv. Immunol.*, 21, 87, 1975.
196. **Talal, N.**, Autoimmunity and the immunologic network, *Arthritis Rheum.*, 21, 853, 1978.
197. **Mackay, I.**, Ageing and immunological function in man, *Gerontologia*, 18, 285, 1972.
198. **Talal, N.**, Disordered immunologic regulation and autoimmunity, *Transplant. Rev.*, 31, 240, 1976.
199. **Howie, J. and Helyer, B.**, The immunology and pathology of NZB Mice, *Adv. Immunol.*, 9, 215, 1968.
200. **McCombs, C., Hom, J., Talal, N., and Mishell, R.**, Functional deficiency of splenic adherent cells in New Zealand Black Mice, *J. Immunol.*, 115, 1695, 1975.
201. **Lehman, D., Wilson, C., and Dixon, F.**, Increased survival times of New Zealand hybrid mice immunosuppressed by graft-versus-host reactions, *Clin. Exp. Immunol.*, 25, 297, 1976.
202. **Papoian, R., Pillarisetty, R., and Talal, N.**, Immunological regulation of spontaneous antibodies to DNA and RNA. II. Sequential switch from IgM to IgG in NZB/NZW $F_1$ mice, *Immunology*, 32, 75, 1977.
203. **Roubinian, J., Papoian, R., and Talal, N.**, Androgenic hormones modulate autoantibody responses and improve survival in murine lupus, *J. Clin. Invest.*, 59, 1066, 1977.
204. **Mellors, R. and Huang, C.**, Immunopathology of NZB/Bl mice. V. Virus-like (filtrable) agent separable from lyphoma cells and identifiable by electron microscopy, *J. Exp. Med.*, 124, 1031, 1966.
205. **Izui, S., McConahey, P., Theofilopoulos, A., and Dixon, F.**, Association of circulating retroviral gp70-anti-gp 70 immune complexes with murine systemic lupus erythromatosus, *J. Exp. Med.*, 149, 1099, 1979.
206. **Lambert, P. and Dixon, F.**, Pathogenesis of the glomerulonephritis of NZB/W mice, *J. Exp. Med.*, 127, 507, 1968.
207. **Yunis, E., Fernandes, G., and Greenberg, L.**, Tumor immunology, autoimmunity, and aging, *J. Am. Geriatr. Soc.*, 24, 258, 1976.
208. **Howie, J. and Simpson, L.**, Autoimmune hemolytic disease in NZB mice, *Ser. Haematol.*, 7, 386, 1974.
209. **Russell, P., Hicks, J., Boston, L., and Abbot, A.**, Failure to transfer haemolytic anemia or glomerulonephritis with cell-free material from NZB mice, *Clin. Exp. Immunol.*, 6, 227, 1970.
210. **Mellors, R. C.**, Immunological and virological aspects of leukemia lymphoma experimental murine model and its clinical relevance, in *Proceedings of the International Conference on Leukemia-Lymphoma*, Lea & Febinger, Philadelphia, Pa., 1968, 203.
211. **Raveche, E., Steinberg, A., Klassen, L., and Tjio, J.**, Genetic studies in NZB mice. I. Spontaneous autoantibody production, *J. Exp. Med.*, 147, 1487, 1978.
212. **Fernandes, G., Yunis, E., and Good, R.**, Age and genetic influence in NZB and autoimmune-resistant mice, *Clin. Immunol. Immunopathol.*, 6, 318, 1976.
213. **Knight, J., Adams, D., and Purves, J.**, Genetic contribution of the NZB mouse to the renal disease of the NZB × NZW hybrid, *Clin. Exp. Immunol.*, 28, 352, 1977.
214. **Murphy, E. and Roths, J.**, A single gene model for massive lymphoproliferation with immune complex disease in new mouse strain MRL, in *Proc. 16th Int. Congr. Hematol.*, Amsterdam, Excerpta Medica, 1976, 69.
215. **Murphy, E. and Roths, J.**, New inbred strains, *Mouse News Lett.*, 58, 51, 1978.
216. **Cerrottini, J., Lambert, P., and Dixon, F.**, Comparison of the immune responsiveness of NZB and NZB × NZW $F_1$ hybrid mice with that of other strains of mice, *J. Exp. Med.*, 130, 1093, 1969.
217. **Stutman, O., Yunis, E., and Good, R.**, Deficient immunologic functions of NZB mice, *Proc. Soc. Exp. Biol. Med.*, 127, 1204, 1968.

218. **Gelfand, M. and Steinberg, A.,** Mechanism of allograft rejection in New Zealand mice. I. Cell synergy and its age-dependent loss, *J. Immunol.,* 110, 1652, 1973.

219. **Krakauer, K., Forrey, S., and Zurier, R.,** Prostaglandin $E_1$ treatment of NZB/W mice. III. Preservation of spleen cell concentrations and mitogen-induced proliferative responses, *Clin. Immunol. Immunopathol.,* 11, 256, 1978.

220. **Talal, N.,** Autoimmunity and lymphoid malignancy in New Zealand black mice, *Prog. Clin. Immunol.,* 2, 101, 1974.

221. **Bach, J., Dardenne, M., and Salomon, J.,** Studies of thymus products. IV. Absence of serum thymic activity in adult NZB and (NZB × NZW) $F_1$ mice, *Clin. Exp. Immunol.,* 14, 247, 1973.

222. **Gershwin, M., Ikeda, R., Kruse, W., Wilson, F., Shifrine, M., and Spangler, W.,** Age dependent loss in New Zealand mice of morphological and functional characteristics of thymic epithelial cells, *J. Immunol.,* 120, 971, 1978.

223. **Teague, P.,** Spontaneous autoimmunity and involution of the lymphoid system, *Fed. Proc. Fed. Am. Soc. Exp. Biol.,* 33, 2051, 1974.

224. **Theofilopoulos, A., Eisenberg, R., Bourbon, M., Crowell, J., and Dixon, F.,** Distribution of lymphocytes identified by surface markers in murine strains with systemic lupus erythematosus-like syndromes, *J. Exp. Med.,* 149, 516, 1979.

225. **Staples, P., Steinberg, A., and Talal, N.,** Induction of immunologic tolerance in older New Zealand mice repopulated with young spleen, bone marrow, or thymus, *J. Exp. Med.,* 131, 1223, 1970.

226. **Izui, S., McConahey, P., and Dixon, F.,** Increased spontaneous polyclonal activation of B lymphocytes in mice with spontaneous autoimmune disease, *J. Immunol.,* 121, 2213, 1978.

227. **McKearn, J., Miller, G., and Quintans, J.,** The immune response in NZB mice of different ages to thymus-dependent and thymus-independent phosphorylcholine antigens, *Immunology,* 34, 1063, 1978.

228. **Barthold, D., Kysela, S., and Steinberg, A.,** Decline in suppressor T cell function with age in female NZB mice, *J. Immunol.,* 112, 9, 1974.

229. **Weigle, W. and Parks, D.,** Effect of aging on immune and tolerant states, *Fed. Proc. Fed. Am. Soc. Exp. Biol.,* 37, 1253, 1978.

230. **Primi, D., Hammarstrom, L., and Smith, C.,** Genetic control of lymphocyte suppression. Lack of suppression in aged NZB mice is due to a B cell defect, *J. Immunol.,* 121, 2242, 1978.

231. **Ohsugi, Y. and Gershwin, M. E.,** Studies on congenitally immunologic mutant New Zealand mice. III. Growth of B lymphocyte clones in congenitally athymic (nude) and hereditarily asplenic (Dh/+) NZB mice: a primary B cell defect, *J. Immunol.,* 123, 1260, 1979.

232. **Cohen, P. and Ziff, M.,** Abnormal polyclonal B cell activation in NZB/NZW $F_1$ mice, *J. Immunol.,* 119, 1534, 1977.

233. **Naor, D., Bonavida, B., Robinson, R., Shibata, I., Percy, D., Chia, D., and Barnett, E.,** Immune response of New Zealand mice to trinitrophenylated syngeneic mouse red cells, *Eur. J. Immunol.,* 6, 783, 1976.

234. **Akizuki, M., Reeves, J., and Steinberg, A.,** Expression of autoimmunity by NZB/NZW marrow, *Clin. Immunol. Immunopathol.,* 10, 247, 1978.

235. **Taurog, J., Moutsopoulos, M., Rosenberg, Y., Chused, T., and Steinberg, A.,** CBA/N X-linked B cell defect prevents NZB B-cell hyperreactivity in $F_1$ mice, *J. Exp. Med.,* 150, 31, 1979.

236. **Nakajima, P., Datta, S., Schwartz, R., and Huber, B.,** Localization of spontaneously hyperactive B cells of NZB mice to a specific B cell subset, *Proc. Natl. Acad. Sci. USA,* 76, 4613, 1979.

237. **Gershwin, M. E., Castles, J., Erickson, K., and Ahmed, A.,** Studies of congenitally immunologic mutant New Zealand mice. II. Absence of T cell progenitor populations and B cell defects of congenitally athymic (nude) New Zealand Black (NZB) mice, *J. Immunol.,* 122, 2020, 1979.

238. **Leventhal, B. and Talal, N.,** Response of NZB and NZB/NZW spleen cells to mitogenic agents, *J. Immunol.,* 104, 918, 1970.

239. **Rodey, G., Good, R., and Yunis, E.,** Progressive loss *in vitro* of cellular immunity with ageing in strains of mice susceptible to autoimmune disease, *Clin. Exp. Immunol.,* 9, 305, 1971.

240. **Teague, P., Yunis, E., Rodey, G., Fish, A., Stutman, O., and Good, R.,** Autoimmune phenomena and renal disease in mice. Role of thymectomy, aging, and involution of immunologic capacity, *Lab. Invest.,* 22, 121, 1970.

241. **Stobo, J., Talal, N., and Paul, W.,** Lymphocyte classes in New Zealand mice. I. Ontogeny and mitogen responsiveness of thymocytes and thymus-derived lymphocytes, *J. Immunol.,* 109, 692, 1972.

242. **Smith, J. and Pasternak, R.,** Syngeneic mixed lymphocyte reaction in mice: strain distribution, kinetics, participating cells, and absence in NZB mice, *J. Immunol.,* 121, 1889, 1978.

243. **Cantor, H., Asofsky, R., and Talal, N.,** Synergy among lymphoid cells mediating the graft-versus-host response. I. Synergy in graft-versus-host reactions produced by cells from NZB/B1 mice, *J. Exp. Med.,* 131, 223, 1970.

244. **Gerber, N., Hardin, J., Chused, T., and Steinberg, A.,** Loss with age in NZB/W mice of thymic suppressor cells in the graft-vs-host reaction, *J. Immunol.,* 113, 1618, 1974.
245. **Gelfand, M. and Steinberg, A.,** Basis of impaired graft rejection of aging NZB/W mice, *Transplant. Proc.,* 5, 145, 1973.
246. **Klassen, L., Zarate, A., Gelfand, M., and Steinberg, A.,** Suppressor cell activation by anti-Thy1.2 in NZB/WF$_1$ mice, *J. Immunol.,* 119, 2067, 1977.
247. **Gershwin, M., Klingerstein, R., Chused, T., and Steinberg, A.,** *In vitro* and *in vivo* cytotoxicity to EL-4 sarcoma in New Zealand mice, *J. Immunol.,* 113, 1968, 1974.
248. **Creighton, W., Zinkernagel, R., and Dixon, F.,** T cell-mediated immune responses of lupus-prone BXSB mice and other murine strains, *Clin. Exp. Immunol.,* 37, 181, 1979.
249. **Hirano, T. and Nordin, A.,** Age-associated decline in the *in vitro* development of cytotoxic lymphocytes in NZB mice, *J. Immunol.,* 117, 1093, 1976.
250. **Theofilopoulos, A., Shawler, D., Katz, D., and Dixon, F.,** Patterns of immune reactivity in autoimmune murine strains. I. Cell-mediated immune responses induced by H-2 identical and H-2 incompatible stimulator cells, *J. Immunol.,* 122, 2319, 1979.
251. **Crocker, B., Zinkernagel, R., and Dixon, F.,** Natural cytotoxic cells in NZB mice: spontaneous *in vivo* and *in vitro* primed activity and structural characteristics, *Clin. Immunol. Immunopathol.,* 12, 410, 1979.
252. **Gershwin, M., Glinski, W., Chused, T., and Steinberg, A.,** Lymphocyte-dependent antibody-mediated cytolysis of DNA-anti-DNA-coated target cells using human and murine SLE effector population, *Clin. Immunol. Immunopathol.,* 8, 280, 1977.
253. **McCombs, C., Hom, J., Talal, N., and Mishell, R.,** Decreased response of cultured New Zealand mouse spleen cells to sheep erythrocytes, *J. Immunol.,* 112, 326, 1974.
254. **Morton, J. and Siegel, B.,** Response of NZB mice to foreign antigen and development of autoimmune disease, *J. Reticuloendothelial Soc.,* 6, 78, 1969.
255. **Roubinian, J., Papoian, R., Pillarisetty, R., Sawada, S., and Talal, N.,** Immunological regulation of spontaneous antibodies to DNA and RNA. III. Early effects of neonatal thymectomy and splenectomy, *Immunology,* 33, 399, 1977.
256. **Hahn, B., Mehta, J., Knotts, L., Ihle, J., and Levy, J.,** The effect of altered lymphocyte function on the immunologic disorders of NZB/NZW mice. Response to anti-thymocyte globulin, *Clin. Immunol. Immunopathol.,* 8, 225, 1977.
257. **Gershwin, M., Castles, J., Ikeda, R., Erikson, K., and Montero, J.,** Studies of congenitally immunologic mutant New Zealand mice. I. Autoimmune features of hereditarily asplenic (Dh/+) NZB mice; reduction of naturally occurring thymocytotoxic antibody and normal suppressor function, *J. Immunol.,* 122, 710, 1979.
258. **Shirai, T., Hayakawa, K., Okumura, K., and Tada, T.,** Differential cytotoxic effect of natural thymocytotoxic autoantibody of NZB mice on functional subsets of T cells, *J. Immunol.,* 120, 1924, 1978.
259. **Goldblum, R., Pillarisetty, R., and Talal, N.,** Independent appearance of anti-thymocyte and anti-RNA antibodies in NZB/NZW F$_1$ mice, *Immunology,* 28, 621, 1975.
260. **Eisenberg, R., Theofilopoulos, A., Andrews, B., Peters, C., Thor, L., and Dixon, F.,** Natural thymocytotoxic autoantibodies in autoimmune and normal mice, *J. Immunol.,* 122, 2272, 1979.
261. **Niaudet, P. and Bach, M.,** Thymic function in NZB mice. I. Duration of thymic function in New Zealand Black (NZB) mice, *Clin. Exp. Immunol.,* 23, 328, 1976.
262. **Morton, R., Goodman, D., Gershwin, M., Derkay, C., Squire, R., and Steinberg, A.,** Suppression of autoimmunity in NZB mice with steroid-sensitive X-radiation-sensitive syngeneic young thymocytes, *Arthritis Rheum.,* 19, 1347, 1976.
263. **Wolf, R. and Ziff, M.,** Transfer of spleen cells from young to aging NZB × NZW F$_1$ hybrid mice. Effect on mortality, anti-nuclear antibody, and renal disease, *Arthritis Rheum.,* 19, 1353, 1976.
264. **Gershwin, M., Steinberg, A., Ahmed, A., and Derkay, C.,** Study of thymic factors. II. Failure of thymosin to alter the natural history of NZB and NZB/NZW mice, *Arthritis Rheum.,* 19, 862, 1976.
265. **Borel, Y., Lewis, R., and Stollar, B.,** Prevention of murine lupus nephritis by carrier dependent induction of immunologic tolerance to denatured DNA, *Science (Wash. D.C.),* 182, 76, 1973.
266. **Parker, L., Hahn, B., and Osterland, C.,** Modification of NZB/NZW F$_1$ autoimmune disease by development of tolerance to DNA, *J. Immunol.,* 113, 292, 1974.
267. **Goldblum, R., Pillarisetty, R., Dauphinee, M., and Talal, N.,** Acceleration of autoimmunity in NZB/NZW F$_1$ mice by graft-versus-host disease, *Clin. Exp. Immunol.,* 19, 377, 1975.
268. **Fernandes, G., Yunis, E., and Good, R.,** Influence of protein restriction on immune functions in NZB mice, *J. Immunol.,* 16, 782, 1976.
269. **Fernandes, G., Good, R., and Yunis, E.,** Attempts to correct age-related immunodeficiency and autoimmunity by cellular and dietary manipulation in inbred mice, in *Immunology and Aging,* Makinodan, T. and Yunis, E., Eds., Plenum Medical Book Co., New York, 1978, 111.

270. **Fernandes, G., Yunis, E., Miranda, M., Smith, J., and Good, R.,** Nutritional inhibition of genetically determined renal disease and autoimmunity with prolongation of life in kdkd mice, *Proc. Natl. Acad. Sci. USA,* 75, 2888, 1978.
271. **Rodger, B., Whittingham, S., and MacKay, I.,** Influence of immunosuppression on antinuclear antibody and survival of WEHI mice, *Aust. J. Exp. Biol. Med.,* 53, 325, 1975.
272. **Gerber, N., Powell, D., and Steinberg, A.,** Therapeutic studies in NZB/NZW $F_1$ mice. V. Comparison of cyclophosphamide and chlorambucil, *Arthritis Rheum.,* 20, 1263, 1977.
273. **Morris, A., Esterly, J., Chase, G., and Sharp, G.,** Cyclophosphamide protection in NZB/NZW disease. Mechanisms of therapeutic regimens, *Arthritis Rheum.,* 19, 49, 1976.
274. **Walker, S. and Bole, G.,** Suppressed heterogeneous antinuclear antibody response in lymphoma-bearing NZB/NZW mice, *Clin. Exp. Immunol.,* 24, 210, 1976.
275. **Zurier, R., Sayadoff, D., Torrey, S., and Rothfield, N.,** Prostaglandin $E_1$ treatment of NZB/NZW mice. I. Prolonged survival of female mice, *Arthritis Rheum.,* 20, 723, 1977.
276. **Zimecki, M. and Webb, D.,** The role of prostaglandins in the control of the immune response to an autologous red blood cell antigen (Hb), *Clin. Immunol. Immunopathol.,* 8, 420, 1977.
277. **Krakauer, R., Waldmann, T., and Strober, W.,** Loss of suppressor T cells in adult NZB/NZW mice, *J. Exp. Med.,* 144, 662, 1976.
278. **Roder, J., Bell, D., and Singhal, S.,** Regulation of the immune response in autoimmune NZB/NZW $F_1$ mice. I. The spontaneous generation of splenic suppressor cells, *Cell. Immunol.,* 29, 272, 1977.
279. **Dauphinee, M. and Talal, N.,** Failure of NZB spleen to respond to prethymic bone marrow suppressor cells, *J. Immunol.,* 122, 936, 1979.
280. **Creighton, W. D., Katz, D., and Dixon, F.,** Antigen-specific immunocompetency, B cell function, and regulatory helper and suppressor T cell activities in spontaneously autoimmune mice, *J. Immunol.,* 123, 2627, 1979.
281. **Chan, Y., Chia, D., Barnett, E., Knutson, D., and Pearson, C.,** Functional impairment of macrophages in old NZB/NZW mice, *Fed. Proc. Fed. Am. Soc. Exp. Biol.,* 37, 884, 1978.
282. **Morgan, A. and Steward, M.,** Macrophage clearance function and immune complex disease in New Zealand Black/White $F_1$ hybrid mice, *Clin. Exp. Immunol.,* 26, 133, 1976.
283. **Finbloom, D. and Plotz, P.,** Studies of reticuloendothelial function in the mouse with model immune complexes. II. Serum clearance, tissue uptake, and reticuloendothelial saturation in NZB/W mice, *J. Immunol.,* 123, 1600, 1979.
284. **Raveche, E. and Steinberg, A.,** Lymphocytes and lymphocyte functions in systemic lupus erythematosus, *Sem. Hematol.,* 16, 344, 1979.
285. **Playfair, J.,** Strain differences in the immune response of mice. III. A raised tolerance threshold in NZB thymus cells, *Immunology,* 21, 1037, 1971.
286. **Datta, S. and Schwartz, R.,** Genetic, viral, and immunological aspects of autoimmune disease in NZB mice, in *Genetic Control of Autoimmune Disease,* Rose, N., Bigazzi, P., and Warner, N., Eds., Elsevier/North-Holland, New York, 1978, 193.
287. **Fabris, N., Pierpaoli, W., and Sorkin, E.,** Hormones and the immunological capacity. III. The immunodeficiency diseases of the hypopituitary Snell-Bagg dwarf mice, *Clin. Exp. Immunol.,* 9, 209, 1971.
288. **Piantanelli, L., Basso, A., Muzzioli, M., and Fabris, N.,** Thymus-dependent reversibility of physiological and isoproterenol evoked age-related parameters in athymic (nude) and old normal mice, *Mech. Ageing Dev.,* 7, 171, 1978.
289. **Morse, H., Steinberg, A., Vchur, P., and Reed, N.,** Spontaneous "autoimmune disease" in nude mice, *J. Immunol.,* 113, 688, 1974.
290. **Fabris, N., Pierpaoli, W., and Sorkin, E.,** Hormones and the immunological capacity. IV. Restorative effects of developmental hormones or of lymphocytes on the immunodeficiency syndrome of the dwarf mice, *Clin. Exp. Immunol.,* 9, 227, 1971.
291. **Hildemann, W., Rathbun, W., and Walford, R.,** Early manifestations of acute transplantation (allogeneic) disease in mice, *Transplantation,* 5, 504, 1967.
292. **Gleichmann, E., Gleichmann, H., and Wilke, W.,** Autoimmunization and lymphomagenesis in parent→$F_1$ combinations differing at the major histocompatibility complex: model for spontaneous disease caused by altered self antigens? *Transplant. Rev.,* 31, 156, 1976.
293. **Lennon, V., Lindstrom, J., and Seybold, M.,** Experimental autoimmune myasthenia gravis, cellular and humoral immune response, *Ann. N.Y. Acad. Sci.,* 274, 283, 1976.
294. **Kajima, A., Tanaka-Kojima, Y., Sakakura, T., and Nishizuka, Y.,** Spontaneous development of autoimmune thyroiditis in neonatally thymectomized mice, *Lab. Invest.,* 34, 550, 1976.
295. **Wick, G., Schwarz, S., and Muller, P.,** No development of experimental autoimmune thyroiditis in nude mice, *Z. Immunitaetsforsch. Immunobiol.,* 154, 162, 1978.
296. **Scheinberg, M., Cathcart, E., Eastcott, J., Skinner, M., Benson, M., Shirahama, T., and Bennett, M.,** The SJL/J mouse: a new model for spontaneous age-associated amyloidosis. I. Morphologic and immuno-chemical aspects, *Lab. Invest.,* 35, 47, 1976.

297. **Barnett, E., Chia, D., Knutson, D., Van Lancker, J., Cheney, K., Weindruch, R., and Walford, R.,** SLE, an accelerated form of aging, in *Immunological Aspects of Aging,* Segre, D. and Smith, L., Eds., Dekker, New York, 1980.
298. **Masi, T.,** Family, twin, and genetic studies: a general review illustrated by systemic lupus erythematosus, in *Population Studies of the Rheumatic Diseases,* Bennett, P. and Wood, P., Eds., Excerpta Medica Foundation, Amsterdam, 1968, 267.
299. **Leonhardt, E.,** Family studies in systemic lupus erythematosus, *Clin. Exp. Immunol.,* 2, 743, 1967.
300. **Block, S., Winfield, J., and Lockshin, M.,** Twin studies in systemic lupus erythematosus. A review of the literature and presentation of 12 additional sets, *Am. J. Med.,* 59, 533, 1975.
301. **Block, S., Lockshin, M., Winfield, J., Weksler, M., Imamura, M., Winchester, R., Mellors, R., and Christian, C.,** Immunologic observations on 9 sets of twins either concordant or discordant for SLE, *Arthritis Rheum.,* 19, 545, 1975.
302. **Brunner, C., Horwitz, D., Shann, M., Sturgill, B., and Davis, J.,** Clinical and immunologic studies in identical twins discordant for systemic lupus erythematosus, *Am. J. Med.,* 55, 249, 1973.
303. **Yocum, M., Grossman, J., Waterhouse, C., Abraham, G., May, A., and Condemi, J.,** Monozygotic twins discordant for systemic lupus erythematosus, *Arthritis Rheum.,* 18, 193, 1975.
304. **Williams, R., DeBoard, J., Mellbye, O., Messner, R., and Lindstrom, F.,** Studies of T- and B-lymphocytes in patients with connective tissue diseases, *J. Clin. Invest.,* 52, 283, 1973.
305. **Moutsopoulos, H., Fye, K., Sawada, S., Becker, M., Goldstein, A., and Talal, N.,** *In vitro* effect of thymosin on T-lymphocyte rosette formation in rheumatic diseases, *Clin. Exp. Immunol.,* 26, 563, 1976.
306. **Rivero, S., Liorente, L., Diaz-Jouanen, E., and Alarcon-Segovia, D.,** T-lymphocyte subpopulation in untreated SLE. Variations with disease activity, *Arthritis Rheum.,* 20, 1169, 1977.
307. **Scheinberg, M. and Cathcart, E.,** B cell and T lymphoxenia in systemic lupus erythematosus, *Cell Immunol.,* 12, 309, 1974.
308. **Hebert, J., Sadeghee, S., Schumacher, H., Zweiman, B., Zmijewski, C., and Abdou, N.,** Null cells in peripheral blood of normals and systemic lupus erythematosus, *Clin. Immunol. Immunopathol.,* 6, 347, 1976.
309. **Wernet, P., Fotino, M., Thoburn, R., Moore, A., and Kunkle, H.,** Blockage of lymphocyte surface antigens and shedding phenomenon in systemic lupus erythematosus, *Arthritis Rheum.,* 16, 137, 1973.
310. **Diaz-Jouanen, E., Bankhurst, A., and Williams, R.,** Antibody-mediated lymphocytotoxicity in rheumatoid arthritis and systemic lupus erythematosus, *Arthritis Rheum.,* 19, 133, 1976.
311. **Diaz-Jouanen, E., Bankhurst, A., Messner, R., and Williams, R.,** Serum and synovial fluid inhibitors of antibody-mediated lymphocytotoxicity in rheumatoid arthritis and systemic lupus erythematosus, *Arthritis Rheum.,* 19, 142, 1976.
312. **Scheinberg, M. and Cathcart, E.,** Antibody dependent direct cytotoxicity of human lymphocytes. I. Studies on peripheral blood lymphocytes and sera of patients with systemic lupus erythematosus, *Clin. Exp. Immunol.,* 24, 317, 1976.
313. **Cooper, S., Hardin, B., Mirick, G., Schneider, J., Quismorio, F., and Friou, G.,** Selective decrease in antibody dependent cell-mediated cytotoxicity in systemic lupus erythematosus and progressive systemic sclerosis, *Clin. Exp. Immunol.,* 34, 235, 1978.
314. **Sagawa, A. and Abdou, N.,** Suppressor-cell dysfunction in systemic lupus erythematosus *J. Clin. Invest.,* 62, 789, 1978.
315. **Fauci, A., Steinberg, A., Haynes, B., and Whalen, G.,** Immunoregulatory aberrations in systemic lupus erythematosus, *J. Immunol.,* 121, 1473, 1978.
316. **Sakane, T., Steinberg, A., Reeves, J., and Green, I.,** Studies of immune functions of patients with systemic lupus erythematosus. Complement-dependent immunoglobulin $M_1$ anti-thymus-derived cell antibodies preferentially inactivate suppressor cells, *J. Clin. Invest.,* 63, 954, 1979.
317. **Talal, N., Pillarisetty, R., DeHoratius, R., and Messner, R.,** Immunologic regulation of spontaneous antibodies to DNA and RNA. I. Significance of IgM and IgG antibodies in SLE patients and asymptomatic relatives, *Clin. Exp. Immunol.,* 25, 377, 1976.
318. **Beaulieu, A., Quismorio, F., Friou, G., Vayuvegula, B., and Mirick, G.,** IgG antibodies to double-stranded DNA in systemic lupus erythematosus sera. Independent variations of complement fixing activity and total antibody content, *Arthritis Rheum.,* 22, 565, 1979.
319. **McDevitt, H. and Bodmer, W.,** HL-A, immune-response genes, and disease, *Lancet,* 1, 1269, 1974.
320. **Svejgaard, A., Platz, P., Ryder, L., Staub-Nielsen, L., and Thomsen, M.,** HL-A and disease associations . . . a survey, *Transplant. Rev.,* 22, 3, 1975.
321. **Brohee, D., Delespesse, G., Debisschop, M., and Bonnyns, M.,** Circulating immune complexes in various thyroid diseases, *Clin. Exp. Immunol.,* 36, 379, 1979.
322. **Tokya, K., Drachman, D., Griffin, D., Pestronk, A., Winkelstein, J., Fischbeck, K., and Kao, I.,** Myasthenis gravis. Study of humoral immune mechanisms by passive transfer to mice, *N. Engl. J. Med.,* 296, 125, 1977.

323. **Wekerle, H. and Ketelsen, U.**, Intrathymic pathogenesis and dual genetic control of myasthenia gravis, *Lancet*, 1, 678, 1977.
324. **Papatestas, A., Mulvihill, M., Genkins, G., Kornfeld, P., Aufses, A., Wang, D., and Bulbrook, R.**, Thymus and breast cancer plasma androgens, thymic pathology, and peripheral lymphocytes in myasthenia gravis, *J. Natl. Canc. Inst.*, 59, 1583, 1977.
325. **Simpson, J., Behan, P., and Dick, M.**, Studies on the nature of autoimmunity in myasthenia gravis. Evidence for an immunodeficiency type, *Ann. N.Y. Acad. Sci.*, 274, 382, 1976.
326. **Buckingham, J., Howard, F., Bernatz, P., Payne, W., Harrison, E., O'Brien, P., and Wilano, L.**, The value of thymectomy in myasthenia gravis: a computer assisted matched study, *Ann. Surg.*, 184, 453, 1976.
327. **Abdou, N., Lisak, R., Zweiman, B., Abrahamsohn, I., and Penn, A.**, The thymus in myasthenia gravis: evidence for altered cell populations, *N. Engl. J. Med.*, 291, 1271, 1974.
328. **Piantelli, M., Lauriola, L., Carbone, A., Ejoli, A., Tonali, P., and Musiani, P.**, Subpopulations of T lymphocytes in maysthenia gravis patients, *Clin. Exp. Immunol.*, 36, 85, 1979.
329. **Naor, D., Bonavida, B., and Walford, R.**, Autoimmunity and aging: The age-related response of mice of a long lived strain to trinitrophyenylated syngeneic mouse red blood cells, *J. Immunol.*, 117, 2204, 1976.
330. **Meredith, P., Kristie, J., and Walford, R.**, Aging increases expression of LPS-induced autoantibody-secreting B cells, *J. Immunol.*, 123, 87, 1979.
331. **Gozes, Y., Umiel, T., Meshorer, A., and Trainin, N.**, Syngeneic GVH induced in popliteal lymph nodes by spleen cells of old C57B1/6 mice, *J. Immunol.*, 121, 2199, 1978.
332. **Hallgren, H., Buckley, C., Gilbertsen, V., and Yunis, E.**, Lymphocyte phytohemagglutinin responsiveness, immunoglobulins and autoantibodies in aging humans, *J. Immunol.*, 3, 1101, 1973.
333. **Lange, A., Garncarek, D., Charzynska, E., and Mydiak, H.**, Diagnostic specificity of autoantibodies. III. Age related changes in appearing autoantibodies serum IgD levels and their association with peripheral blood lymphocyte profiles, *Arch. Immunol. Ther. Exp.*, 26, 887, 1978.
334. **Hackett, E., Beech, M., and Forbes, I.**, Thyroglobulin antibodies in patients without clinical disease of the thyroid gland, *Lancet*, 2, 402, 1969.
335. **Whittingham, S., Irwin, J., Mackay, I., Marsh, S., and Cowling, D.**, Autoantibodies in healthy subjects, *Aust. Ann. Med.*, 18, 130, 1969.
336. **Pandley, J., Fudenberg, J., Ainsworth, S., and Loadholt, C.**, Autoantibodies in healthy subjects of different age groups, *Mech. Ageing Dev.*, 10, 399, 1979.
337. **Kipshidze, N.**, Quantitative changes in lipid, protein, and carbohydrate metabolism in relation to age, *Cancer and Aging, Thule Int. Symp.*, 2, 49, 1967.
338. **Mathews, J., Hopper, B., Whittingham, S., Mackay, I., and Steinhouse, N.**, Association of autoantibodies with smoking, cardiovascular morbidity, and death in the Busselton population, *Lancet*, 2, 754, 1973.

# INDEX

## A

## D

## E


Ecological niche, 31, 36, 80, 82, 85

## H



## I

## M

## N



## O

## P

## Q



## R



## S

## T



## U

## V



## W



## X